Getting Tough On
Gateway Drugs

A   Y

DATE DUE		

Getting Tough On Gateway Drugs

A GUIDE FOR THE FAMILY

By *Robert L. DuPont, Jr., M.D.*

WITH A FOREWORD BY
Ann Landers

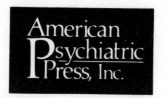

American
Psychiatric
Press, Inc.

1400 K Street, N.W.
Washington, D.C. 20005

Cover Design by Sam Haltom
Text Design by Tim Clancy and Richard E. Farkas
Typeset by Unicorn Graphics
Printed by R. R. Donnelley & Sons Co.

Library of Congress Cataloging in Publication Data

DuPont, Robert L., 1936–
  Getting tough on gateway drugs.
  Includes index.
  1. Drug abuse—United States. 2. Youth—United States—Drug use.
HV5825.D95   1984   362.2'92'0973   84-14595
ISBN 0-88048-035-1
ISBN 0-88048-046-7 (trade pbk.)

To my parents, Bob and Martha, who continue to
teach me the good things family means;

To my children, Elizabeth and Caroline, who
continue to show me the satisfaction of
being a parent; and

To my wife, Helen, who helps me manage my life so
it works, reasonably well, and who makes it
all worthwhile

Contents

Foreword

BY ANN LANDERS

The impact of drugs on family life is a frequent and painful concern expressed by my readers. In answering letters from people who are struggling with problems created by drugs and alcohol, I have often consulted Dr. Robert L. DuPont, Jr., one of the best in the field.

In his new book, *Getting Tough On Gateway Drugs: A Guide for the Family*, Dr. DuPont comes down hard on the three drugs which are gateways into the drug experience—alcohol, marijuana, and cocaine. Dr. DuPont calls these the GATEWAY DRUGS because they are mistakenly considered to be easy to control and harmless.

At last, here is a book for the family that explains how to deal with drug problems and the reasons for the drug epidemic of the last two decades.

Dr. DuPont helps families answer the central and frustrating question asked by kids: "What's wrong with trying a drug just to learn for myself?" He explains why addicted drug users can never safely use drugs "now and then—for recreational purposes." Total abstinence is imperative for rehabilitation.

Dr. DuPont suggests family solutions to the problem. He outlines the changes within the family that are necessary to help young people achieve healthy adulthood free of drugs. In a separate and particularly useful chapter, he offers a superb and realistic guide to drug abuse treatment.

This is a personal, family book. It has some strong medicine expressed with uncompromising clarity. When Dr. DuPont argues that teenagers should *not* use alcohol and marijuana, he rejects the popular (and dangerous) idea that drug experimentation is a "normal" and even a "healthy" part of growing up in America today. When Dr. DuPont says *no* intoxicating drugs are acceptable in schools, on the highways, or at work, he cuts close to the nerve of many—from the pot-smoking youth, to the cocaine-sniffing young executive, to the alcohol drinker driving home from a party.

Dr. DuPont argues that we must see beyond the controversies to basic principles about the way we want to live in families and in communities. We must recognize that drug and alcohol use is a major threat to the quality, and the very existence, of life. We must also be tough and united if we are to solve the problem.

In this book, Dr. DuPont offers a balanced, reasonable approach based on solid scientific findings. He stresses that the nation's best defense against the menace of drugs is the family. During the last 20 years, the family has been at a terrible disadvantage against drugs, because families have lacked clear guidelines for solving the drug and alcohol problem. In fact, many so-called experts have undermined family struggles against drugs with arguments that drugs like cocaine and marijuana are "not addictive," that "abuse is the problem, not use," and that to interfere with the use of drugs violates one's "civil rights." Dr. DuPont's book will enable families to see through this nonsense and successfully combat the drug problem with clear principles.

This book grows out of Dr. DuPont's long professional and personal interest in drug abuse prevention in this country and around the world. I was pleased to find in reading the book that the content and tone have stayed at a practical level. This, I suspect, reflects Dr. DuPont's long and direct involvement with drug abuse patients and their families. It may also reflect the fact that he and his wife have two teenage children.

Armed with the facts in *Getting Tough on Gateway Drugs*, families need no longer feel incompetent and ill-equipped to deal with a drug or alcohol problem. This book says it all.

Ann Landers

Acknowledgments

This book exists as the result of the support, encouragement, and even the direction of many people during the four years it took me to write it. I am particularly indebted to Verne Powers, who saw in my first notes the possibility for the book, and who began, and ended, the editing process with skill, dedication, and limitless patience. Patricia Carson, a friend, neighbor, and mother of two teenagers, assisted as typist and editor during the difficult final stages of the process.

Ron McMillen, the General Manager of the American Psychiatric Press, gave valuable support and guidance. Evelyn Stone brought confident, experienced professionalism to the task of editing and saw beyond the controversies stirred by the book to its potential to help families. Jean McMillen, a longtime friend in drug abuse prevention, was a strong supporter and expert editor. I owe a special debt of gratitude to my professional colleagues who generously read and criticized the book. These colleagues include Sidney Cohen, Edward Senay, George Russell, Joyce Nalepka, Richard Hawley, and Keith Schuchard.

Ann Landers, with her generous Foreword to this book and her strong support for my work over many years, has earned a unique place in these acknowledgments. This is an appropriate place to express one further indebtedness. Ann Landers says in her Foreword that she has often consulted me. The street runs both ways. Many have been the mornings when my wife and daughters have greeted me at the breakfast table with the latest quote from our ultimate authority on family life, Ann Landers. She has been a steady and strong voice for the family and against drug use for many years. Her ideas have helped shape my thoughts and this book.

My own family contributed not only to supporting me during the many months it took to write the book, but by helping me think and live through the process of family-based prevention of drug and alcohol problems. The many groups I have spoken with during the last five years have helped me focus my thinking. None has been more useful than the group of parents and teenagers I met with in an eight-week course in 1983 at my own church, St. John's, of Norwood Parish in Bethesda, Maryland.

Finally, my most valued collaborators, whom I cannot acknowledge by name, were my patients. They have taught me by their courage and their pain to respect, if not to fear, the deadly threat drug dependence is for individuals, families, and communities.

Robert L. DuPont, Jr., M.D.

About the Author

Dr. Robert L. DuPont, Jr. has been one of the nation's leaders in drug abuse prevention since the late 1960s when he developed the Narcotics Treatment Administration, the comprehensive program that treated over 15,000 heroin addicts in the District of Columbia between 1970 and 1973 while he was Director. He then moved to the federal government, where he became the first Director of the National Institute on Drug Abuse, serving in that capacity from 1973 to 1978. From 1973 to 1975 he was also White House Drug Chief. As NIDA Director, Dr. DuPont visited more than 20 nations to study their drug problems. He represented the United States at five consecutive meetings of the United Nations Commission on Narcotic Drugs, and he was Chairman of the Section on Drug and Alcohol Abuse for the World Psychiatric Association.

Since leaving the government, Dr. DuPont has been President of the nonprofit American Council for Drug Education in Rockville, Maryland. Dr. DuPont directs the Center for Behavioral Medicine, which provides clinical psychiatric services from offices in Baltimore, Rockville, Richmond, Norfolk, and Raleigh. He is Vice-President of Bensinger, DuPont, and Associates, Inc., a national firm with offices in Chicago and Rockville, providing consultation on drug abuse prevention in the workplace.

A graduate of Emory University and the Harvard Medical School, Dr. DuPont is Clinical Professor of Psychiatry at Georgetown Medical School and Visiting Associate Clinical Professor of Psychiatry at Harvard Medical School. He is a Fellow of the American Psychiatric Association.

Dr. DuPont maintains an active clinical practice of psychiatry, having worked directly with hundreds of drug-dependent people and their families during the last 15 years. He is married and has two teenage children.

About This Book

This book is written for people who live, love, and suffer in *families*. It is intended to help parents prevent drug problems from crippling their children, before problems occur. It is intended to help parents of children who already have drug problems and who are seeking ways to solve these problems. It is intended for family members, of any age, who are concerned about drug problems in other members of the family. It is also intended for the large number of children who are concerned about the drug problems—and most often the alcohol problems—of their parents. It is written to help degreed and nondegreed professional therapists who work with drug- and alcohol-dependent people and their families. Finally, this book is intended to be helpful to those people concerned about their own drug use and the problems it may cause or already has caused.

My experience has convinced me that this last group of drug users, surely the most urgently in need of assistance, is the group least likely to benefit directly from reading this book. They are less likely to make the effort to read it, or having read it, they are less likely to apply its lessons to themselves. And, if they try to put the book's principles into action, they are less likely to succeed unless they are supported strongly and consistently by other members of the family who do not use drugs. Thus, the reader to whom this book is primarily directed is the concerned family member who is not personally dependent on drugs.

This is not a "cookbook" which will tell you what to do in *every* specific situation. It is my best effort to help you understand the principles underlying the drug problems you face and to help you understand what you can do to solve these problems. The goal of the book, in other words, is to bring *understanding* which you can translate into *action* within your family to prevent or solve drug problems.

The book is a guide for the family, a survival guide for the most urgent problem facing American families today: drug and alcohol abuse.

This is a practical, a personal book. While I have included a few statistics and some recent scientific findings, the heart of the book is neither theoretical nor political. This book as a whole is based on my experience for more than a decade as a physician working directly with drug abusers and their families.

While I worked for many years as a government official, first at the local and later at the national level, my primary commitment there was to the individual people I saw on a day-to-day basis. It was their personal struggles which educated me about drug abuse. My government work did, of course, give me a chance to participate in many policy debates. It also afforded me a unique opportunity to visit more than 20 other nations and to study their drug problems.

This book grows directly out of my private clinical practice of psychiatry and out of hundreds of talks on prevention of drug abuse that I have given in communities and schools in all parts of the United States during the years since I left the government. Initially, my clinical work and my talks about drug abuse prevention were tentative and indirect. As I have gained experience—and as my work and my views have become more sharply focused and perhaps (as some have said) even dogmatic—I have increasingly felt the need to communicate my battle-tested ideas to others by way of the printed word. *Getting Tough on Gateway Drugs: A Guide for the Family* offers me a unique opportunity to communicate more broadly and in greater detail than I can in either psychotherapy or in any number of one- or two-hour speeches.

Drug use in America today is a major threat to our health, productivity, and quality of life. Drugs, including alcohol and tobacco, now cause 30 percent of all Americans to die prematurely. Drug use costs the national economy over $100 billion a year, with much of that cost attributed to lost productivity. Among America's young adults ranging in age from 18 to 25, which is the segment of our population that uses drugs most heavily, 41 percent used marijuana, 20 percent used cocaine, and 84 percent used alcohol during 1982. Nationally, we have 57 million people who have used marijuana at least once; 20 million of them are now regular, current users of a drug which was a rarity in the United States 20 years ago. Nearly two million Americans will use marijuana for the first time next year, with over 80 percent of them 17 years of age or younger. Twenty-two million Americans have used cocaine, and of this number, about four million are regular, current users. Nearly two million more Americans will first use cocaine this year.

America's teenagers, polled by George Gallup in 1983, were asked to name the leading threat to their generation. They ranked "Drug Abuse" number one. Twice as many picked "Drug Abuse" (35 percent) as picked the second most frequently named threat, "Unemployment" (16 percent). The number three threat was "Alcohol Abuse," while "Peer Pressures" was listed as number four. Gallup found that teenagers in 1977 also picked "Drug Abuse" as the number one threat to their generation. Between 1977 and 1983, the percentage which identified "Drug Abuse" as the leading threat *rose* from 27 percent to 35 percent.

How can a danger of this magnitude be so commonly overlooked? The answers are not easy. First, most of the more than one million American families who will be hit by a drug problem for the first time this year will experience the tragedy in silence, believing it to be the result of personal failures and a unique and shameful family experience. Second, many of our nation's opinion leaders in medicine and in politics—but especially in the intellectual community—have written off the drug problem as a quirky social issue to be relegated to the right-wing fringes of our society. Third, drugs are so commonly used that it is hard for us to fully grasp the devastation they are causing us. We tend to lose our fear of anything we see about us every day. Fourth, drug-caused problems such as auto fatalities and overdose deaths typically occur long after the initial drug use has begun; furthermore, these problems are often, from the perspective of the individual drug user, uncertain and unpredictable. If every heroin user had a fatal overdose within a few days after initial use of the drug, heroin use would disappear. If every alcohol drinker got cirrhosis of the liver within a few weeks of beginning to drink, alcohol use would stop. But, for the individual heroin user, overdose death is an unpredictable, usually long delayed, and not too common occurrence. The same is true for cirrhosis of the liver among drinkers. Finally, there are large numbers of users of drugs who seem to "get away with it." They use drugs, from heroin to alcohol, apparently without ill effects. Whether these individuals represent the majority or the minority of all users, this apparently invulnerable group exerts a powerful attraction to potential users; they hold out the hope of a "safe high."

These and many other factors contribute to the greatest obstacle preventing effective personal, family, and community response to drug abuse: *denial*. We all engage in the psychological process of denial of the simple reality of the drug abuse tragedy. If we are to overcome our drug problems, we have to get beyond denial to constructive, realistic solutions. That is what this book is about: seeing the drug abuse tragedy for what it is, and developing positive, active coping strategies.

The only hope of a winning strategy is clear: say *no* to drugs. Public and personal acceptance of the reasonableness of "trying" drugs and of "social," "controlled," or "safe" use is a step toward drug dependence. Furthermore, the initial decisions to use all dependence-producing drugs (except prescription drugs) is virtually limited to the ages of 12 to 20. Thus, the specific goal of drug abuse prevention is to help young people grow up to adulthood free of drugs. In achieving this goal, there are positive roles for schools, churches, health care professionals, law enforcement officials, employers, and all other parts of our community.

The key to successful drug abuse prevention is closer to home: *the family*. Drug abuse prevention succeeds or fails primarily in the family. This book is designed to help families cope better, to prevent drug use before it begins, and—if it begins—to solve the drug problem effectively and permanently. To achieve this goal takes understanding and hard work.

For those families already suffering from a drug problem as well as for those who now do not have a drug problem in their family and who seek to prevent one from occurring, I ask you to make the effort to understand the problem and to do what is necessary to say no to drugs. It is not easy, but it is possible. The goals are to keep drug problems from occurring in the first place and, once they have developed, to stop them. Here are two keys to achieving these objectives. First, understand the phenomenon of drug dependence so you know what you are up against. Second, structure your family life so as to discourage drug use. These two basic concepts are the stuff of this book.

The book as a whole is divided into three parts. Part One answers the question "What Is the Drug Problem?" by defining in practical terms the nature of the Drug Dependence Syndrome. Part Two, "What Are the GATEWAY DRUGS?" deals with the Big Three among drugs: marijuana, alcohol, and cocaine. This special treatment is necessitated by two unfortunate facts: (1) *alcohol, marijuana, and cocaine are used far more widely than any other mind-altering or psychoactive drugs* and (2) *these three substances are the GATEWAY DRUGS to the use of all other drugs.* These are the GATEWAY DRUGS through which virtually all Americans who become dependent on drugs enter the Drug Dependence Syndrome. They are dangerous because they are mistakenly thought to be harmless. They are likely to produce full-blown dependence partly because use of these drugs is widely—and wrongly—thought to be easily controlled.

Part Three, "How Can Families Prevent and Treat Drug Problems?" is a guide for the family. In these final chapters, we take a positive look at several principles as they operate in the family context, with special emphasis on interactions between parents and teenagers. We look, too, at how to make drug abuse treatment work, and how self-help groups can be used effectively by individuals and families. Drug use among specific groups of people and prevention of drug dependence in various community settings such as schools and the workplace are also discussed.

Some readers—because of impatience, lack of time, or even acute distress—may be anxious to hurry right to the most important parts of this book. Although I recommend that you eventually read it in its entirety, if you do need to grasp the main ideas quickly, let me point you directly toward the two most important chapters, Chapters 2 and 6. Chapter 2 outlines the fundamental processes of drug dependence. It is the key to understanding the source—the solution—of the pain caused by drug problems. Building on this understanding, Chapter 6 offers the family-based approach to preventing and treating drug dependence by structuring family life in ways that say no to drugs.

According to the most recently available statistics, about 101 million Americans currently use alcohol—about 55 percent of the entire U.S. population over the age of 12—and 57 million Americans have used marijuana at least once. Excepting cigarettes (which are used by 58 million, but which are not intoxicating), the third most widely used drug is cocaine, used at least once by about 22 million Americans. No one would deny that alcohol and marijuana are, when it comes to intoxicating drugs, the Big Two, and that cocaine, in the 1980s, has joined them as a national threat.

Alcohol is the first psychoactive drug used by most American youth. Alcohol use is the GATEWAY to the taking of intoxicating drugs for relaxation and pleasure or, as some have called this unfortunate behavior, "recreational pharmacology." The earlier and more intensively a young person uses alcohol, the more likely that person is to use other drugs, including marijuana. Conversely, those relatively few American teenagers who do not drink alcohol are virtually immune from use of any other intoxicating drugs, from marijuana to heroin.

Marijuana is aptly named a GATEWAY DRUG for two reasons. Its use is powerfully related to the age of its victims, beginning usually in the very early teens or even sooner. Nearly three million adolescents between the ages of 12 and 18 use it. Of high school seniors who have ever used marijuana, 35 percent first used it *before* the ninth grade. And, of equal concern, marijuana use is *the* GATEWAY to all illegal drug use. It is rare for young people ever to use any other illegal drug without having first used marijuana. Thus, these two intoxicants—alcohol and marijuana—are not only the most widely used drugs in America today, but they also open the gates to virtually all other drug taking and drug dependence. It is for these reasons that they have come under heavy fire in this book.

Cocaine is singled out because of its recent rise to common use and because its current, undeserved image as safe and chic makes it the most likely of all other illicit drugs to show big rises in use in coming years. Unlike the situation with regard to alcohol and even marijuana, most Americans remain ignorant of even the most basic facts about cocaine. That it is, for example, the most powerfully reinforcing of all commonly used drugs, and that it can kill users, even when it is just snorted up the nose. Cocaine has also, in recent years, become a GATEWAY DRUG in another tragic way. Millions of Americans begin using cocaine by snorting it and then move on to injecting the drug intravenously, thus opening the gates to intravenous drug use. This has become a new path to heroin addiction.

After reading this book, you will have the basic tools to understand and cope with the drug problem in its many forms, ranging from its possible occurrence in your own behavior or in the behavior of your loved ones to the larger drug-related dilemmas confronting our nation today.

I do not have the illusion that you will agree with all of my suggestions or that, even with your increased understanding, all conflicts about drugs will disappear. After reading this book, I believe you will be able to see beyond the confusion, controversy, and often the pain, to the core experience of drug dependence, and you will be able to see constructive solutions for you, your family, and your community.

Of these levels, the most important to me is the most personal: If you feel you understand your own drug use or the drug use of some member of your family, and if you feel you know better how to manage the problems this use creates, then I will be more than satisfied. Indeed, my satisfaction will be equal to that which I experienced recently when a high school student came up after one of my talks and handed me a note which read:

I thought it was an excellent presentation, and I think you might like to know you've helped me reach an important decision—not to experiment with drugs. I just wanted to say thanks and I enjoyed the talk.

Some readers, jaded by the apparent sophistication of much writing about drugs in recent years, may find such a simple, direct statement to be naive. They may conclude that my emphasis on the importance of drug-free living is simplistic and even outdated. My contention is that this "sophisticated" view, which often translates into an almost casual acceptance of illicit drug use, is itself substantially responsible for the American drug abuse epidemic of the last two decades. I believe that a commitment to simple, family-based values of drug-free love and hard work is the best hope of ending that epidemic. When it comes to solving the drug problem, the family is the place to start.

PART ONE

What Is the Drug Problem?

CHAPTER
ONE

The Drug Epidemic
and Related Disasters

I NDIVIDUAL CHOICES—decisions we make about our lifestyles—are the primary determinants of our health. Health is more than merely living, but since death is easier to define and measure, I will start by citing some death rates from a report recently published by the Surgeon General of the United States. Two of the trends are good news; one is distinctly bad news.

HEALTH IN THE UNITED STATES: GOOD NEWS—AND BAD

First, the good news: Americans are now living longer than ever before. The average life expectancy of a newborn American is now 73 years, having increased a total of 26 years since the turn of the century. Quickly, I must point out, however, that this good news is better for women than for men. Today, a newborn girl has a life expectancy of 77 years, whereas a newborn boy in today's America has a life expectancy of only 69 years. This is a gap of eight years between male and female life expectancy. At the turn of the century, the gap, which then also favored women, was only two years. The second good news statistic is that, although during the 1960s Americans added only *one* year to the life expectancy of the average newborn, during the 1970s we added nearly *three* years. During that decade our nation did a good job of lengthening the average life expectancy.

The third statistical trend I want to highlight: throughout the twentieth century every segment of the American population—*except one* —has shown an improvement in its health as measured by a decrease in the death rate. That exception is the bad news: Americans between

4

the ages of 15 and 24 years were dying in 1982 at an 8 percent greater rate than they were in 1960. Other age segments of our population have, since the turn of the century, been healthier at the end of each successive decade than they were at the beginning. Let there be no doubt about it—what happened to the health of Americans in the 15- to 24-year age bracket since 1965 was unique in the health history of this country.

Vital—Really Vital—Statistics

The amazing 26-year lengthening of the life span since 1900, the puzzling eight-year longevity gap between the sexes, the tragic eight percent acceleration in the death rate of the young . . . what do these three statistics, these three trends, mean? How do they relate to drug abuse? Let us go back to the first one: the increase in life expectancy from 47 to 73 years and to the enormous gap in life expectancy between men and women. The major reason for this welcome increase in the length of life since 1900 has been the conquest of infectious diseases, particularly among children. Today, in contrast to 1900, 30 percent of all deaths occurring in the United States are *premature* for two reasons: alcohol drinking and cigarette smoking. Think of it. Thirty percent of all of the people who will die in the United States this year will die early because of the use of tobacco and alcohol.

Furthermore, most of that eight-year difference in life expectancy between the sexes can be attributed to the difference in rates of heavy consumption of alcohol and tobacco, as they exist between men and women. When the death rates of nonsmoking and nondrinking men are compared with those of nonsmoking and nondrinking women, the life-expectancy gap between men and women almost vanishes.

My second statistic, remember, pointed toward the big increase in general life expectancy occurring during the 1970s. As a physician I wish I could say that this was the result of some new miracle drug or some inventive improvement in medical care. Such was not the case. The major reasons for this jump in life expectancy are to be found in the increased understanding of those diseases which are presently killing vast numbers of the people: heart disease and cancer. Roughly 50 percent of all deaths occurring in America today are the result of either heart disease or stroke; almost 20 percent of all deaths are the result of cancer. Even so, heart disease and stroke deaths in this country decreased by about 25 percent during the 1970s. Talk about some really good news—an astounding, if still incomplete, triumph was achieved over our major killer in just one decade.

How and why did this happen? It happened because of changes in our diet, with decreased consumption of saturated fats and cholesterol; increases in physical exercise (a 100 percent increase in only one decade in the number of Americans who exercise on a regular basis); and decreases in smoking, particularly among men over the age of 40. These were the main reasons for the improvement in the health of our overall population during the preceding decade.

The "Danger Zone": Ages 15 to 24

Now, what about the one segment of our population in which health is deteriorating? The leading causes of death, in order, for Americans from ages 15 to 24 are accidents, suicides, and homicides. These three killers cause three-fourths of the deaths among American 15- to 24-year-olds.

During the last two decades, as we have seen an increase in adolescent accidents, suicides, and homicides, we have seen also an enormous increase in adolescent alcohol problems, drug problems, unwanted pregnancies, sexually transmitted disease, and crime. Consider a few examples:

- The suicide rate among adolescents has roughly doubled in the last two decades.
- The accident rate among adolescents has gone up substantially, as has the homicide rate.
- The percentage of teenagers who come to school drunk at least once a month has doubled, going from 10 percent in 1964 to 20 percent in 1979.

Most of these problem-measures for youth have increased between 50 and 200 percent during this two-decade period. Bad as these increases are, there is one which is even more shocking: the drug use rates are up many, many times, not just 50 to 200 percent. *Drug use rates among adolescents have risen 10 to 30 times between the early 1960s and today.* That means that drug use rates have risen 1,000 percent to 3,000 percent during the last 20 years. In addition, all the other teenage problems I mentioned, from teenage pregnancy to dropping Scholastic Aptitude Test (SAT) scores and homicide, are strongly associated with drug use. Kids who use drugs have lower grades, more delinquency, and higher rates of suicide and homicide, for example, than do kids who do not use drugs. A further irony: as American adults during the last decade were exercising more and smoking fewer cigarettes, American teenagers were exercising less and smoking more cigarettes. American teenagers were, on the average, less physically fit in 1984 than they were in 1965.

HEALTH VERSUS DRUGS

If you needed convincing, then this picture should strongly persuade you that one of the most important segments—probably the *most* important segment—of our population stands in danger. That segment is our youth, and that danger is a wide range of behavioral problems, especially drug use. Having pinpointed the area and the age of greatest vulnerability in terms of personal and national health—young people between the ages of 15 and 24—and having identified the principal destroyer of that health, we can benefit by taking a close, hard look at what we are up against. *Health versus drugs*—that is one of the major concerns of this book. By health, I mean not only physical health, but also *mental* well-being. The two are almost inseparable. Furthermore, both physical and mental health translate directly into work capacity—what economists call "productivity."

For both teenagers and their parents, the shared tasks loom clear and imperative: to prolong lives, to enjoy life more, and to live more productively.

To achieve a satisfying and enduring life is to reduce and, to the greatest extent possible, to eliminate forces which wreck the health and well-being of both children and parents. Make no mistake about this. If teenagers take up drug use, they will not be the only ones to suffer. Parents will suffer, too—in less physically painful ways, perhaps—but they will be faced with a formidable array of repugnant realities and agonizing uncertainties. As a nation, over the decade of the 1970s we lost many vital battles as a result of the drug-abuse epidemic among the young.

A WORKING VOCABULARY FOR TALKING ABOUT DRUGS

As a first step toward understanding the drug problem, we need to develop a *working vocabulary*. A classification with a list of the names of the major drugs and their hazardous effects on human health is shown below. Take time to study and familiarize yourself with the names and characteristics provided in this list and in the descriptions which follow it. Since, throughout, I will be referring often to specific drugs and drug effects, the sooner you encounter and familiarize yourself with relevant terms, the more understandable and informative your reading will become as we go along. Sometimes I will be using the technical or scientific names; at other times I will employ their "street" names.

Equally sound and practical, I believe, is the *communication* reason for being able to recognize and use the nomenclature of drugs. Parents and teenagers cannot expect to communicate and interact successfully unless they have a working—a "talking"—knowledge of the *language* of drugs. When parents listen to their children—and they must listen if they are to understand and help them—they must know what their children are talking about. Use of terms such as "space cadet" and "rocket fuel" could reflect a genuine interest in interplanetary travel, but it could also mean that the adolescent speaker is already far out on a "spaced-out" trip to drug dependence. Whether you are a parent or a teenager, acquiring an enlarged understanding of drugs means, among other things, an enlarged and continuously enlarging *familiarity* with key words, terms, substances, subterfuges, and behaviors related to the drug epidemic. A mutual agreement to listen to one another is a valuable starting point to some truly productive communication, "a bridge over troubled waters," and a shared vocabulary will help that process of communication.

In other words, knowing at least the names of the specific drugs being used in America today, knowing how and why they are classified as they are, recognizing some of the "street" terminology, and being aware of the drug-taking "accessories" is basic to parent-teenager interactions about drugs.

MAJOR CLASSES OF DRUGS AND THEIR MAJOR EFFECTS

With that sobering prologue, let us take a moment to examine the major classes of drugs in order to see their major effects. I list eight major classes of drugs. They are opioids, depressants, stimulants, hallucinogens, phencyclidines, cannabinoids, inhalants, and alcohol. In terms of pharmacology, or the "science of drugs," alcohol fits in the depressant classification. However, because of the pattern, extent, and consequences of alcohol use in America, it is treated as a separate category.

Note that three of the eight drug categories are unique to particular drugs: phencyclidines, cannabinoids, and alcohol. Although these drugs have properties similar to drugs in other classes (phencyclidines and cannabinoids, for example, produce some effects similar to those of both hallucinogens and depressants, and alcohol has many properties in common with depressants), each one is sufficiently unique and is used with sufficient frequency to warrant a separate classification.

CLASSIFICATION OF DRUGS OF ABUSE

Drugs of abuse can be classified in several ways. Some of these are best for research purposes and others are more clinically useful. *They are classified in this book according to their most prominent effects on the brain or the central nervous system.* The various classes, with examples of the most frequently abused drugs in each class, are presented below.

Drug Classifications

Class	*Examples*
Opioids	Heroin, morphine, methadone
Depressants	Barbiturates, methaqualone
Stimulants	Amphetamines, cocaine
Hallucinogens	LSD, mescaline
Phencyclidines	PCP, ketamine
Cannabinoids	Marijuana, hashish
Inhalants	Acetone, benzene, ethyl acetate, nitrous oxide
Alcohol (ethanol)	Beer, wine, whiskey, etc.

ABOUT THE DRUGS THEMSELVES

Opioids

Also called "narcotic analgesics," these drugs are often used medically to decrease pain. This class includes morphine and other alkaloids of opium. Narcotics—opium, its derivatives, or synthetic substitutes—are used medically to relieve intense pain, suppress coughs, remedy diarrhea, and induce a drowsy, euphoric state. These drugs are used nonmedically for their intense euphoric effect—a dream-like sense of well-being and relaxation.

Heroin

Users' Names:

horse   "H"
boy

Depressants

These drugs depress excitable tissues at all levels of the brain. The central nervous system depressants include almost all antianxiety drugs (such as Valium) and sleeping aids (such as Seconal). These drugs have been called "solid booze" because their effects are similar to alcohol. This characterization is more typical of barbiturates than of antianxiety drugs, such as Valium, because this latter group produces less generalized sedation in typical therapeutic doses. Depressants relax the body's muscles and bring on sleep by slowing down messages to the central nervous system.

Barbiturates

Users' Names:

downers   sleeping pills
reds   yellow jackets
barbs   red devils
beans   Christmas trees

Methaqualone

Quaalude   "Q"
"Ludes"   "sopor"

Tranquilizers

Valium   "V's"

Stimulants

The most prominent effect of these drugs is their ability to stimulate the central nervous system, producing euphoria, hypersensitivity, insomnia, and appetite suppression. The stimulants most commonly encountered are cocaine and the amphetamines—often taken to suppress sleep, tiredness, and appetite.

Stimulants increase a person's alertness, activity, and excitement by speeding up messages to the central nervous system. The aftermath of stimulant use is depression—exhaustion of the drug-stimulated nervous system. The higher the high, the lower the subsequent low.

Amphetamines

Users' Names:

uppers	crank
speed	dexies
bennies	meth
black beauties	black mollies
crossroads	jelly beans
hearts	greenies
brownies	wakeups

Cocaine

coke	snow
toot	"C"
girl	happy dust
flake	ice

Hallucinogens

These substances produce hallucinations, usually of a visual nature, but sometimes of sound or smell. The hallucinogens, which have no accepted medical use, include LSD, mescaline, and psilocybin. Hallucinogens are natural or synthetic drugs which can produce great changes in the mind. To hallucinate means to misperceive reality—to see, smell, or hear things that really are not there. This occurs because of the poisoning of the brain which produces profoundly abnormal thinking.

LSD

Users' Names:

California sunshine	acid
red, green, and	purple haze
orange dragon	micro-dots

Philocybin/pilocyn Mushrooms

buttons

Phencyclidines

Phencyclidines are related, pharmacologically, to hallucinogens and produce somewhat similar effects. However, a number of researchers believe that these drugs constitute a separate class because they produce different symptoms of tolerance and withdrawal. Users of phencyclidines speak of "floating" and being cut off from their feelings.

Phencyclidine (PCP)

Users' Names:

flakes	green
dust	hog
busy bee	angel dust
peace pills	rocket fuel
white powder	killer weed (K.W.)
embalming fluid	DOA (Dead on Arrival)
elephant tranquilizer	superjoint (when laced
lovely	with marijuana)

Cannabinoids

Marijuana and hashish (derived from the *Cannabis sativa* plant) as well as their principal active ingredient, delta-9-tetrahydrocannabinol (THC), produce an intoxicated state marked by altered time sense, euphoria, and—at high doses—hallucinations.

Marijuana and derivatives act most similarly to hallucinogens, but possess also the elements of stimulation and depression.

Marijuana, Hashish

Users' Names:

grass	Mary Jane
Maui Waui	pot
weed	Panama Red
joint	THC
reefer	cannabis
herb	Colombian
California Sinsemilla	Acapulco Gold
hash	hashish oil

Inhalants

This class of drugs includes solvents that are widely used in cleaning compounds, aerosol sprays, fuels, and glues. As drugs of abuse, inhalants are used to induce altered states of consciousness, primarily lightheadedness and confusion associated with general depression of brain functioning.

Nitrous Oxide

Users' Names:

laughing gas   nitrous

Isobutyl Nitrite

poppers	snappers
locker room	discoroma
bolt	rush

Alcohol

This drug is consumed in a variety of forms: beer, wine, and distilled spirits or liquor. The active agent in all of these forms is ethanol, or ethyl alcohol, a general, nonspecific central nervous system depressant.

The foregoing classification of the major drugs and their principal effects is largely "brain-based": it focuses on the effects of these classes of drugs on the user's one target organ—the brain. This is a useful classification for our purposes because it is the brain the drug user seeks to affect, and it is the particular drug's effect on the brain which produces dependence. Keep steadily in mind, however, that most of these drugs affect many parts of the body, in addition to the brain. Marijuana, for instance, produces severe lung damage after repeated use. Alcohol and marijuana have profound effects on reproduction and hormone levels. Thus, the entire spectrum of the physical effects of each drug is often more widespread and varied than this brain-based classification suggests.

DRUGS AND DRUG USE: SOME "STREET TALK"

Dope: A slang term for marijuana and other drugs.
Joint: A marijuana cigarette. Cost: about $1.00.
Roach: The end or "butt" of a marijuana cigarette.
High: An intoxicated feeling—an altered feeling after taking a drug. When "high," a drug user's brain is impaired. Thinking is less effective. Some common slang descriptions for this state of intoxication:

wasted	ripped	stoned
wired	buzzed	blown away
out of it	loaded	spaced out

Head: A person who uses drugs, such as "pot head" and "acid head."
Toke: A puff or "hit" of a marijuana cigarette. To "toke" is to smoke pot.
Burnout: A state of apathy, deadened perceptions, and reduced intellectual capacity that can result from regular or habitual use of marijuana and other drugs.
Space Cadet: The habitual marijuana user whose senses have become dulled.

DRUG PARAPHERNALIA: "TOOLS OF THE TRADE"

Drug paraphernalia are often called smoking accessories—especially as they are used with marijuana. In a broader sense, however, they are anything—instrument, device, tool, implement, portable hiding place—used in conjunction with taking drugs or preparing them for use. The following items are typical:

Bong: A water pipe designed to cool marijuana smoke, to increase its potency (some users believe), and to cool the smoke in order to reduce lung irritation. Cost: $4.50 to $150.00.

Marijuana Pipe: The pipe used for smoking marijuana or hash, which usually has a short stem and metal bowl with a screen inside it. Marijuana burns hotter than tobacco, thus ordinary tobacco pipes are often ruined by marijuana smoking. Marijuana pipes have a smaller bowl than tobacco pipes. Cost: $5.00 to $50.00.

Roach Clip: A clip designed to hold the end of a marijuana cigarette (a roach) to prevent burning the tips of fingers while the joint is being smoked down to its very end. Roach clips are often disguised as other objects: felt-tipped pens, car keys, earrings, necktie clips, lipstick containers, and similar accessories. Cost: $3.50 to $20.00, depending on the complexity of the device.

Rolling Papers: A type of paper used for rolling marijuana cigarettes which is wider than rolling papers used to make tobacco cigarettes by hand. They are wider to permit looser packing of more material than is common in tobacco cigarettes.

Cocaine Spoons: Called "coke spoons," these small utensils frequently take the form of necklaces, bracelets, earrings, and other jewelry and are used to measure and snort or sniff cocaine.

Tooter: A small, hollow tube used to snort or sniff cocaine from a flat surface into the user's nose.

Cocaine Cutting Kits: These kits contain various items used for diluting ("cutting") and taking cocaine. Typical contents: a cutting implement, such as a razor blade, a polished surface, a small container, a tooter, and—sometimes—a very small spoon.

Free-Base Kits: A kit containing solutions and chemicals used in purifying cocaine so that it can be smoked.

Mannite, Mannitol: Promoted as being natural and organic, these substances are used to cut or dilute cocaine. Cost: about $2.00 per ounce.

Stash Can: This is a comparatively small and, usually, portable container in which to conceal drugs from parents, employers, school authorities and police. Examples: Coca-Cola bottles,

Campbell Soup cans, Coors Beer cans, Sears Motor Oil containers, Kodak film canisters, Benzedrex inhalers, and Chapstick (for sniffing cocaine). Because stash cans rarely are what they appear to be, the cost can be high—$12.00 to $25.00.

PEOPLE USE DRUGS BECAUSE THEY LIKE THE FEELINGS THEY GET WHEN THEY USE DRUGS

It is easy to review even such an abbreviated account of various drugs of abuse and wonder, "Why does anyone use drugs at all?" Similarly, the more a person understands the unique and complex properties of individual drugs and even of classes of drugs, the more he may ask, "What do they have in common—why these drugs?" The simple answer, more fully explored in Chapter 2, is that these drugs are chemicals which produce feelings the users like or, more realistically, learn to like. They, as a group, take away bad feelings and produce good feelings. They do this in a variety of apparently unrelated biologically based ways through their effects on the human brain. Drugs, in a word, *work*. Of course, few drug users use all of these drugs, and even those users who do try all or most of these drugs tend to specialize in one or two of them over time. Why? The short answer is, "No one knows." The longer answer is that availability, social support (or lack of it), and complex biological and psychological processes all affect the user's "drug of choice."

Three other frequently used terms should be defined at the outset. *Dependence* refers to complex biological adaptations to prolonged drug use which get expressed, for the drug user, as the feeling after prolonged, frequent use as he craves the continued use of the drug. It also describes the behavior of continuous use of the drug. Finally, dependence implies the pain of *withdrawal* experienced by the user when he attempts to stop using the drug. Dependence has replaced the earlier term *addiction*, which was often narrowly applied to dependence on opiate drugs such as heroin. Thus, a regular marijuana user is dependent on the drug if he has a hard time stopping his use of it. When he tries to stop, he feels a craving for more of the drug; he therefore seeks out the drug to continue use. If he does stop, he feels irritable and has trouble sleeping (withdrawal symptoms).

The precise symptoms produced by withdrawal from each drug differ; and while the symptoms are affected by the dose of the drug used, the frequency and duration of that use, and by still poorly understood individual characteristics of the user, the general pattern of withdrawal symptoms described here is common to all the drugs listed in my classification.

Tolerance to a drug means that the more a drug user takes of that drug, the less effect he gets from each dose. Because the body adapts over time to the presence of the drug, the long-term, high-dose user must take more and more of the drug to produce the desired effect. This is commonly seen with alcohol, where a heavy alcohol user experiences little effect from a single beer, whereas a novice user of alcohol will get a relatively strong drug effect from drinking the same amount. These three words—dependence, withdrawal, and tolerance—are important to understanding the drug experience.

From the point of view of drug abuse prevention and drug abuse treatment, the specifics of which drug the user becomes dependent on and the exact nature of the pharmacological effects of that drug are far less important than are the general characteristics of drug dependence. These constitute the central reality of drug dependence: the pattern of using a chemical (a "drug") to feel good or to stop feeling bad and the willingness to risk health, job, and family in the pursuit of that chemical pleasure. This, of course, is not to say that other facts are not important. For example, alcohol use is legal (over the legal minimum drinking age), and thus becoming dependent on alcohol is quite different from becoming dependent on heroin, the most universally condemned dependence-producing drug. To be hooked on heroin is more than a pharmacological reality; it is, in contemporary America, almost invariably a statement about the heroin user's willingness to inject a drug intravenously several times a day, every day, and a statement about his or her willingness to participate in a criminal subculture.

The reason why individual drug users become dependent on specific dependence-producing drugs is an interesting and unresolved research question. Answering this question is not, in my experience, likely to help the user, his concerned family members, or his therapists. Similarly, I have included information about specific drugs, drug-using language, and paraphernalia to permit a more general and effective communication about drug habits, not because I believe effective prevention or treatment rests on developing a drug-using connoisseur's familiarity with the minutiae of drug use. The opposite is closer to the truth—it is more useful to have a clear view of the forest of drug dependence as a process than to get lost in preoccupation with the individual trees of specific drug characteristics.

FACTORS AND ATTITUDES CONTRIBUTING
TO "THE DRUG EPIDEMIC"

For most Americans over the age of 35—that is, those who passed through their drug-vulnerable teenage years before the drug epidemic of the late 1960s and 1970s—drugs like tobacco and alcohol are so familiar they are hardly considered to be "drugs." The "new" drugs, introduced for the first time to the majority of American youth only in the last two decades, are not new in any sense other than that they were not previously familiar to most Americans. Cocaine is now enjoying its third run as a drug of mass use and dependence (the earlier cocaine infatuations occurred in the 1880s and the 1920s). Marijuana has been around, and generally viewed quite negatively, in other cultures for thousands of years. Opiates, such as heroin, as well as many stimulants, depressants, and hallucinogens are also not new. Only our mass exposure is new. Here the simple, tragic fact is that American youth, in the last 20 years, have made themselves guinea pigs in a national "experiment" of unprecedented proportions. Never before in world history has so large a segment of a national population used such a large number of dependence-producing drugs—and become so hooked on them. When the full impact of this "experiment" is assessed, it will, I am convinced, be seen as a national tragedy of immense proportions.

Safe-Seeming Drugs Are Uniquely Dangerous

Another key to understanding which drugs emerged as major drug problems during the last two decades is the *image* each drug had. Drugs that were perceived as "safe" and "fun" shot ahead of drugs considered "dangerous." Thus, marijuana, cocaine, and—to a lesser extent—Quaaludes and stimulants like amphetamines shot far ahead of scarier drugs such as heroin, LSD, PCP, and even barbiturates. These safe-seeming drugs I have called GATEWAY DRUGS, because they are the drugs most Americans now use to enter the world of drug dependence. The "gate" is attractive to millions of American youths precisely because these drugs are seen as harmless.

During the past two decades, young people doubted their elders on everything, but on nothing so profoundly as on drugs. Often the attitude was, "What do *they* have to teach *me*?" The fact that adults had little personal experience with these new drugs added to this conviction of the unique wisdom of young people. There was a widespread sense among youth that "you must find out for yourself," and that meant experimenting with drugs—lots of them. For many American youths during the last two decades, the outcome of all that experimenting was that they liked the drugs. They continued to use them, and they encouraged their friends to do the same.

In this vacuum of adult authority, many hoped the scientific community could be relied on to provide persuasive reasons for youth not to use drugs, including alcohol and tobacco as well as marijuana and other illegal drugs. There was no strong voice committed to helping adolescents avoid drug use. In fact, the scientists' repeated assertions that "We don't know yet" or the apparent conflict of experts' opinions in many ways fed the drug epidemic. Tens of millions of young people, as a result, concluded that in this, too, adults had little to teach them. Adult use of alcohol and tobacco often was seen by teenagers as revealing the hypocrisy of adult authority when it came to drug abuse prevention: "Pot's no worse than booze!"

One of the lessons I learned early in my medical training was suggested by the words of the old-time bank robber, Willie Sutton. When the cops finally caught up with him, they asked him why he robbed the banks. "Because," said Willie, "that's where the money is." Now, if we are asking ourselves, "Where is the 'health bank' of this country?" we might well paraphrase Willie's words a bit and say, "Youth is where it's at." If we are seeking ways to improve the health and prolong the lives of the young, we should realize that the payoff has much to do with lifestyles. While the teenage years are not the only years during which decisions involving lifestyles threaten an individual's health, they are the years when lifestyles—and hence health-preserving or life-destroying habits—are established in ways destined to affect all the days of each person's time on earth. During the teenage years, to cite but one example, people make lasting decisions about what they are going to do about the use of tobacco, alcohol, and other drugs. In fact, it is unusual (though not quite rare) for a person to begin drug use before the age of 12 years or after the age of 20.

Primarily, here, we are talking about vulnerability between the ages of 12 and 20—a uniquely vulnerable opening stage between childhood and adulthood. Standing in this opening, often with unseeing eyes, young people make personal decisions about the use of alcohol and other drugs that will deeply affect the rest of their lives. After the age of about 20, the vulnerability dramatically falls. New drug use after the age of 20 is almost as uncommon as it was before age 12.

Once, someone who heard me speak on these matters asked, "Do you mean that if we stop smoking, if we stop drinking, if we end our

overeating and start exercising, then we may live longer?" "Yes," I
said, "you got my message." "Well," he said, "I'm not sure whether I
would live longer if I did all that, but I know it would *seem* a lot
longer." Subtract the humor and you are left with a sense of sadness
for the flippant cynicism that covers the close-to-the-surface fears of
the young and the not-so-young among us: the awareness, often
avoided, that when it comes to avoiding illness and premature death,
we are usually our own worst enemy.

The Extent of American Drug Use

Look for a moment at some of the specifics of drug use and the
extent to which it pervades the lifestyles and the health of young
Americans. From Table 1 (Annual Drug Use: 1972–1982), we see
both the extent of the current use of various drugs and the trends
over the last decade. Here we see the percentages of all Americans
who reported use of each particular drug during the year prior to the
taking of the annual survey. Overall, the table covers 11 classes of
drugs, including alcohol and tobacco. From it, certain conclusions are
readily apparent. All drug use is highly *age-related*, with peaks of use
of all drugs (including tobacco and alcohol) occurring between the
ages of 18 and 25 years. Only three drugs—alcohol, tobacco, and
marijuana—are used by massive segments of the American population. The drug that is now making a strong move on the leaders, and
which is presently in fourth place, is cocaine.

Use of drugs other than tobacco and alcohol was uncommon, if not
rare, prior to 1960. The last two decades, however, saw an unprecedented rise in the use of such drugs as LSD, cocaine, heroin, and
marijuana. Indeed, the drug abuse epidemic occurred during this two-
decade era. Centered on America's youth (some of whom are no
longer young), this epidemic is powerfully related to a variety of other
lifestyle problems: teenage crime, teenage suicide, teenage sexually
transmitted disease, and early teenage pregnancy. These problems
are all results of loss of self-control and of family and community
control of impulsive, pleasure-seeking behavior.

Why Do We Have a Drug Epidemic?

While there is no easy answer as to why this epidemic has occurred
during the last two decades, there are several reasonable and mutually reinforcing explanations. When we understand these reasons, we
can more clearly understand what has caused the epidemic and what
needs to be done to end it.

TABLE 1. Annual Drug Use: 1972–1982

Age group, drug	1972	1974	1976	1977	1979	1982
Youth (12–17)						
Marijuana	...	18.5%	18.4%	22.3%	24.1%	20.7%
Hallucinogens	3.6%	4.3	2.8	3.1	4.7	3.6
Cocaine	1.5	2.7	2.3	2.6	4.2	4.3
Heroin	<0.5	<0.5	<0.5	0.6	<0.5	<0.5
Nonmedical Use of						
Stimulants	...	3.0	2.2	3.7	2.9	5.5
Sedatives	...	2.0	1.2	2.0	2.2	3.6
Tranquilizers	...	2.0	1.8	2.9	2.7	3.0
Analgesics	...	...	...	...	2.2	3.8
Any Nonmedical Use	...	...	...	...	5.8	8.2
Alcohol	...	51.0	49.3	47.5	53.6	46.9
Cigarettes	...	...	...	...	13.3	14.2
Young Adults (18–25)						
Marijuana	...	34.2	35.0	38.7	46.9	40.7
Hallucinogens	...	6.1	6.0	6.4	9.9	7.3
Cocaine	...	8.1	7.0	10.2	19.6	19.5
Heroin	...	0.8	0.6	1.2	0.8	<0.5
Nonmedical Use of						
Stimulants	...	8.0	8.8	10.4	10.1	11.0
Sedatives	...	4.2	5.7	8.2	7.3	8.4
Tranquilizers	...	4.6	6.2	7.8	7.1	5.9
Analgesics	...	...	...	...	5.2	4.6
Any Nonmedical Use	...	...	...	...	16.3	16.1
Alcohol	...	77.1	77.9	79.8	86.6	83.5
Cigarettes	...	...	...	...	46.7	41.1
Older Adults (26+)						
Marijuana	...	3.8	5.4	6.4	9.0	10.8
Hallucinogens	...	<0.5	<0.5	<0.5	0.5	0.8
Cocaine	...	<0.5	0.6	0.9	2.0	3.9
Heroin	...	<0.5	<0.5	<0.5	<0.5	<0.5
Nonmedical Use of						
Stimulants	...	<0.5	0.8	0.8	1.3	1.8
Sedatives	...	<0.5	0.8	<0.5	0.8	1.4
Tranquilizers	...	<0.5	1.2	1.1	0.9	1.1
Analgesics	...	...	...	...	0.5	1.0
Any Nonmedical Use	...	...	...	...	2.3	3.0
Alcohol	...	62.7	64.2	65.8	72.4	68.5
Cigarettes	...	...	...	...	39.7	37.3

Note: Numbers are percentages based on any reported use of the listed drugs during the preceding year in repeated national surveys; ... indicates "data not available."

Source: National Household Survey on Drug Abuse, 1982. National Institute on Drug Abuse.

The period 1960 to 1980 was a time of many changes in the United States. The most fateful for the drug epidemic was the rise in the number of youths in the population. The last two decades saw the post–World War II Baby Boom pass through adolescence.

Other changes occurred, although many of them were derived from, or at least reinforced by, this demographic tidal wave. We saw the flowering of the "youth culture," which all but overturned the traditional forces restraining the reckless behavior that has long been characteristic of adolescence. Virtually all of the "reforms" of the last two decades were reductions in controls over individual and group behavior and also reductions in expectations for youths. This was the era of reduced requirements in schools and at home and reduced limitations on what was previously considered deviant behavior (including the lowering of the drinking age in many states during the 1970s). There was a widespread, romantic belief that went something like: "Let the kids have fun. They'll figure it out for themselves." Parents, teachers, and employers were everywhere in retreat as the onslaught of the "youth culture" peaked in the mid-1970s.

Note that I have placed the words "youth culture" and "reforms" in quotation marks. I am not suggesting that all of the changes in America during the last two decades, let alone all aspects of changed roles for youth, have been dangerous. Rather, I am calling your attention to several specific aspects of these changes, aspects that are almost a caricature of many truly positive changes that have occurred. These specific aspects have had a profoundly negative impact on American youth.

The "Me Generation" flowered beyond youth. Adults were caught up in the winds of change and began to ask, "What about me?" The more traditional expectations and responsibilities of each of us were undercut, and we wondered, "When do I get mine?" Job changes, divorce, and alternate lifestyles were "in." Adults who, for generations, were convinced they had the answers to the problems of their children, over the last two decades grew suddenly hesitant. The Vietnam War, the Civil Rights Movement, the War on Poverty, and the Women's Movement all raised serious questions about the wisdom of the "older generation" and traditional guidelines for individual behavior. It seemed that the new generation had little to learn from their elders, except not to live the way they did. What rules youth needed they would, it seemed, "learn for themselves." "Problems" were not the fault of youth or of the pursuit of pleasure, but of the "no-saying authorities."

What an irony that the generation whose values were crystalized in the austerity of the Great Depression and the sacrifices of World War II and who were so remarkably successful in providing material comforts and quality education for their children (often beyond their most optimistic hopes) discovered that many of their children rejected these prized values, seeking instead the self-gratifications of personal and frequently reckless pleasure.

There is another dimension to this personal pursuit of pleasure. One of the principal characteristics of the "youth culture" is the focus on the present tense. If it is not *now*, it is not, period. That was one of the essential messages of the last two decades. For American youth, earlier ideas about delay of gratification—doing something unpleasant now so that at some later time one could feel good—became as unfashionable as it was to do something "for someone else." Any attempt to suppress personal, present-tense pleasure was seen, in this view, as a "cop-out," a failure of courage or as hypocritical and "other directed."

Drugs fit nicely into this value scheme since the drug-induced pleasure is *now* and the drug-caused problems tend to come later on— often years after the drug use has become habitual. Similarly, since intoxicating drugs tend to obscure the drug user's critical judgment as an early and characteristic effect, the drug user's own self-awareness of drug-caused problems was restricted.

Over this period of 20 years, the legitimacy of *others* in controlling personal behavior was progressively eroded. Whether these others were rooted in religion, law, school, work, or the family, they were all seen as irrelevant or even hostile to the pursuit of personal needs. This, too, fueled the drug epidemic. One poignant aspect of this historical experience is that these others were often acting in the best interests of the youth themselves: they were essentially saying "No" to dangerous but pleasure-producing behaviors because they were concerned not about the pleasure but about the youth.

One of the long-term, painful consequences of this historical process is the difficulty now experienced by many young people between the ages of 20 and 35 in making commitments and even, paradoxically, in finding pleasure in many everyday activities of life, from work and sex to raising a family and participating in religious activities. As the expectation for pleasure rose, as the restraints on pleasure-producing behavior were seen ever more negatively, as intense drug-induced pleasures became the standard against which all pleasure was measured by many in this generation, the "normal" pleasures seemed like "work," and they seemed, somehow, insufficient. Sex, for example, once it became cheap, lost a lot of its excitement. While previous generations complained about impotence and frigidity (often associated with viewing pleasure as bad), young people between 20 and 35 now complained most often of a total lack of interest in sex (often associated with early, extensive sexual activity).

The national economy, too, played a role in the drug epidemic. Throughout the 1960s and the early 1970s, the sustained, unprecedented prosperity made it seem as if material plenty was an entitlement rather than a reward to be earned by hard work. For children of the middle and upper economic classes, growing up in the 1960s and 1970s was accompanied by a shower of economic plenty given to them by their well-meaning, depression-surviving parents. The earlier values of planning for the future, and even sacrificing one's comfort for the opportunities of one's children, became old-fashioned or, even worse, ridiculous. Indeed, such values were rapidly replaced by the new *now* values. "If it feels good now, do it now" became the new motto. To many Americans, young and old, it seemed that the era of the proverbial "free lunch" had arrived.

There were other factors at work, as well—many of which specifically affected the family life of teenagers. There was an unprecedented rise in divorce, producing a ballooning number of single-parent families. Women entered the work force in unprecedented numbers, thus further eroding the effective parenting power in millions of homes. For the young especially, travel and communications became all but universal. Behaviors and experiences—including drug use—which heretofore had been relatively isolated by time, space, and cultural barriers, were suddenly and easily available to huge numbers of American young people. To a greater or lesser extent, a whole generation followed the advice of the self-appointed high priest of drugs, Timothy Leary: "Turn on, Tune in, Drop out!" Although this advice was given initially about hallucinogens, it rapidly was generalized to all illegal drugs.

The Electronic Revolution—instant communication, instant excitement, instant everything, seemingly made possible by the advent of television—profoundly reinforced and extended these trends. This drug-using youth population, born after World War II, was the first generation raised on television. What exists between TV viewing and drug use is no accidental relationship. Television-watching has many elements in common with drug-taking. Both tend to be mindless, passive, and ultimately isolating. Fascination with a television screen, like fascination with a drug, can produce a dependence requiring someone else—a nonuser—to set limits on the user. Television can be, in fact, a plug-in drug.

And the ``Contagion'' Will Spread . . .

In the United States during the last two decades, many things changed, not all of them bad and not all of them permanent. The hula hoop came and went. Hair styles changed as many a youth concluded, "If you can see his ears, you can't trust him." The more optimistic among the oldsters comforted themselves by saying, "Not to worry. These things are mere fads."

Drug use, however, is not like a passing fad: once a person becomes dependent on any drug, that person is likely to have a long and painful experience either in living with or living without the drug. This confusion, especially in the minds of many youths, about the unique seriousness of decisions concerning drug use played a central role in the sweeping drug epidemic.

Playing an almost equally important role is the inescapable fact that drug use in a population acts like a contagious disease. The new drug user tends to proselytize or recruit nonusers, thereby spreading drug-taking behavior. This chain reaction, this epidemic spread of drug use, was encouraged in the United States by the large demographic and social changes described in this chapter. Many observers of these trends, having had no experience with drug use, even now fail to judge accurately the seriousness and persistence of drug-using behavior. This failure is surprising in view of the increasingly widespread recognition among public health experts of the devastating social and health impact of alcohol and tobacco use by Americans. The so-called newer drugs, while once thought to be less likely to produce long-term harm to health and/or less likely to produce dependence, are now increasingly understood to have all the negative effects of alcohol and tobacco, plus many additional problems unique to themselves.

Another factor often overlooked by observers of the drug epidemic is that all drug use is *linked*. Those who use one drug are *more* likely to use each of the other drugs and are not, as many earlier observers assumed, *less* likely to use other drugs. Thus, the same epidemic that carried marijuana and cocaine, as well as LSD and PCP, to unprecedented new levels of use in the United States also produced a sharp rise in the use of tobacco and alcohol among our youth population. Many early observers thought marijuana, for example, might displace alcohol or, in more recent years, that the rise in alcohol use might lead to falling levels of marijuana use. The facts proved to be exactly the opposite: *rising marijuana use leads to rising alcohol use and vice versa.* This linkage inherent in all drug use also helps to explain the

puzzling rise in cigarette smoking by adolescents during the last two
decades when cigarette smoking by adults was declining. Among the
young, cigarette smoking rates were pushed up by the general rise in
drug use.

Finally, we must not overlook the significant fact that all drug use is
positively correlated with each of the other problems—including delinquency, unwanted pregnancy, murder, and suicide—experienced by
young people at unprecedentedly high rates during the last two decades. All of these problems, most noticeably those involving drug
use, were both the direct and the indirect results of reductions in the
societal, familial, and personal control over the pleasure-producing
behaviors of the young.

. . . UNLESS Strong ''Remedies'' Are Promptly Taken

During the last few years, countertrends have begun to emerge.
Schools have begun, slowly and often ambivalently, to strengthen
discipline and to raise standards of basic performance and behavior.
When it comes to defining what acceptable adolescent behavior is, it
is growing more fashionable to speak of "parents' rights" and somewhat less fashionable to talk of "children's rights." However, if we
are to manage these new trends to help reduce drug abuse and other
behavioral problems, while not abandoning the real improvements our
society has made during the past two decades—especially, real improvements in civil liberties and opportunities for women—we must
understand more specifically what the drug problem is and what can
be done about it directly.

We can also look at the sharp rise in the life expectancy of almost
all Americans during the 1970s for guidance in our efforts. During
those years, the rise in life expectancy came from real and important
changes in the lifestyles of millions of Americans, changes which had
a prompt and profound impact on health. The most recent information about adolescent health suggests that the lessons learned during
the 70s may be more directly relevant to today's teenagers than even
the most optimistic observers would have predicted only three years
ago. In the chapters ahead, I will explore these themes and possibilities and, in so doing, help to achieve the aim of this book as a whole.
That aim is to provide you with an understanding of the drug problem
and also of some of the more urgent, related problems it creates, and
to build a firm foundation for positive actions which can be taken to
solve drug problems in families and in communities.

SUMMING UP

Drug problems are part of a larger challenge facing Americans today: the explosive increase in personal choices available to all of us. This has created a health crisis because many choices are dangerous and unhealthy. Particularly deadly are choices which produce pleasure in the short run and hazard in the long run. Particularly vulnerable have been Americans from 15 to 24 years old. Drugs are the most dramatic of these new dangers.

Drugs which produce intoxication, or a high, all cause physically based dependence. They can be classified into eight groups based on their effects on the human brain. The basic language of drugs, from the research laboratory to the street scene, must be mastered before effective communication about drugs is possible.

During the last two decades, the United States and much of the rest of the world have experienced an unprecedented drug abuse epidemic. It has uniquely affected Americans who were teenagers during these years. This group, the drug epidemic generation, is now 16 to 35 years old.

The factors which caused this epidemic include the huge increase in the youth population—the post–World War II Baby Boom hitting adolescence—plus complex and mutually reinforcing cultural forces such as a reduced respect for authority and an increased reliance on self-determination of personal behavior. Additional causes of the current drug epidemic were increased communication and travel, as well as the remarkable economic prosperity during the beginning decade of the epidemic.

The safe-seeming drugs, particularly alcohol, marijuana, and cocaine, became the GATEWAY DRUGS for American youth entering into drug dependence. These are all dangerous addicting drugs, despite their popular images. Although there is evidence of a leveling off of drug use in recent years for most dependence-producing drugs, the drug epidemic is continuing on an historically unprecedented scale.

An understanding of the drug epidemic and related problems suggests many likely solutions, including education about the health hazards of all drugs, particularly the GATEWAY DRUGS, and about the Drug Dependence Syndrome itself. More directly, it encourages greater use of the family as an effective control over individual behavior. These solutions will be explored in later chapters.

CHAPTER
TWO

The
Drug Dependence
Syndrome

T HE MOST DIFFICULT PART of solving the drug abuse problem is knowing what the problem is. One cynic observed that "a drug is a chemical used for fun by someone you don't know or don't like." During the last two decades, many people have been unable to see the drug problem through the political smoke. Great mystery is introduced by trying to separate "drug abuse" from "drug use," trying to label the latter safe and the former dangerous. Many people have all but abandoned hope of understanding the drug problem, thereby reinforcing the already strong tendency to deny the seriousness or even the existence of drug dependence in our society.

WHAT A DRUG IS—A "WORKING" DEFINITION

To help chart our way we need to start with a simple, comprehensive definition of a drug. In this book, when I use the word *drug*, I am referring to a chemical or a group of related chemicals which, when taken into the body, produce feelings the user likes. Such feelings are sometimes called an altered state of consciousness. As a direct result of the drug affecting the user's brain, it produces intoxication, an altered, "feeling good" mental state. These chemicals can also be called "self-reinforcing substances." They produce pleasure—either by making the user feel good or by taking away bad feelings. They work on the user's brain to produce the feelings and thoughts which can best be translated as "Do It Again!"

To be more concrete, this definition of a drug includes alcohol as well as heroin, cocaine, and marijuana. This definition also includes most stimulants, most sleeping pills, and many of the painkillers and tranquilizers. For example, Valium and codeine are drugs in this sense because they produce good feelings; Thorazine and aspirin are not drugs according to the definition I am using here, because they do not make users feel good or "high." Nor can insulin and penicillin be properly classified as drugs in the sense I am using the word. People do not use aspirin or penicillin to get high. These chemicals—medicines—are not part of the drug problem as I am defining it because they do not produce pleasurable feelings.

Similarities Among Drugs Are
More Important Than Differences

While thinking about drugs generally, it is important not to be confused by the differences between the effects of the various drugs or by their different histories and legal status in our country. Primarily to avoid confusion, these are the significant general facts to keep in mind: All of the chemicals I call drugs have a *pleasure-producing effect*, and they all create drug problems.

Simplicities and Complexities

Some drugs, as we saw in Chapter 1, are single, relatively simple chemicals. Alcohol and cocaine are examples. Others are vastly complex mixes of different chemicals related only because they are produced by a single natural chemical factory: a plant. Marijuana is a good example. Understanding the effects of the single-chemical drugs is an unfinished research challenge. Understanding the *full* range of biological effects of complex drugs such as marijuana will be beyond our reach for many years to come. This does not mean, however, that much is not already known about these complex drugs. It does mean that what we know now is only the beginning of the story. Later, I will focus on some of the important differences among various drugs. But, before doing so, we must first consider some common patterns and progressions because they will help us keep our bearings as we deal with the complexities of drug problems and their impact upon our lives.

A SPECIAL NOTE ABOUT TOBACCO DEPENDENCE

Tobacco use has long been considered a habit. In recent years, research has shown that tobacco use is more than a habit; it is a drug

addiction. The same basic brain mechanisms which produce dependence on drugs from alcohol to heroin also work to hook the tobacco
user.

The connection between tobacco and other dependence-producing
drugs goes deep. Addicts who are allowed to inject nicotine intravenously often compare the experience to heroin use. Cigarette smoking
usually precedes marijuana and other illegal drug use in adolescence,
often by introducing the teenager to smoking as a way of getting a
drug into the body.

Twelve- to 17-year-olds who are current smokers of cigarettes,
when compared to youths of the same age who do not smoke, are
twice as likely to be current users of alcohol, nine times as likely to
make illegal use of pills such as stimulants and tranquilizers, 10 times
as likely to smoke marijuana, and 14 times as likely to use cocaine,
heroin, or hallucinogens. Thus, current smoking of cigarettes is a
strong predictor of other drug use among teenagers. One conclusion:
prevention of cigarette smoking is a high priority in the prevention of
dependence on all drugs.

In this book, I have not singled out cigarettes as a GATEWAY
DRUG, and I have not highlighted tobacco dependence because tobacco use—unlike the use of the other drugs considered in the
book—is *not intoxicating*. For the same reason, I have not focused on
caffeine or sugar dependence, or upon such nondrug addictions as
television watching or gambling. These behaviors are all related. They
all create biologically reinforced, pleasure-producing behavior disorders. To have included these behaviors, I believe, would have significantly complicated and confused the central messages of this book.
However, it is important to see the similarities between these
behaviors and drug dependence, and especially to recognize the
unique place of tobacco dependence as the most common and deadly
of all addictions. Tobacco use claims about 320,000 American lives a
year, far exceeding the death toll from all other drug addictions
combined.

Although I do not specifically highlight tobacco dependence in this
book, I will often illustrate my points by using the tobacco addiction
example. I do this partly because I recognize the unique and tragic
place tobacco plays in the drug dependence problem, but also because tobacco dependence is the most publicly visible of all drug
habits. Thus, tobacco dependence is—for the user and the nonuser
alike—a particularly useful model of the Drug Dependence Syndrome.

THE DRUG DEPENDENCE SYNDROME

A *syndrome*, according to *Webster's Dictionary*, is "a group of signs and symptoms that occur together and characterize a particular abnormality." Often the signs and symptoms occur in an identifiable pattern or sequence—a *progression*.

At the outset, too, it is important to understand what I mean when I say drug dependence. The term *drug dependence* has replaced and, to a large extent, incorporated the meaning of two previously much-used terms, *addiction* and *habituation*. According to the World Health Organization (WHO), "Drug dependence is a state, psychic or also sometimes physical, resulting from *the interaction between a living organism and a drug, and characterized by behavioral and other responses that always include a compulsive desire or need to use the drug on a continuous basis in order to experience its effects and/or avoid the discomfort of its absence*." The concept of *tolerance* lies at the root of drug dependence, and it means that the user of a particular drug—in order to continue to experience the same pharmacological effects—must take in increasing quantities of that drug. Once dependence on a drug develops, the user experiences a "craving" which, if not promptly satisfied by more use of the drug, proceeds to painful *withdrawal* symptoms.

Although earlier research into drug dependence focused on the unique characteristics of heroin and other opioid dependence, the most recent research has focused on the pleasure/pain centers in the mid brain and, more specifically, on the neurotransmitters, the chemicals by which one nerve cell in this part of the brain passes information on to another nerve cell. It now appears that all dependence-producing drugs have the capacity to trigger pleasure signals in these specific centers in the brain. Thus, the most fundamental biological effect of dependence-producing drugs is not withdrawal, as was previously thought, but pleasure. Any drug which produces pleasure—a good feeling—produces dependence. The new research gives a firm, biological foundation for the common clinical experience that these chemicals which seem to be so different from each other are, in real-life human drug abuse, closely related. They all produce stimulation in the same brain areas.

Not all people who try a particular drug go on to full-blown dependence upon it. Some drugs appear to be easier to use without developing dependence than are others. Also, the setting in which a drug is used significantly affects the consequences of its use. Consider the contrast between the effects of drinking communion wine in a church and the effects of drinking alcohol in a barroom.

The circumstances of the drug taking are important in other ways, too. Codeine or Valium, if taken in small quantities and used under effective medical supervision, is not likely to cause a drug problem. However, these same chemicals can produce real dependence when the user, in pursuit of pleasure, self-administers them outside close medical supervision. The attitude of the user toward taking the drug, as well as the size of the dose, also affects the outcome. Someone using morphine to treat the pain of a heart attack has a vastly different experience from the opiate addict who is using the same drug in similar quantities to avoid withdrawal pains.

The specific consequences of using any particular drug differ from the consequences of using other drugs. Cocaine, a stimulant, is quite different from alcohol, a depressant, for example. Nevertheless, despite specific variations in effects from drug to drug, we can better understand the drug problem by taking note of the four stages of the Drug Dependence Syndrome as the basic underpinning of all human self-administered drug taking. (See Figure 1 for a diagram of this process.)

The Four Stages of the Drug Dependence Syndrome

The most observable aspect of the Drug Dependence Syndrome is the *pattern of use* and the sequence or progression of the signs and symptoms resulting from that use. In the use of any drug, there are four basic stages. Whether the user is taking alcohol or marijuana or heroin, this basic pattern can be observed.

Stage One: Experimentation and First-Time Use. The first stage of the syndrome is experimental use. This is the stage that is central to an understanding of our current problem with adolescent drug use. Too many of our youth apparently believe that experimentation with drugs is safe and for certain drugs—especially alcohol— even normal. But, in point of fact, not only is experimentation unsafe, but it is also *the first step toward drug dependence.*

In the case of most drugs, at the stage of initial use or experimentation the user often finds the experience a negative one. The first-time cigarette smoker is likely to cough, wheeze, and suffer burning eyes. The new alcohol user must either dilute the drink or take it with a heavy dose of sugar. The beginning heroin user often vomits.

Unfortunately, these initial ill effects fail to deter most novice users, many of whom are socialized into drug use by more experienced users who reassure them that these symptoms will soon pass as use of the drug continues. A tolerance for these initially negative experiences quickly develops, and the progress toward dependence proceeds.

On the other hand, some novice users take these almost universal initial negative symptoms as a sign that they are allergic to the particular drug and stop using it. Novice drug users also seldom feel good after use of a dependence-producing drug. If they do not feel sick when they first use a drug, they often report, "It did nothing for me." Many never try the drug again. Like those who conclude they are allergic to a drug when they have an initially bad experience, these one-time drug users are saved from further drug use by their misunderstanding of the Drug Dependence Syndrome. To love a drug, as to love a person or an activity, takes much repetition—real practice. I am not, of course, encouraging anyone—young or old—to work to "love a drug." The opposite is my suggestion: Stay away

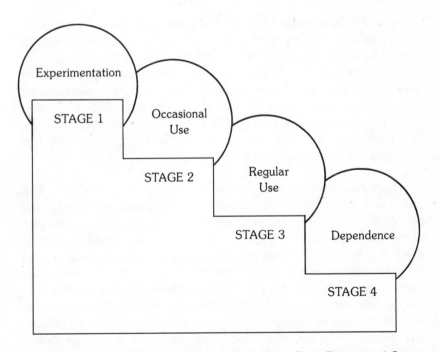

FIGURE 1. The Drug Dependence Syndrome: Four Downward Steps to Drug Dependence.

from that kind of chemical infatuation. It can do worse than break your heart—it can kill you.

Stage Two: Occasional or "Social" Use.   During this stage, as in the experimentation stage, the drug user is essentially passive. He accepts the drug—often from proselytizing friends who are already users of the drug themselves. Educated by them, he continues on past his initial negative experiences. The neophyte usually does not seek out the drug, but simply responds by taking it when it is made available. Large numbers of youths who eventually try drugs turn them down the first few times they are offered. Only after repeated exposure do most young people decide to try any particular drug. Therefore, even initial drug refusal is not a secure sign of success for drug abuse prevention: it can be a phase of the incubation process of drug dependence. During this stage, use is usually less frequent than once a week, and the pleasure produced by the drug use is often modest. This stage of the Drug Dependence Syndrome seems to confirm the novice user's belief that he or she can handle the drug, saying, in effect, "Look, I can take it or leave it."

Stage Three: Regular Use.   In this stage, drug users actively seek the chosen drug and try to maintain their own supply, making sure of continuing access to it. In settings where the user has decided to take the drug regularly, he or she makes sure the desired drug is readily available. Use at this stage is typically once or twice a week. Some drug users progress rapidly from Stage One to Stage Three. Usually, they are strongly motivated to get high on drugs in general and have little inhibition in their use of drugs. Others who progress quickly just like a particular drug right away.

Stage Four: Dependence—On the Road to Nowhere.   The fourth and final stage of this process is *dependence* or addiction. At this stage, use of one or more particular drugs becomes a major part of the user's life, and any effort to separate the user from the drug or drugs will be met with substantial resistance. When dependence has been established, many drug users will, in fact, give up almost all other things in life to maintain the connection with the chosen substance. The extreme priority given to drug use is commonly seen in dependent users of tobacco and alcohol, as well as in users of cocaine and heroin. They will, if a choice must be made, buy drugs rather than food. In the earlier stages of the syndrome—experimentation, occasional use, and even regular use—the decision to use a drug is, for example, usually far more responsive to such factors as price, supply, and family disapproval of use. However, once dependence has developed, almost no price is too high for most drug users to pay.

Because alcohol and tobacco are so inexpensively available and because use is so widely accepted even for youth in the United States, the full extent and irresistible pull of the dependence at Stage Four of the syndrome is not obvious except among the very poor. It is not obvious because it is generally easy for the alcoholic or tobacco user to keep using those drugs without sacrificing other needs or desires. The intense compulsion to use drugs is, however, quite evident among the users of the more expensive drugs such as cocaine and heroin. Users of these drugs frequently will give up almost anything to keep using the drug once they are hooked. At all ages, as soon as drug dependence has set in, it is commonplace for drug users to continue the drug taking even when threatened with jail, loss of job, and expulsion from family life.

The user seldom faces directly the facts of his or her decision to use drugs. Not long ago, an alcoholic physician whose wife and children had left him and who had lost his job as a senior researcher because he would not stop drinking, said to me, "My problem is that they just don't understand me. I need some time to think this all over." It was easier, apparently, for this formerly successful doctor to blame his predicament on the conflicts in his relationships with others than to face the central fact of his dependence on alcohol. Such denial of utter dependence is usually obvious to the nonuser of drugs, who is often puzzled by the distorted priorities of those who take them. What the nonuser misses, and what leads to puzzlement, is the power of drug dependence to take over and control the mind and thoughts of the user, no matter how intelligent that user may be.

While readers may be shocked by many statements in this book, I expect none will be more shocking to readers than my assertion that *the first use of a drug is the first step to drug dependence.* For most of the last two decades, an assumption has been widely made that trying a drug is safe and even desirable. Once the Drug Dependence Syndrome is clearly understood, then trying a drug is seen to be not only unsafe but as the most important step in the entire dependence process. Looked at this way, it becomes clear that the prevention of drug problems means stopping experimenting with drugs. Trying to stop the dependence process, the syndrome, at any other stage is more difficult, more expensive, and far more likely to fail. After nearly two decades of working in drug abuse treatment, I am painfully aware of just how hard and uncertain is the cure, once the Drug

Dependence Syndrome has begun. By contrast, prevention—stopping dependence *before it even begins*—is relatively easy, cheap, and effective if the goal is clearly understood.

Trying to stop the drug dependence process between the stages of Regular Use and Dependence is horribly hard. Heedless to this reality, so often confirmed in the experience of drug-abuse treatment, many people stubbornly cling to the idea that "a little drug use is okay" and that "the problem is addiction, not use." Much more to the point is the simple question: "What is the benefit from trying drugs?" What is the gain one seeks which can possibly offset the risk of life-long drug dependence? The steps down to dependence are slippery once the drug use begins. The pharmacology of pleasure-producing drugs works against success in this effort. Remember, *drug problems are easier to prevent than they are to cure.*

Some Progressive Consequences of the Drug Dependence Syndrome

As drug users go down these four steps or stages of the Drug Dependence Syndrome, they encounter a regular progression of consequences, both physical and psychological. In the initial stages, there are few consequences; frequently, in fact, there are no major consequences. There may, of course, be negative consequences in one or more of the earlier stages, but they are less common and more easily shrugged off by users as accidental. Examples of these earlier adverse drug reactions include panic-anxiety attacks after marijuana use, paranoia following cocaine use, asthma following the smoking of marijuana, and motor-vehicle collisions and other accidents resulting from intoxication of users who may or may not yet be totally dependent on alcohol or other drugs.

The most serious consequences of drug use, especially physical consequences, predominate and become all but inescapable only in the late stages of the Drug Dependence Syndrome. Most people have observed one of the more familiar of these consequences: the painful and often ambivalent struggle of drug-dependent individuals to become free of their dependence once it has become definitely established. They want to stop having problems, but they do not want to stop using the drug. Or they want to cut down their use of the drug, but they do not want to stop using it.

As a clinician, I know that this struggle to stop drug use is probably the hardest task the drug-dependent person will ever face. When dependent on a drug, the user is unlikely ever to break free of it without making an enormous effort. A drug-dependent person must make this effort to become drug free the most important activity in his or her life—at least for a period of time. And even if successful, former users are likely to spend the rest of their lives in a struggle to maintain their "sobriety"—their status as a nonuser. This pattern is insistently obvious and is repeated over and over again by all confirmed users of all drugs, including alcohol.

The fact that we can recognize and identify the stages of the basic Drug Dependence Syndrome does not mean that everybody who tries a drug will necessarily progress through all four of the stages. Some users quit in one or another of the first three stages, whereas others who use drugs never actually stop using them; but for some as yet unknown reason, they do not move on to the next stage, at least not for long periods of time.

WHAT MAKES A DRUG PROBLEM?

The Pleasure/Pain Principle and Adaptive Behavior

While much remains unknown about causes of the drug problem, some answers have emerged. The brain and our behavior are organized around the simple principle of maximizing pleasure and minimizing pain. We all depend on a brain-reward system that is finely tuned to the adaptive needs of the individual and of the society. This pleasure/pain orientation—and our adaptational capacity for it—is biologically based. It can be seen in all animal species. Take away a close linkage between pleasure and pain on the one hand and adaptive behavior on the other, and no individual or species can long survive in a competitive environment.

This linkage between pleasure and pain and its significance becomes clearer when we think about what motivates our behavior, individually and collectively. A college student, a patient of mine, recently attempted to describe the motivational connection between behavior and the pleasure/pain principle when he succinctly stated, "The pleasure system represents the three F's: Food, Fear, and Sex." Although his description lacks a certain measure of accuracy (to say nothing of elegance), he had nevertheless grasped something of the fundamental role played by the pleasure/pain principle in human existence.

How does drug dependence fit into this pleasure/pain reality? Drug dependence can be viewed as a subversion of the adaptational capacities of the brain-reward system. Essentially, the chemicals in the drug which produce dependence preempt the healthy pleasure system of the brain. These chemicals serve as short circuits to that basic adaptive experience in the early stages of use of any drug. The drug "tells" the brain to produce a high of pleasure (before the pleasure burnout occurs in the late stages of drug dependence). The almost instantaneous pleasure produced by drugs is reproducible, easy, and intense. Natural pleasures, such as success in school, athletic pleasure, or sex, are all, by contrast, more difficult to achieve and generally less intense. Recent research has shown that such natural, and potentially healthy, pleasure-producing experiences cause the release of the same neurotransmitters in the same pleasure centers of the brain as does the use of dependence-producing drugs.

The early adolescent who is most vulnerable to drug dependence is experiencing the awakening of the brain's pleasure system: it seems to get turned on, or at least turned up, at puberty. This helps make understandable other pleasure disorders of adolescence arising from such eating problems as anorexia nervosa, bulimia, and obesity, and from sexual excesses. The instant pleasure produced by drugs over the short haul almost surely will—in the long haul—produce increasingly prolonged intervals of pain and very possibly not a few life-long regrets. These things, despite their intensity, are often insufficient to overcome deep drug dependence. While the search for a good feeling starts the process, it is often sustained by the hook of physical dependence, which is both no fun and terribly hard to break free of. This is a sad paradox of addiction: drug dependence which begins as a search for pleasure progresses to an increasingly unsuccessful effort to avoid the pain of withdrawal. To an impartial observer, few chronic drug-dependent people seem to be happy. In fact, most of them look miserable as their brain-reward systems fail as a result of unnatural, excessive stimulation.

The "Social User" and the "Addiction Switch"

There is still another striking feature of the drug-dependence problem which requires special attention, and that is the relationship between the social or casual user of drugs, on the one hand, and the "addict" on the other. This relationship is seen most often in the contrast between the social drinker and the alcoholic. The same distinction exists between drug use and drug abuse. Some people seem to use drugs casually and have few resulting problems, while others center their lives around a drug and literally follow its pleasures, however hapless or harrowing, to their graves. When I talk with drug-dependent people about this distinction, I emphasize that the users themselves always underestimate the intensity and consequences of their addiction.

I also stress that dependence, once established, is unlikely to permit the addict ever again to be only a *social* user. Clinically, it is as if there is an "Addiction Switch" which gets thrown in the user's brain. Once it is thrown to "on," it cannot be returned to "off," even after years of abstinence from drug use. However much the addicted person may yearn for the earlier state of social drug use and however envious the dependent user may be of others who appear to use the particular drug occasionally without developing dependence, it is virtually impossible for the current or former addict to use his drug again without being engulfed in a run of active addiction.

Becoming addicted to a drug is much like falling in love. There is a period in the relationship of two people during which they are just getting to know each other, when they are just fooling around. Then, after a highly variable period of time, one (but not necessarily both) falls in love. Love is not an easy state to describe, but it surely means one is "hooked." Judgment is shot; the person in love is crazy in the sense that he or she is unable to make sensible judgments about the true characteristics of the loved one. Imperfections vanish, and every trait is elevated to perfection. Work, food, shelter—everything—is forgotten in the pursuit of the loved one. Some people fall quickly; others take a long time. Some fall hard; others never really do fall in love in this sense. It can happen at almost any age; but, for most of us, falling hard is related to youth: the fervor of the 15-year-old in love makes the 50-year-old's passion seem pallid.

The analogy goes further. For falling in love to take and to last, it usually requires a sexual reinforcement and a complex social reinforcement over a period of time. This sexual pleasure is like the drug-induced pleasure; it is repeated often over the duration of the relationship. But love, at least in this intense sense, commonly does not last. With drugs, the honeymoon high is soon replaced by the experience of dependence. The drug user begins by seeking and usually finding intense pleasure. He rapidly moves to using drugs to avoid pain, especially withdrawal pain.

Finally, as the song suggests, once in love, always in love. Let us suppose, for example, that you had at one time been in love, but you have not seen that person for 20 years, and then suddenly you find yourself again alone with that person you once loved so fervently. What is likely to happen? The chances are very good that you will reexperience the full passion of your earlier relationship. You are unlikely to be able to resist the pull of those feelings. Many people handle this kind of response by turning love to anger in order to protect themselves from the pain of loss of control, or they just avoid exposure to their former loves. Just as it is true that one can seldom become friends with a former lover, it is also true that one who has been dependent on a drug cannot again become a casual or social user of that drug. The brain does not forget the original passion. As I have emphasized, the Addiction Switch, once turned on, is never again turned off, even after years of no exposure to the loved one or to the drug.

Why is an Addiction Switch thrown for some but not others? And why, for some, is it thrown early in their drug use, while for others the switch is thrown to "on" only after years of apparently safe drug use? Much is still unknown, but—again clinically—I am convinced that the most important reason why the switch goes on is a pattern of prolonged, frequent use of the drug. By this I mean that if a person is willing to use a dependence-producing drug at intoxicating doses on a daily or near-daily basis over a period of months, he is likely to become dependent on that drug. In contrast if, for whatever reason, a person is unwilling to use the drug at such a frequency, then dependence is less likely. This may seem to be a circular definition, since regular, heavy use is associated with dependence, and infrequent, low-dose use is not. The point I am making is more basic. The experience of loss of control of drug use, which I describe as the Addiction Switch going on, is more than simply an act of using a drug frequently. It is a hook; it is addiction. Users who become drug-dependent often can, in retrospect, identify this change. It is common among heavy drug users. It has a profound effect on their drug use and on their entire lives. It is far more than a simple bad habit. This is a biologically based behavior disorder. It is drug dependence, and it is primarily caused by a period of prolonged high-dose drug use.

While there are almost certainly biological and even genetic differences in vulnerability to drug dependence, the two most important practical considerations are (1) heavy use of any dependence-producing drug ensures addiction for almost all users, and (2) the nonuser of any particular drug runs no risk of addiction to it. These two almost self-evident observations have profoundly practical implications for individuals, families, and communities. While drug dependence is difficult to cure, it is easy to prevent: *Do not use a dependence-producing drug!*

In addition, regular heavy use of a dependence-producing drug is likely to cause physical dependence in most, if not all, users. Such frequent use—more than several times a week, for instance, especially if large, intoxicating doses of the drug are used each time—is likely to lead directly, and often quickly, to full-blown drug dependence.

Much has been made by some of my medical colleagues about particular psychological vulnerabilities to drug dependence. Troubled people, they theorize, are more likely to use drugs in the first place, and, once they use them, they are more likely to become addicted than are their psychologically healthier peers. This theory is often carried to the family level: drug-using kids come from troubled families. Sometimes this concept is even carried to the point of concluding that the drug user in the family uses drugs *because* his family members *need* him or her to be a drug user. In this view, the drug user is a *victim* of family problems. A related view, less often heard today than it was 10 years ago, is that drug use is a symptom of economic or racial problems.

While I certainly cannot completely dismiss these apparently sophisticated formulations, I can say without hesitation that they are clinically crippling to patient and therapist alike. They are also misleading.

The typical drug-using youngster in America today comes from a typically healthy family and is himself a typically healthy teenager. That does not mean that he, or his family, has no problems. It does mean that no marker of deviance in him or his family can reliably predict dependence on any specific drug or on drugs in general. It also means that drug dependence is a *primary* disorder, and not merely a symptom of some other, presumably more serious or fundamental, disorder. Finally, my view—increasingly shared by physicians and others who work directly with drug-dependent people—is that the drug user himself is the problem, and even more specifically that the user's drug use is the problem. This straightforward view is important to all treatment efforts. Any other view is likely to perpetuate the drug dependence by excusing it and by focusing prevention and treatment efforts on practically unsolvable problems.

While some experts talk of the addictive personality as if a particular individual were generally vulnerable or invulnerable to drugs or to pleasure-producing behavioral disorders, I see only limited clinical evidence for this. Many people have desperately serious problems with one drug and seem relatively immune from dependence on others. On the other hand, like all clinicians, I have seen more than a few people who seem to fall into dependence on many pleasure-producing chemicals in a poly-addiction or, less elegantly but more accurately, a "garbage-head" syndrome. My point here is that theories, however attractive and sophisticated they may be, can often get in the way of both drug prevention and drug treatment. The best guideline to keep in mind is this: We are all vulnerable to drug dependence, and that vulnerability is most likely to be revealed if we use any drug regularly and heavily for a prolonged period of time.

NATURAL PLEASURES VERSUS DRUG PLEASURES: BASIC DIFFERENCES

To understand drugs and drug-use problems, we need to recognize some basic differences between natural pleasures, on the one hand, and drug pleasures on the other. Four distinctions, in particular, merit our attention:

1. The Active/Passive "Work" Requirement. One important distinction is that natural pleasures, by and large, take work. By natural pleasures, I am referring to such enjoyments as food, exercise, and sex, as well as the more complex pleasures that motivate us: a sense of self-respect, a feeling that people around us feel good about us, and the like. An *active effort* is required for the enjoyment of most natural pleasures.

Drug pleasures, in contrast, tend to be *passive*. I recently talked with a young man who was dependent on marijuana. He said that as he became progressively more dependent on this drug, he found his interest in sex diminished for a variety of reasons, not the least of which was that it was "just an awful hassle." There was, he said, too much work involved in his sexual relationships.

2. The Intensity of the Experience. A second significant difference between natural pleasures and drug pleasures is the intensity of the sensations or feelings generated by the experience. Natural pleasures tend to be subtle; drug pleasures tend to be relatively intense in the sense that drug-induced sensations and feeling states—initially, at least—often seem strong and exciting to the user. Depending upon the drug, the size of the dose, and the setting, regular and dependent drug takers, for instance, experience an intense feeling of euphoria or great happiness. This may be mixed with intense excitement, a joyful disarrangement of ideas, a decrease in impulse control, a disassociation from reality, and a distorted sense of time and distance. Such a feeling may be followed by a severe onset of anxiety or other painful feeling, but for many, the memory of the high persists. Contrast the intensity of experiencing that type of chemically produced pleasure with the subtle satisfactions of experiencing the natural pleasure of an approving glance, an intimate smile from a loved one, or the warm handclasp of a friend.

3. The Frequency of Occurrence. A third difference between natural pleasures and drug pleasures lies in the frequency with which they are likely to occur and the degree of personal control over when they can be made to happen. The natural pleasures—the good feelings that keep us going in the face of daily disappointments, discouragements, and drudgeries—occur in our lives with relative infrequency. Drug pleasures, by contrast, can be scheduled and are therefore less spontaneous, but more frequent and repetitive in their patterns of occurrence. They are far more easily controlled by the pleasure-seeking individual than are natural pleasures.

4. The Aftermath of the Experience. The fourth and perhaps the most important difference between the two types of pleasure is *what happens afterward*: the aftermath of the enjoyment. Following the experiencing of natural pleasures, by and large there is a sense of fulfillment, a sense of being truly energized. Generally, after a drug-induced pleasure, there is a sense of exhaustion, even dullness, that can be traced directly to the over-stimulation of the brain-reward mechanisms. This helps explain why most drug users start taking drugs for the purpose of seeking pleasure. By the time dependence—and heavy, regular use—develops, drug users no longer look, act, or feel happy. Their capacity to experience pleasure, be it natural or drug-induced, is exhausted, and they ingest drugs more to avoid pain, especially withdrawal pain and the pain caused by their drug-weakened lives.

Other Differences Unique to Specific Drugs

There are, admittedly, limits to the "natural pleasures versus drug pleasures" model I have outlined. Not all drugs are alike, by any means. Alcohol is a special drug because it is the only one that has calories. This unique characteristic has a number of important implications, including some that are related to nutrition rather than to drug abuse. Today, we Americans get about eight percent of our total caloric intake from alcohol. When we talk disparagingly of empty calories and go after the doughnut or the candy bar, we ought rather to think about the fact that alcohol, the ultimate junk food, is a far larger supplier of nutritionally empty calories in the average American diet than are other junk foods.

Drugs that produce dependence differ in other important ways as well. Tobacco, especially in cigarettes, is unique in that relatively few people are able to stabilize their frequency of use at any level other than either abstinence or constantly dependent usage. There are, in drug lingo, few "chippers" among users of cigarettes. By way of contrast, alcohol has a large percentage of users who persist at Stage Two (occasional use) and Stage Three (regular use) without going on to Stage Four (dependence). Recent data suggest that this seeming stability of alcohol use is more unstable than many of us would like to believe. One recent study found that more than 13 percent of American adults have, at some point in their lives, been diagnosable as alcohol abusers or alcoholics. For purposes of comparison, this was almost three times as many as reported having ever suffered from a major depression. In this study, alcoholism and alcohol abuse were found to be the most common single mental disorder in the United States.

Marijuana use seems, in this regard, to be more like tobacco than alcohol: among marijuana users, there is—over time—a strong tendency toward either daily use or toward nonuse. About one-third of all people who use even one marijuana cigarette in their lives progress to a period of *daily* pot use.

DENIAL OF DRUG USE

The biggest problem in dealing with the Drug Dependence Syndrome, however, is not the limitation or complexity of the model of the syndrome; it lies in *denial*. Drug users, as I have pointed out, seldom are willing to face directly the facts of their dependence. When, as a medical student, I studied hypnosis, I learned a useful lesson which later helped me understand the phenomenon of denial. If a person is hypnotized and told that, on waking, he will open a certain window at a precise time, and if he is also told that he will not remember the instruction given under hypnosis, he will perform exactly as told under the force of hypnotic suggestion. If this person is asked, when wide awake, "Why did you open the window?" he will answer by saying something like "I . . . I felt it was too stuffy in here." That is, he rationalizes his behavior because he cannot call up the real reason for it.

This closely resembles what happens to many drug users when they are confronted with a demand that they stop drug use, when they are asked to consider the consequences of their drug use. They rationalize and excuse their behavior by denying the connection between the consequences and their drug use. For example, if the drug user misses work on Monday because of a heavy weekend of drug use, he may say, "I had the flu and didn't feel I could work." When drug-caused automobile accidents occur, they are similarly rationalized: "The turkey pulled in front of me without warning! That's why I hit his car." Part of this is simple lying. But often, in my experience, the drug user is as unaware of the connection between his drug use and its consequences as the hypnotized subject was unaware of the real reason why he opened the window during the experiment.

One of the unique and extremely unfortunate features of the Drug Dependence Syndrome is that people simply do not want to know the facts about drug dependence. To discover the reasons why this is so, we need to look at certain cultural and biological factors, at the misleading assumptions about the seeming lack of ill effects from initial drug-taking, and at monetary motivations. These factors of denial pervade the thinking of the country as a whole and appear to be quite firmly rooted in the consciousness of both users and nonusers of drugs.

Cultural Factors in Denial

There is an American tradition of individual liberty rooted in 18th-century idealism and reinforced in the last two decades by the crude caricature of the youth culture, "You do your thing and I'll do mine." This attitude underlies the individual user's strong resistance to admitting his or her own dependency and seeing the consequences of that drug dependence while, at the same time, obviously providing a significant reinforcement for denial. The turning over to the individual of key decisions about his or her own drug use increases the risk of drug dependency by the same mechanism that the involvement of others in one's drug use decisions reduces the risk of drug dependence.

Put simply, pleasure in one's brain distorts one's judgment: A drug-dependent person rationalizes the drug use to keep the pleasure, thereby diminishing his or her usual powers of judgment. Reducing total reliance on one's self in the making of decisions to use or not to use drugs and increasing reliance on the judgment of nonusers help the drug user overcome denial. All too often, unfortunately, this does not occur. Today, cultural factors promoting total self-control and

discouraging family and community control of individual behavior in-
hibit this solution and thereby promote drug dependence. Again, to
put it simply, one whose judgment is not distorted by drug-caused
pleasure can more easily see the connection between the drug use
and its consequences, and can more easily conclude that the drug use
should stop.

While few alcoholics or other drug-dependent people recognize
their dependency, at least in its early stages, without forceful intervention by someone who is not drug dependent, the tendency to deny is
not limited to the user alone. Most families, physicians, teachers, and
employers prefer not to know about drug use in their midst. To know
is to have to face a painful situation; to ignore drug dependence is to
hope it will just go away or that someone else will deal with it. Much
of this kind of denial in those around the drug user is also prompted
by guilt feelings, and some of it by misplaced love. After outright
denial by the user, the most common distortion of the involved nonuser is to minimize the drug problem and to try to make peace with
the user's drug taking.

Frequently, nonusers try to shrug off the drug problem by saying,
"He will handle it for himself" or "It is just a temporary phase she's
going through." Typically such denial persists until the tragic end
stages of the drug dependence process, after the costs have mounted
high and after easier interventions are no longer possible.

We can see how this type of denial can be reinforced when we look
at another facet of our contemporary culture: smoking cigarettes. The
tobacco industry, having virtually abandoned its earlier contention
that smoking has not been proved to be a health hazard, has now
settled on a strategy of defending the smoker's right to smoke. In the
process, the industry is making some previously impoverished civil
rights lawyers wealthy. The marijuana lobby has recently adopted a
similar strategy, the activation of which has been, so far, much less
generously funded. In sum, these and similar cultural varieties of
denial and acceptance of drug use by both users and nonusers contribute perniciously to the drug problem in our society.

Biological Factors in Denial

The second factor behind the denial of the Drug Dependence
Syndrome is *biological*. Who wants to have pleasure taken away?
Freud observed that no person willingly gives up a pleasure. The best
anyone can do, in this view, is to substitute one pleasure for another.
Without necessarily going as far as Freud did, giving up any pleasur-

able activity is, at best, difficult. I remember being touched by the example of one of the leading authorities in the field of drug addiction. He was an older man who had a dependence on smoking a pipe that rivaled Freud's own notorious dependence on cigars. At a conference on drug abuse, I talked with this physician's wife about the impact of this tobacco dependence on her husband's health, because his lung function was obviously diminishing. It was clearly evident that *not* smoking that pipe would be good for his health. She told me, literally with tears in her eyes, that she and their children had once begged him to stop smoking. Here was a man who had studied heroin addiction all of his working life, a man who was one of the great theoreticians in the field of addiction. And yet, for him to think about giving up his pipe was, he had told his wife, like giving up life itself. His wife had concluded that even bringing up the issue was so upsetting to her husband that she would never do it again.

The "Deceptive Absence of Bad Effects" Factor

The third factor supporting the drug user's denial lies in the nature of the dependence process itself. Understanding this process is necessary in dealing with young people because, at the outset of drug use, there are relatively few negative consequences, and this apparent absence of bad effects reinforces denial. The typical teenager considering the use of marijuana, for example, has been told alternately, "There is nothing wrong with marijuana" and "It is the scourge of the modern age." Which is he to believe? Today many American teenagers try a drug and find out that nothing much happens—at least nothing bad. This picture is not universal. Sometimes initial drug use causes severe, even fatal problems. For most youths, however, initial use of marijuana does appear to be what John Lennon once called "a harmless giggle." The novice user finds a similar lack of problems among most of his new-user friends. This tends to reinforce denial that marijuana use creates any problem and that there is such a thing as marijuana dependence. Among initial users, this type of denial is often advanced for other drugs as well.

The Smell of Money as a Factor in Denial

A fourth factor promoting denial of the Drug Dependence Syndrome is *money*. There are literally tens of billions of dollars made every year in the United States by selling intoxication, especially to the most heavily drug-using segment of our population, our youth.

There is good reason for many people—the farmer working in the field to grow tobacco and the people working in the alcohol industry, to cite merely two examples—to encourage drug users not to know what they are already eager not to know. The sellers of illicit drugs are, of course, even less concerned by their personal responsibility for drug-caused problems. Who wants to know, after all, that his or her product, whether farm-produced or manufactured, whether legally sold or not, is killing tens of thousands of people each year? Such an idea is not likely to be greeted with much enthusiasm, especially when product liability is considered. People in drug industries are usually willing to accept the reality of dependence in relation to *other* drugs, but not their own. They deny the obvious evidence to the contrary by blaming the dependent user, not the drug: "The *alcoholic* causes the alcoholism, not the alcohol."

It is urgent that we realize that the user of a drug—captured for reasons of culture, biology, the initial absence of ill effects, and the financial greed of drug sellers, among other reasons—is in a poor position to observe the dependence process or its long-range consequences. In my experience with drug-dependent patients, it is a routine finding that users themselves are the last to know they are dependent. Users are also the last to see the negative health consequences of their drug use.

To overcome this almost universal denial by drug-dependent people requires, probably more than anything else, "loving others": people who care enough to say and, often, to do something honest and meaningful about the destructive consequences of the dependence process. The drug experience itself distorts the user's ability to think, thereby making it hard for him to be realistic about his drug dependence and its consequences. Those who know the drug user, and whose brains are not affected by drugs, are in a far better position to properly identify the extent and consequences of drug dependence. The drug-induced pleasure in the user's brain makes him deny the negative reality of his own use.

Who are these "loving others"? They are family and friends. The alcoholism experience demonstrates that they are often, in addition, such people as policemen, doctors, bosses and coworkers, teachers, and others whose commitment includes a concern for the individual's well-being. Frequently, there is a concern for the productivity of that individual in the larger society. This theme of productivity drastically reduced, on both a personal and public level, by a heedless, headlong pursuit of drug pleasure is a factor to be reckoned with in any successful attempt to achieve drug abuse prevention.

VARIETIES OF DRUG EXPERIENCES

An Example: Experiencing the Many Effects of Alcohol

Having examined the core problem, the Drug Dependence Syndrome, we are now better prepared to consider some of the varieties of drug experiences. When thinking about the ways different drugs affect different people at different times and in different doses, we can start with one of the simplest and most common of drug experiences: the effects of alcohol.

Even a brief reflection on our personal experiences with alcohol use, either by ourselves or by people we know, reveals much of the difficulty in trying to summarize the effects of this or any other drug. Here we have a single, simple chemical, alcohol, which produces effects ranging from excitement to lethargy, from casual relaxation to fatal overdose. From observation, even if not from personal experience, we are aware that alcohol affects different people differently and that even the same person can have markedly different experiences with alcohol at different times. Some of these differences are specific to particular people. Some of the differences relate to dose: a little alcohol produces one effect; a lot produces another quite different effect.

Most of us are unlikely to have noticed that the particular emotional state which the alcohol user brings to any given drinking episode has much to do with the effect of the drug. For example, a person may, with no ill effects, consume several drinks when calm and carefree, but can—when disturbed or angry—drink the same amount of the same drug with devastating results.

Think about the complex, changing effects of drinking over the lifetime of an individual. Levels of alcohol use and their respective consequences often change markedly for many reasons, including biological as well as psychological ones. Think, too, of the way drinkers of alcohol hold strong feelings about the form and circumstances in which they will consume the drug. Some people would rather fight than switch brands of whiskey or beer even though there is virtually no pharmacological difference. Some people will drink at a friendly cocktail party, but not at a formal affair.

I have reviewed this complexity of the effects of alcohol to suggest that the experiences and attitudes of users of other and (for most of us) less familiar drugs are just as complicated as the many varieties of alcohol use.

Some Basic Commonalities of the Drug Experience

Space limitations dictate that this excursion into the specifics of drugs must be brief. For our present purposes, however, I want to stress the *commonalities* of drug experiences rather than the unique properties of any specific drugs or, even more specifically, the effects of any drug used by any person at any time. These commonalities include, as we have noted, the following tendencies or themes:

- All nonmedical use of dependence-producing drugs tends to occur first during adolescence in a peer setting in pursuit of pleasure and recreation.
- Initial drug use, often after a brief negative experience, produces pleasure with few, if any, apparent negative consequences.
- Use of any drug, once begun, tends to progress for many, but not all, users through four clearly defined stages—from initial use to final dependence—in a predictable pattern.
- The common themes of the end stage or final dependence include a progressive escalation of negative social, personal, and physical consequences, leading commonly to death.

Dramatizing the Concept of Drug Dependence:
The Tobacco Example

When I speak with young people about dependence, I often focus on *tobacco* as a model. I do this with full recognition that tobacco use is unique because, although it causes drug dependence, it is not intoxicating. Tobacco dependence does not directly interfere with the user's work or personal relationships (at least until the physical consequences such as emphysema, heart attacks, and lung cancers disrupt, and ultimately end, many smokers' lives). Precisely because of this unique place of tobacco among the drugs of dependence, its use is the most public of drug-using patterns. I always encourage my young listeners to do some personal research on tobacco smoking by asking certain *questions* of their smoking peers and of their adult friends and family members who smoke. The following lines of inquiry are typical:

"When did you start to smoke?"
"By what stages did your tobacco use progress over time?"
"When did you first know you were addicted?"
"Did you know you were going to become addicted when you started?"

"Have you tried to quit smoking?"

"What happened when you tried?"

"What advice would you give me, based on your experiences, about whether I should try just one cigarette or not?"

When the students have had a chance to gather answers to these questions and related data, we pool the findings in the classroom to develop a rough but serviceable natural history of a drug habit. The most useful outcome of this exercise is that it highlights the fateful nature of the decision to "try" smoking. Persons who try smoking cigarettes may or may not go on to addiction, but when they start, they do not know—nor do they later fully control—the outcome of that experiment.

I also ask students to get to know other young people and adults who have become dependent on mind-altering, and thus more typical, drugs. Alcohol and marijuana are the most accessible examples. Once these students have the basic conceptual tools to understand the Drug Dependence Syndrome, they can see—in others—the dependence process in its successive stages. One of the most telling questions they can ask their drug-using peers (most of whom deny their dependence on the drugs they use) is this: "Okay, you say you're not hooked. Why don't you stop using that drug for three months, and then let's see what you think about it?" The nearly universal response to this invitation is, "I could stop if I wanted to, but I don't want to." For those students who understand the insidious and destructive workings of drug dependence, this answer has a chilling impact. After a review of the results of the research project I have just described, a 13-year-old said, "I don't want to try cigarettes, even once, because I might like smoking!" She got my message.

The more general framework for understanding drug dependence, as I am presenting it in this chapter, has another benefit: it helps explain why it is vital—literally vital for survival—for nonusers to act to reduce drug use by others. It makes clear why the widespread attitude of "You do your thing and I'll do mine" is devastating when it comes to drugs. A whole broad and, at first blush, unpleasant set of responses to drug use becomes understandable and even essential. These anti-drug responses range from informal to highly formal controls on drug use, some of which involve religion and law. Among these responses, family-based prevention is the most important. It also makes the tough stance taken by many schools and employers against drug use and even against drug experimentation understandable.

SPECIAL PROBLEMS IN UNDERSTANDING
DRUG DEPENDENCE

Of all the responses I have received from teenagers regarding this approach to understanding drug dependence, however, two of them center upon problems which are the most difficult for me to deal with: (1) teenagers with drug-dependent parents, and (2) teenagers with drug-dependent siblings and peers.

Teenagers with Drug-Dependent Parents

The first of these problems is the great difficulty many newly drug-educated teenagers have in dealing with the use of alcohol and other drugs by their parents. When we recognize that today roughly 10 percent of the adults in the United States are actively alcoholic, we begin to glimpse the dilemmas faced by many teenagers. Recognizing that some teenagers do indeed have alcoholic parents and that a few have parents dependent on illicit drugs, the majority of kids who bring up this point in discussion, or in therapy, are attempting to rationalize their own drug use by pointing out what they are quick to call adult hypocrisy. Distinguishing between the genuinely troubled teenager and the merely argumentative drug-using youth is seldom difficult in practice. The first deserves real help. The second needs education. Adult drug use does not excuse teenage drug use, under any circumstances: it is, for the kids, a cop-out.

Nonusing Teenagers with
Drug-Dependent Siblings and Peers

The second related problem, and one that is the most painfully difficult for me to deal with, is that of the nonusing adolescent who has to cope and interact with his or her drug-using siblings and peers. In our society, the concerned teenager is in a poor position to take action which restricts the freedom of his or her peers. Teenagers who do not use drugs and try to protest their use by others are frequently admonished to mind their own business when it comes to personal choices. This, unfortunately, is how most people still approach drug use.

The two problems I have just described are both common and difficult manifestations of the drug epidemic. I want to sketch some basic guidelines for dealing with them. First, the concerns of teenagers about the drug and alcohol problems of their peers and parents need to be taken seriously. Simply to turn away from such concerns is not only wrong from a humanitarian point of view, but it also undermines the significance of a much-needed message of concern for the drug problem: if you cannot help a child deal with these concerns, is there any help for him or for her in preventing or treating *any* drug problem? Second, it is important to open the problem up to possible solution by finding adults who will help the teenager deal with the problem. Adults must be found who can and will act as adults. In terms of dealing with drug and alcohol problems in the home, using other adult family members and family physicians can often help resolve the problem. For drug-using peers, involving parents, teachers, and adult counselors can often produce good results.

Finally, teenagers who are concerned about these problems can be referred to Alateen, the teenage affiliate of Alcoholics Anonymous, a subject explored in depth in Chapter 7. In Alateen young people find a youth community which on the one hand helps them understand their own painful experiences with alcohol and other drugs, and on the other hand provides guidance and support for effective action.

In the teacher-student interaction in which we were seeking a personally researched understanding of drug dependence, as I described it a moment ago, young people often ask perplexing questions, and they do not always respond the way one might want them to. Many times, however, I have found the interchange to be mutually informative and rewarding. People of all ages, and especially adolescents, are intensely curious about drug dependence. If they can be helped to see beyond what many of them perceive as a power struggle between adults and kids, they will enthusiastically enter into a frank, educational, and sometimes heart-rending exploration of the facts of drug dependence. Once they understand this process, even power struggles—so often resented initially—become comprehensible; these conflicts can be seen as useful, even if they still seem unpleasant.

Teenagers need to grasp one fact in particular: Beginning drug use is virtually limited to the teenage years. They need to be encouraged to understand that once they reach the age of 20 or so, they are unlikely to initiate the use of a new drug except for the purposes of medical treatment. At the same time, they should recognize another specific threat: the younger the user and the more intensive the youthful drug use is, the more likely are dependence and tragedy. When teenagers can be helped to realize that time is on their side, the goal of getting through the teenage years free of drug use can often make sense and work to their self-interest. Awareness of this self-interest in staying drug free greatly reduces the adult-teenager power struggles over drug use.

TWO UNIQUE VARIATIONS OF DRUG-TAKING PATTERNS

Substitution of "Medical" Drugs for "Street" Drugs

Before leaving our consideration of the Drug Dependence Syndrome, I call your attention to two additional and quite different patterns of drug use. One is the medical substitution (often on pretended medical grounds) of prescription drugs such as tranquilizers and sleeping pills for earlier use of purely illegal drugs. Many prescription drugs, including opiates such as morphine and Dilaudid, are frequently taken by users of nonmedical drugs in much the same pattern as marijuana or heroin are taken. Frequently, these drugs are ingested as a part of a multiple drug- or polydrug-using pattern with little or no distinction drawn between whether or not they have come from legal or illegal sources. This pattern of purely illicit use of prescription drugs fits the general description provided earlier in this chapter for the use of pleasure-producing drugs outside of medical supervision.

Excessive Use of Medically Prescribed Drugs

The second and quite different pattern involves people who do not use "street" drugs and whose eventual dependence grows out of taking prescribed drugs for specific medically diagnosed problems. Unlike the other drug-use patterns, this particular route to dependence on drugs usually starts in mid- or late life, and typically begins not in a peer, pleasure-seeking setting, but in a physician's office. This pattern and its attendant problems are treated in depth in Chapter 7.

ANOTHER VIEW: "CHEMICAL" DEPENDENCE AND THE "DISEASED" CONCEPT

In concluding our examination of the Drug Dependence Syndrome, one concept which has gained increasing recognition in recent years should be explored. This is the "disease concept" of dependence. The words *disease concept* come from the experience with alcoholism and from the impressive achievements of the Alcoholics Anonymous program. Put simply, the idea is that many individuals can use drugs without becoming dependent, while others are different in that, from an early stage in their drug use (or even before the first use), they show signs of the disease. Thus, in this view, there are healthy drug users and sick drug users. Those who are healthy can use drugs with impunity; those who are sick, who have the disease—now often called Chemical Dependence—can never use any dependence-producing drug. One dangerous defect of this concept needs to be identified.

The disease concept is useful for the addicted individual seeking to understand what is wrong with him or her and to solve this problem. It has great explanatory power, and it directs the dependent person to the one goal which will permit his life to make sense: to become and remain totally drug free. When it comes to drug abuse prevention, however, the disease concept is a disaster. It implies that some people can use drugs safely. Thus, the disease concept is, from the prevention perspective, a positive reassurance to those who experiment with drugs. My suggestion is this: for those in drug abuse or alcohol abuse treatment, the disease concept makes sense, so use it. For those concerned with prevention, emphasize how one catches the disease of chemical dependence. One becomes chemically dependent by using dependence-producing chemicals. While there may be differences of relative vulnerability between one person and another, some of which is probably biologically or genetically determined, the only sensible assumption is that everyone is vulnerable to drug dependence. One catches the disease by using drugs. One cures and, even more importantly, one prevents the disease by not using drugs.

SUMMING UP

Since the Drug Dependence Syndrome, as I have described it in this chapter, is the foundation of the entire book, it is appropriate that we review these central points:

1. A drug is a chemical which makes users want to use it again—on a purely biological basis. Examples include alcohol as well as heroin and cocaine.
2. Most drug use begins between the ages of 12 and 20 years. Once begun, it progresses in four stages: Experimental Use, Occasional Use, Regular Use, and Dependence.
3. Negative consequences of drug use can occur at any stage, but physical consequences are most common in the late progression toward dependence, often after many years of use. By contrast, most initial drug use appears to confirm the user's wishes that his or her high is safe—that is, that the user can take the drug without adverse consequences.
4. Denial is the greatest barrier to clear thinking about drug use.

Denial is widespread among users as well as many people who come in contact with users.

5. Overriding all other needs today in combatting drug use are (1) clear, hard-hitting information about the hazards of drug use— including the substantial and, for each individual user, unpredictable progression to dependence and (2) greater action and even militancy from the nonusers who relate to the user. This will require more aggressive action from parents and other family members, more action from employers, physicians, the criminal justice system, and others who have a stake in the behavior of drug users.

A clear understanding of these principal features of the Drug Dependence Syndrome is essential to the development of effective drug abuse prevention. A comprehension of this concept should be kept well to the front in our thinking as we move ahead into succeeding chapters.

PART TWO

What Are the
Gateway Drugs?

CHAPTER
THREE

Marijuana:
The Dumb High

MARIJUANA PLAYS A SPECIAL ROLE in the drug dependence process. It is almost universally the first illegal drug a youngster uses. The adolescent who avoids marijuana use is unlikely ever to use any other illegal drug, including cocaine or heroin. In contrast, if young people use pot, they run a substantially increased risk of using other dangerous and illegal drugs. Up to 50 percent of regular users of marijuana also use heroin, for example. Marijuana use has become the GATEWAY to all illicit drug use in America. Recent studies also have shown that fully one-third of all Americans who try marijuana even once progress on to a period of daily use of marijuana.

THE NOT-SO-INNOCENT, NOT-SO-NORMAL DRUG OF ADOLESCENCE

One of the disastrous drug myths is that marijuana is a "soft" and therefore unimportant drug. Largely because of this myth, during the last two decades marijuana has been added to the use of alcohol and tobacco as one of the leading threats to the health of our nation. It poses, in my view, the single biggest *new* threat to our national health. Making this threat even more ominous is the fact that the contemporary marijuana epidemic has occurred in a nation pathetically unprepared to deal with it.

For two decades many Americans have been saying that marijuana is a relatively harmless drug. During the last decade in particular, many experts have been advising parents and children that marijuana use has become a normal part of adolescence. One teenager succinctly summed up this prevalent "marijuana is harmless" fallacy when she added: "Parents and teachers should stop being so uptight about marijuana. It's no big problem for kids. Using pot is just a

normal phase for kids who need to find out about it for themselves."
Another teenager told me, "Marijuana is not a drug. It's like blue
jeans—just part of life." Even more disturbing, the Presidential Commission on Marijuana and Other Drugs issued its first report in 1971
under the unfortunate title *Marijuana: A Signal of Misunderstanding.*
The clear implication was that the marijuana problem was merely a
difference of opinion between parents and their teenage offspring—a
generational "misunderstanding"—rather than the rapidly escalating
drug epidemic with far-reaching destructive consequences. These twin
ideas—that marijuana is harmless and that its use is a normal part of
adolescence—are among the most dangerous pieces of misinforma-
tion in our society.

I share some responsibility for this dismal state of affairs because
10 years ago I supported decriminalization for marijuana possession. I
supported it under the mistaken assumption that marijuana use was
not a big problem and that we did not have to employ the legal threat
of prison to oppose marijuana use.

In 1974, while serving as the White House Drug Abuse Advisor, I
spoke at the annual convention of the National Organization for the
Reform of Marijuana Laws (NORML). After a lengthy (and hostilely
received) discussion of the health hazards of marijuana use, I outlined
a then popular concept called "decriminalization": remove criminal
penalties for marijuana possession while keeping its sale illegal,
thereby sparing the innocent, marijuana-using youth the trauma of
arrest and criminal records. It was, I then argued, possible to discourage marijuana use by nonlegal means such as health education. This
public support for decriminalization, delivered at the meeting of the
nation's principal pro-marijuana lobby, made headlines in virtually
every paper in the nation and was carried on all the television network news programs. To my embarrassment, the fact that I had
spent most of the speech describing the health dangers of marijuana
use was ignored. My plea for discouragement of marijuana use was
also judged to be not news. All that came across was "White House
Drug Chief Supports Decriminalizing Pot." That was my first painful
lesson about the symbolic importance of anti-marijuana laws. If you
favored removing criminal penalties, then—in the public view, at
least—you favored pot. I now *reject* decriminalization as a dangerous
concept. After 13 years of government service, the single biggest
regret I carry is my naive support for decriminalization of marijuana.
As I watched the marijuana-use figures double between 1974 and
1978, I felt the pain of regret with ever greater force. Of course, I
was not alone in those days. Many people in public and private life

shared this concept—and this responsibility. Many of us have also had some responsibility for similar errors of the past decade, errors which have fostered the unwise, unexpected, and unwanted increase in marijuana use.

The Scope of Marijuana Use—and Its Younger, Increasing Number of Victims

How big, specifically, is the problem of marijuana use? By 1982, 57 million Americans had used marijuana at least once, and more than 20 million were regular users of the drug. Of these 20 million, 2.6 million were 17 years of age and under. Among Americans 12 to 17 years of age, 2.8 million smoked tobacco cigarettes in 1982, barely more than those who smoked marijuana.

Numerous health indicators for adolescents—suicide, accidents, sexually transmitted disease, and premature pregnancy, for example—have shown a deterioration ranging, roughly, between 50 percent and 200 percent since 1960. In trying to assess the accelerating rate of the use of marijuana, we find that in 1962 only one percent of Americans aged 12 to 17 had ever smoked marijuana; by 1982 the figure was 27 percent—more than a 30-fold increase in a 20-year period. Among the 18- to 25-year-olds, only four percent had used marijuana in 1962; but by 1982, 64 percent had used it.

Many people are justifiably concerned about the age at which the young begin to use marijuana. Recent surveys make it clear that the peak ages for first-time use or incidence of marijuana use is 14 to 16 years—that's eighth grade to tenth grade. Thirty-five percent of high school seniors who have ever used marijuana first used it in the eighth grade or earlier. To pinpoint the age level where the biggest change is occurring, we must focus our attention on students in grades six through ten.

- Among American sixth and seventh graders, eight percent have already used marijuana, and four percent are regular users by the time they complete the seventh grade.
- Among American eighth and ninth graders, 32 percent have used marijuana, and 17 percent are regular users.
- Among tenth and eleventh graders, 51 percent have used the drug at least once, and 28 percent are regular users.
- Among 18- to 21-year-olds, 69 percent have used it, and 40 percent are regular users.
- As age increases beyond those years, the rates of marijuana use go

down until, beyond the age of 35, only 10 percent of the American population as a whole have ever used the drug during their lives, and only two percent are continuing to use it.

When we look at just the *daily use* of marijuana in 1983, we find the most disturbing statistic of all: among high school seniors in the United States, 5.5 percent smoked marijuana every day of their senior year. Fully 20 percent of high school seniors report smoking marijuana daily for at least a month at some time during high school. For purposes of comparison, an identical 5.5 percent of high school seniors drank alcohol every day, and 21 percent smoked tobacco cigarettes every day.

A few years ago, people said, "Well, marijuana users just use it *occasionally*." Or they tried to dismiss marijuana use, saying, "It is used only by healthy young adults." This relatively comforting picture, if indeed it ever was true, is *not* true today. We are now witnessing a strong movement among marijuana users toward very frequent use: *Over five percent of all high school seniors smoke an average of three and one-half marijuana joints per day*. We also know that dropouts (about 20 percent of the high school age group have already dropped out before the end of their senior year) are even heavier users of marijuana and other drugs.

What all this adds up to is that two very unhealthy facts about marijuana use are now inescapably evident: (1) *marijuana use on a large scale has grown rapidly since 1960*, and (2) *marijuana is smoked frequently by millions of Americans, especially by many of the young*.

Marijuana use has been the leading edge of an intertwined, unprecedented rise in the use of dozens of other illegal drugs ranging from LSD and cocaine to PCP and heroin.

The data on marijuana use levels from the 1980s are more difficult to sort out. They show a modest but hopeful change in trend. Daily use of marijuana among high school seniors rose from six percent in 1975 to 10.7 percent in 1978. In 1983 it fell back to 5.5 percent. Similarly, the inexorable steep rises in the rates of use of other illegal drugs that characterized the 1970s ended in the early 1980s as use rates leveled off and, for some drugs, declined slightly. In no case, however, was a sharp and sustained fall recorded for any illegal drug. Even alcohol and cigarettes showed a leveling off of use rates in the most recent years. For daily use of cigarettes, there was a significant drop among high school seniors from 29 percent in 1977 to 21 percent in 1983. From 1975 to 1983, daily use of alcohol remained about level—at about six percent—among American high school seniors. The drug epidemic may have peaked, but it is still continuing, and it is massive.

Focusing on the most recent trends in marijuana use specifically, the percentage of high school seniors who had ever smoked pot rose from 47 percent in 1975 to a peak of 60 percent from 1979 through 1981, with a tiny fall to 57 percent in 1983. The percentage of high school seniors who used marijuana at least once in the last month rose from 27 percent in 1975 to a peak of 37 percent in both 1978 and 1979, with a fall to 27 percent in 1983.

The reason for the fall in the regular use of marijuana, and the much smaller fall in the rate of experimentation with marijuana, is clear from the high school survey. An increasing percentage of American students now believe regular marijuana use poses a great threat to their health. The percentage holding this view rose from the 1978 low point of 35 percent to 60 percent in 1982. Thus, for every five percent rise in health concerns, there has been a one percent fall in the daily marijuana use rates among high school seniors. This clearly shows the positive impact of health education. Nevertheless, the tragedy of ignorance continued in 1982 as 40 percent of high school seniors still do not know that regular marijuana use poses a direct, personal, and severe health threat.

I have included many statistics in this examination of the marijuana problem because, more than with any other drug problem, the simplistic focusing on only a few numbers can be misleading when it comes to marijuana. I am especially concerned that the modest declines in some marijuana numbers may mislead us to the comforting, but wrong, conclusion that the marijuana problem is over. Before turning away from these numbers, I want to emphasize again that the marijuana epidemic is still raging. The best estimates are that 1.7 million Americans will try marijuana for the first time this year, and 84 percent of these first-time pot users will be 17 years old or younger.

Made by ``Mother Nature'': Complex
Chemicals from a Complex Plant

"But," you might ask, "just what is this stuff called marijuana? Is smoking a few joints of marijuana really so bad?" To answer these questions, you must first know that marijuana is not a chemical in the sense that alcohol is—alcohol being a relatively simple chemical, albeit one with complex effects on the human body. The marijuana that is smoked in the United States consists of the dried top leaves and flowers of a plant called *Cannabis sativa*. And, like every plant, the marijuana plant is a chemical factory. Marijuana, in its unburned state, contains over 400 separate chemicals, 60 of which are unique to the marijuana plant. These special chemicals are called cannabinoids. As the dried plant is burned to make smoke, it produces more than 2,000 chemicals which, with every puff, are brought into the smoker's body and distributed to every cell.

Pause and think for a moment about what 2,000 uniquely different chemicals may possibly do to the human body. Imagine, if you can, the prodigious research task required to identify and understand the far-reaching effects of such an intake. Think especially about the problem of understanding the *long-term* effects of prolonged use of this multichemical drug. Weigh also the challenge of understanding the combined effects of multiple drug use, since most marijuana users also use other drugs in combination with cannabis.

Any thinking we may do about the hazardous effects of marijuana on humans is complicated by another worrisome fact: Over the last decade we have had tremendous increases in the potency of marijuana. As I pointed out earlier when describing the classes of drugs in Chapter 1, the major ingredient causing the "high" for marijuana smokers is delta-9-THC or, as more commonly called and more easily remembered, THC. Ten years ago the average or typical marijuana drug had a THC content of about 0.2 of one percent. Today, the content averages about five percent: a 25-fold increase in the potency of marijuana in the last 10 years.

In sum, the frequency of marijuana use is up, the age of first use is down, and the potency of the drug is up—well up. Taken together, these significant trends spell out a message that is loud and clear: The benign image of marijuana and its use as painted for us by the experts 10 years ago is outdated and irrelevant to today's marijuana problem. Old data and old attitudes are not only wrong; they are dangerous.

Trapped in the Human Body, It Stays—and Stays

In what ways, specifically, is marijuana so detrimental to the human body? We can, I believe, more easily find some clear and understandable answers to this question by first taking a closer look at THC. THC is, as I have pointed out, the chemical that produces the euphoria or "high" in the marijuana user. But it also has another highly unusual propensity—and potentially a very dangerous one: *THC is soluble in fat, but not soluble in water.*

Our bodies have a water-based waste disposal system of blood, urine, sweat, and feces. When we take in chemicals that do not dissolve in water, they remain trapped in our bodies. Most people are more familiar with DDT, another chemical which tends to be retained in the body. THC, like DDT, is retained in the body tissues that have a high fat content, including the brain, the lungs, the liver, and the reproductive organs. One puff of smoke from a marijuana cigarette, when taken into the body through the lungs, delivers an appreciable quantity of THC, one-half of which stays in the body for as long as a week or more. In other words, if a person smokes one joint of marijuana, about one-half of the THC taken into his or her body will still be there as THC (or one of its breakdown products) a week later, and measurable amounts will be there a month later.

For those confronted with the argument, "Well, alcohol is as bad as marijuana," the persistence-of-residue effect of marijuana is one of the telling facts you should know. Alcohol does not stay around in the body the way THC does. Even people using marijuana only once each month are continuously exposing their brain, lungs, liver, and other vital tissues to the poisonous effects of THC. If a person is using marijuana more often than once a month, as most users in America today obviously are, then the residue levels of THC are not only retained, but also build up in the user's body.

THE CONSEQUENCES OF USING MARIJUANA

What Marijuana Does to the Lungs

Few marijuana smokers know that marijuana smoke contains more tar and more known cancer-causing chemicals than tobacco smoke. Marijuana smoke also has more carbon monoxide. Condensate from marijuana smoke, when painted on the skins of laboratory mice, produces cancer, and that is the test for the cancer-causing properties of any smoke.

Marijuana smoke has more chemicals known to be harmful to human lungs than does the smoke of an old-fashioned and highly toxic unfiltered ordinary cigarette. Marijuana smoke does not have nicotine, which is primarily toxic to the circulatory system. On the other hand, tobacco smoke does not have THC, which is toxic to the lungs as well as to other human organs. Some marijuana apologists argue that cigarette smokers smoke more cigarettes per day than marijuana smokers do; therefore, tobacco smoking is worse than marijuana smoking. Although cigarette smokers do smoke more cigarettes, you should know that many marijuana smokers also smoke many marijuana cigarettes or joints every day. Also, modern tobacco cigarettes are manufactured in ways that reduce tar and toxic agents.

Marijuana cigarettes, on the other hand, have no such "safety" manufactured into the product. In addition, the marijuana smoker smokes all the way to the end of his cigarette or joint, while the tobacco smoker usually puts out his cigarette before he gets to the end of it. Toxic agents are concentrated in the filter portions of the modern tobacco cigarette.

Remember, too, that the typical marijuana smoker inhales and holds his breath after each puff—to maximize exposure of his lungs to the smoke. Bear in mind that more than 80 percent of marijuana smokers also smoke tobacco cigarettes, thus exposing themselves more dangerously to both nicotine and THC than to either drug alone. In other words, whatever tobacco smoke does to human lungs, marijuana smoke does more and does it more quickly.

Marijuana smoke harms the lungs in other ways as well. The respiratory irritants in the smoke of one marijuana joint causes about 20 times the narrowing of the air passageways caused by the smoke of one tobacco cigarette. This is especially important for anyone with asthma or other respiratory problems. Marijuana smoke paralyzes the anti-infection white blood cells of the lungs, the pulmonary alveolar macrophages. Lung infections are more likely when health defenses are knocked out. Marijuana smoke is almost universally contaminated with the spores of the common soil fungus, *Aspergillus*. This fungus can cause a serious lung disease that is very hard to treat. These fungus spores are quite hardy: they are not killed by being burned in the process of smoking.

Because of the respiratory harm caused by marijuana smoke, pot smokers usually have a "smoker's cough." Studies have shown that marijuana smokers develop serious lung diseases much earlier and more severely than do tobacco smokers. All of this is, of course, not meant to exonerate tobacco smoking—the leading cause of preventable deaths in the United States today. It is meant to show that when it comes to protecting healthy lungs, marijuana smoke is fully as hazardous as tobacco smoke. In recognition of this fact, the prestigious American Lung Association ("The Christmas Seal People") has recently developed a national campaign to educate young people about the specific threat of marijuana to the lungs. Their slogan, "Don't let your lungs go to pot," points out marijuana smoke as a grave new threat to the lungs of millions of Americans.

What Marijuana Does to the Reproductive System

For males who smoke marijuana, there is decreased testosterone (the male sex hormone), decreased sperm production, and increased production of abnormal sperm. For normal human females who smoke marijuana, hormonal upsets produce increased menstrual irregularities. In laboratory studies using female rhesus monkeys treated with marijuana in doses comparable to common human doses, there was a fourfold increase in fetal loss through miscarriage and stillbirths for the monkeys that were given marijuana compared to those that were not. Some ask if there is any specific genetic damage or deformity resulting from marijuana use. On the basis of very limited research, the answer appears to be no, but there are some data to the contrary.

The effects of marijuana on female reproduction, at least in terms of what is known at this time, seem to be a general decrease in the maternal capacity needed to support the unborn but rapidly developing fetus, rather than the causation of any specific deformity. However, research has shown that monkeys born to marijuana-using mothers tend to be smaller and more often irritable and hyperactive than the offspring of the drug-free monkeys. There are also some disputed studies which show that marijuana smoking produces broken chromosomes. Recent laboratory studies using mice have shown abnormalities resulting from either maternal or paternal marijuana exposure that extend for up to three generations, even if the offspring were themselves never exposed to marijuana.

There is, furthermore, evidence that marijuana use may adversely affect human reproduction in somewhat the same way alcohol does. Although alcohol use has been common for thousands of years, only within the last decade have we recognized the devastating "Fetal Alcohol Syndrome," the specific set of physical and psychological deficits which afflict a newborn child whose mother drank appreciable amounts of alcohol during her pregnancy. Similarly, it has been only within the last decade that many people have become aware of the harmful effects on children born to women who smoke tobacco cigarettes. Recent research studies show that the use of marijuana by mothers-to-be produces more severe damage to infants than does their use of either alcohol or tobacco. This tragedy is compounded and made all the more painful by the realization that most pregnant marijuana smokers also drink alcohol heavily and smoke tobacco heavily. Thus, their children are subject to multiple, interrelated threats to their health and well-being.

What Marijuana Does to Brain Functions
and the Central Nervous System

On the basis of research to date, the brain is the most susceptible and, therefore, the most important organ in terms of the effects of marijuana smoking. A few years ago, high school students laughed skeptically when I spoke about marijuana's deleterious effects on the brain. "Marijuana," they said, "is not so bad." Now teenage audiences do not laugh, because in every high school in the country the students easily and frequently see drugged "burn-outs": young people who have lost their mental sharpness and motivation as the result of supposedly "harmless" drug use.

This miserable condition, in its late stages, is perceived by the users themselves and by their friends as the result of drug use and, most often, marijuana use. This perception is further strengthened by studies of rhesus monkeys: When these monkeys had been given marijuana for only six months and had then been entirely cut off from their supply of it, physical changes in their brains could still be found six months after their last intake of marijuana.

I have worked with many former marijuana users who did not feel normal, behave normally, and think normally for at least three and sometimes six months after they had completely given up their use of the drug. One young man with whom I worked recently has not used marijuana for six months but, even so, he and I wonder whether his brain functioning will ever come back to its level before marijuana use. Neither of us is certain that it will.

After a recent appearance on a nationally televised program, I received a letter from a disturbed former marijuana smoker from San Francisco. He wrote, in part:

> I smoked marijuana for about one year, but not very often. I felt sometimes that I needed it, so I smoked it. But what is bothering me is that I have been changed completely in my personality and behavior.
>
> I stopped smoking marijuana completely four months ago. But still my behavior is the same. I forget a lot. I do things I know are wrong, and afterwards I feel sorry. I am a third-year civil engineering student. I study hard, even harder than before I became like this, but I forget what I study. Before, it was different.
>
> Please help me know if this will stay forever, or will I change by continuing to be away from marijuana? I am very disappointed, and I am not optimistic any more. I think there is no need to continue to go to school. Please answer my letter, and I will be grateful to you.

On the air, on the same television show, a caller had this to say:

> Yes, my name is Michael, and I am calling from Detroit. What Dr.
> DuPont is saying is that marijuana does have an effect on things, on
> the mind, so you get off track, you lose sight of things, and I've been
> smoking marijuana for 20 years myself, and I am just now trying to get
> off of it. It has effects, and it leads to other drugs. Just like you say,
> some smokers stay stable, but the majority of them move on to heroin
> or pills, because they get tired of that dumb high.

Another caller, a self-admitted marijuana user, said:

> The point you're making is that people have considered marijuana to
> be harmless, but it's really addictive and it's definitely serious business.

It is one thing, of course, to say that a particular drug harms, or
may harm, the brain, but that doesn't help us very much unless we
know something of the *specifics* of what is at stake. So let's review
what the brain is, what it does, and why possible damage to it can be
extremely dangerous.

   The Brain and Its Functions.   Enclosed within the skull and continuous with the spinal cord, the human brain is often referred to as
the home of its owner's intelligence and intellect—"the house of the
mind." In the more specific terms of *Webster's Dictionary*, the brain is
"the portion of the . . . central nervous system that constitutes *the
organ of thought and neural* [nerve] *coordination*" and "includes all
the higher nervous centers *receiving stimuli* from the sense organs and
interpreting and correlating them to formulate the motor [movement-
causing] *impulses.*" When an alien, disruptive, or even destructive
chemical—like marijuana—is introduced into such a finely tuned,
delicately balanced, and important organ, the brain's whole carefully
orchestrated performance will be at the least upset, and at the worst
thrown into alarming disarray.
   What does the brain *do*? From our definition, we can put together
a useful picture of at least six of its *major* tasks or functions: (1) the
brain is *the organ with which we do our thinking*; (2) it is the *controller
of nerve coordination*; (3) it is the *receiver of stimuli* sent to it from all
parts of the body; (4) it is the *interpreter of these stimuli*; (5) in
meaningful ways, *it relates one stimulus to another* or one set of
stimuli to another set; and it thereby becomes (6) the *generator of the
individual's mental activities* and the *formulator of the body's neuromuscular actions.*

As you can readily see, when we consider only a few of the brain's major functions, we get into complicated territory. So, to simplify our considerations, I will try to be more specific about a *very limited* number of tasks which the brain is principally and primarily responsible for "helping" us with. Bear in mind that this list barely scratches the surface of a vast catalog:

memory	thinking	decision making
speaking	thought formation	reading comprehension
listening	concept formation	choice-reaction time
attending	problem solving	spatial location
time location	motor coordination	sensory perception
academic performance		

The *order* in which I have listed these brain functions—most of which are called "cognitive" (a term I shall explain in a moment) and a few of which are called "sensory-perceptual"—is of no special significance. What is significant is that each item represents *an area of human mental or motor activity on which scientific experts have conducted diligent research studies in efforts to ascertain the possible impact of marijuana use upon a person's ability to function intelligently in his or her environment and in relationships with others.*

The listed functions or tasks are also important because the learning and/or mastery of most, if not all, of these mental and motor activities should normally be nurtured and developed during the formative years of adolescence—the years during which young people are most vulnerable to all drug taking, including marijuana. For these and other reasons, a familiarity with these brain functions will be useful not only in this chapter but also later, as we move to a consideration of alcohol use and of family relationships in Chapters 4 and 6, respectively.

To emphasize further the possible hazards imposed by marijuana use on the brain and the rest of the central nervous system, look more closely at the unique nature of these few functions. In other words, when you allow the insidious chemistry of drugs, legal or illegal, to interfere with the normal functioning of the brain, here are some of the vital human processes, abilities, and skills you are fooling with.

A good place to start is with *memory*, the "storehouse" of things, images, impressions, and pieces of information we learn from experience or from contact with our environment and the other people in it. We say we "remember" something if we recall or recognize it, if we can associate it with something else. Memory, described as being either short-term or long-term, is one of the basics to all human learning and to all educational endeavors. Without it, we could not think or speak or even survive for long, either as individuals or as a society. Senility and Alzheimer's disease—as well as the mental functioning of the "punch drunk" former boxer and the postalcoholism disease, Korsokoff's syndrome—are all medical conditions characterized primarily by profound loss of memory. Of all the patients I have worked with in my medical career, none has been more helpless or pathetic than the people, normal in most other ways, who cannot remember. Speech, relationships, and activity all grind to a halt without the ability to remember.

Memory—or remembering—is one of the first steps toward "knowing." Through memory, we become aware and we judge or evaluate. This is the process by which we "come to know" something: a process psychologists call *cognition*. Put in somewhat oversimplified terms, our cognitions are our "knowings." When memory is disrupted—as it often is, even in so-called normal circumstances—or when memory fails, as not infrequently happens with continued use of drugs, the result is a failure or breakdown in cognitive functioning: a "cognitive *dys*function." Because the brain's normal function has been interfered with, we have a flaw in our ability to know. We cannot add appropriately to our storehouse of knowledge.

Among the many cognitive functions handled by or directly involving the brain and the rest of the central nervous system are the following:

- *Speaking:* The principal means of establishing and maintaining contact with other human beings; one half of the act of communicating.
- *Listening:* The other half of the act of communicating; involves hearing, but goes far beyond that.
- *Attending:* Paying attention; to apply the mind to a stimulus, image, or idea for a necessary time; also involves bodily attitudes.
- *Thinking:* To consider; to weigh; to reflect; to size up; to examine, reject or accept, and correlate ideas; to devise; to invent; to call up a mental image; to originate an idea, allowing it to enter and to be turned over and over in the mind. Thinking is also organizing; the separation and reordering or realignment of images or ideas so as to derive a meaningful interpretation of the whole.
- *Thought formation:* An integral "product" of thinking; the capability to generate ideas and to organize them around one major focal point or central thrust.

- *Concept formation:* The ability to remember a particular instance or image and to generalize it into an abstract or, sometimes, even a visionary idea. A slogan, for example, usually requires concept formation.
- *Problem solving:* Ideally, a five-step process: (1) identifying or defining the problem; (2) analyzing the problem in terms of "the way things are now," "the way I would like to have things," and "the things or obstacles I will have to change if I'm to have what I want"; (3) suggesting possible solutions to the problem; (4) evaluating the possible solutions; and (5) choosing the "best" or at least the most "workable" solution for all concerned.
- *Decision making:* Regarded by many as the equivalent to the fifth step in problem solving; also the ability or capacity to make judgments that are, if not always the ultimate in wisdom, at least reasonably intelligent and to make them as promptly as circumstances may allow or as conditions dictate.
- *Reading comprehension:* The capacity to be informed, instructed, and/or even intelligently persuaded by what you read. Using your intellect in combination with your visual acuity to grasp the meaning and import of what you see in printed matter.
- *Choice-reaction time:* How long it takes you to "make up your mind" in a critical, crucial, or, oftentimes, hazardous situation; the split second between sensing a danger and reacting to avoid it; the interval between making a decision and acting upon it. Equal parts of quickness and accuracy are prime requirements.
- *Spatial location:* The ability to sense or to know how far one object is from another object, to know unerringly "where it's at," to judge distance(s) quickly and accurately; the capacity to comprehend spatial relationships—especially changing spatial relationships—promptly and accurately.
- *Time location:* To locate or place an event or happening in time; to sense or to know how much time has elapsed or is likely to elapse between one event and another; to be able to estimate the "time" between two objects moving on a collision course; to not "lose track of time."
- *Academic performance:* Individual achievement in overall school performance, as measured in grades, involving at least one of the above processes, procedures, or skills and, not infrequently, involving several or a great many of them.

As I have said, the foregoing are far from being a complete catalog of the *cognitive* functions of the brain, but they suffice to provide a measure of their vast significance and to bring us back to our starting point: A failure of any of the brain's functions can happen when the memory is disrupted or if memory is temporarily wiped out for any reason, including—especially—drug use.

The second part of our definition, you will recall, described the brain as the great controller of bodily action. Figuratively (but quite accurately) speaking, the brain is charged with the high priority of making sure that the eye and the hand work together to do exactly what they are told to do. In other words, the brain "supervises" the working together of nerves and muscles to achieve what I have listed as "motor coordination."

Helping to ensure that this goal is achieved are sensory perceptors. Among these, of course, are the eyes, ears, nose, tongue, tastebuds, the body skin, and the appendages facilitating our sense of touch or feeling: fingers, hands, arms, legs, feet, and toes. If any of the perceptual "passages" or "routes" over which perceptual "messages" travel to and from the brain are interfered with or damaged, our perceptions become distorted. Thus, in crucial situations especially, we may get frustrating or dangerous distortions in what and how we see, hear, touch, taste, or smell. This, in turn, puts us out of touch with the realities in our environment. In such a condition, we can no longer interpret appropriately what is happening to us and to others around us.

When our perceptual apparatus is distorted by marijuana or other drugs, or when our perceptions are thrown into disarray because of fear, fatigue, emotions, or plain thoughtlessness, our behavior may go haywire. We may run off the track or, literally, off the road and into a ditch or worse because a lack of proper motor coordination has prevented us from acting as we should. Misjudgments of spatial location or time location are essentially distortions of sensory perceptions; that is, they result when our sensing equipment is jammed up or out of touch with the way things really are.

Motivation and the Power of the Will. Finally, although all may not agree that it resides in the brain, there is the power of the will, which some call motivation. One of the saddest aspects of drug dependence is its eating away of the will: the urge, the desire, the drive, the dreaming, the wanting to do what you had once hoped to do, to be or to become what you once aspired to. Many of the different drugs, and this includes marijuana, can throw you into a state in which you no longer care about your former hopes, ambitions, plans, and goals. You are no longer *motivated.* Despite all that is known about motivation and all that may yet be discovered, the one thing we can be sure of, the one thing that is self-evident, is that motivation—the drive to grow, to learn, to solve problems—is deeply imbedded in the fabric of life itself. It is persistent but fragile in all stages of the human life cycle, but it is particularly vulnerable during adolescence when the demands of life outside the family are growing rapidly. Motivation and the power of the will are especially vulnerable, too, at a time when the adolescent is feeling powerful pressures to become "adult," and when the physical and emotional changes being experienced by the adolescent threaten the still-tender sense of personal identity.

Into this picture put marijuana, an intoxicating drug: a potent and seductive chemical "pleasure." Those teenagers who listen to its siren song and succumb to its inviting lure find that marijuana use is a way to hide out from pain, to feel that they "belong" without having to work for real friendship. They see it as a way to dampen the painful fires of ambition and shut down goal-driven behaviors; it makes them feel, "My world's okay the way it is." For me, as a clinician, the saddest outcome of this destructive drug taking is to see the gradual, progressive fading of ambition clearly evident in the lives of pot-smoking teenagers. Thanks to pot, their vision of personal achievement is progressively restricted. Academic goals plummet. Sports and other extracurricular activities requiring work are casually abandoned. Once-cherished personal goals weaken and vanish. The desire to be married and have a family, like the ambition for college and a career, often go up in puffs of pot smoke.

By the time the young person is effectively confronted with this sad state of affairs or by the time he awakens to the realization that his use of marijuana has become a barrier to goals once fervently sought, he is typically in his 20s or even 30s, and his range of opportunities has drastically narrowed. Now even the motivation of wanting to be self-supporting is elusive, whereas five or ten years earlier—in his pre-marijuana days—such higher goals seemed easily possible. Unfortunately, many of these young people never awaken, at least not fully. They remain dimly, if at all, aware of their loss of motivation and all it could have meant to them. As they have drifted, they have shifted their criteria for success from achievement to chemically in-duced pleasure. Their ambition, if it can be called that, now is only to avoid "hassles" rather than to climb mountains. If, by age 25 or so, the records and accomplishments of these marijuana-using youths are compared to those of their nonusing siblings and former friends, or to those of their parents when they were this same age, the contrast is usually appalling. The achievements of most pot smokers—especially if use of drugs has continued with any frequency—are tiny by comparison to the achievements of their peers who don't smoke pot. Perhaps it is a godsend for many of these victims that they do not fully realize the magnitude of all they have lost. As a therapist, I find the realization inescapable—and infuriating.

Not many years ago, this failure of motivation, this eroding of the will, was given the name *amotivational syndrome*, and research has since established that smoking marijuana can, in fact, produce this syndrome. There are, moreover, worrisome indications, frequently supplied by users themselves, that a lack of motivation is either a particular reason why young people start using the drug, or that—by becoming dependent on marijuana—they then fall victim to the syndrome. In the "Diary of a Teen-Age Drug User," which appears later in this chapter, there is some unusual testimony which may help you to form certain judgments about this problem.

What Scientists Say About the Effects of Marijuana Use on the Central Nervous System. Against the background of possible cognitive failures and sensory distortions I have just described, I call your attention now to a number of relevant and significant conclusions reached by a panel of distinguished research scientists. Following through on a request from the National Institute on Drug Abuse and the National Institutes of Health, the Institute of Medicine of the prestigious, nongovernmental National Academy of Sciences prepared a comprehensive study on the health effects of marijuana use. The report, released in February 1982, represents a cautious, conservative review of the scientific evidence presently available. In a section on the "Effects of Marijuana Use on the Central Nervous System," the panel commented—in essence—as follows:

- Acute effects of marijuana smoking include feelings of euphoria, but use can also cause disturbing mental experiences, including short periods of anxiety, confusion, or psychosis.
- Marijuana impairs or interferes with short-term memory, slows the learning process, interferes with oral communication, and may trigger temporary confusion and delirium. These effects are of special concern because high school students who use marijuana tend to use it during school time. The learning defect in particular persists for hours after the euphoria or high has worn off.
- Chronic, heavy use of marijuana is associated with behavioral and mental disorders in people.

- Marijuana has worrisome and sometimes harmful short-term effects on reflexes, physical effectiveness, and vision.
- Marijuana use significantly impairs motor coordination and the perceptual ability to follow a moving object and to detect a flash of light—factors which pose a substantial risk when driving a motor vehicle and operating other machines, including industrial machinery. These impairments and perceptual deficits can last four to eight hours after the actual high.
- The panel of experts, as a group, found it difficult to determine whether marijuana use is a cause or an effect of the so-called "amotivational syndrome," which produces apathy, poor school work, and poor job performance. The rise in marijuana use during the last two decades, however, closely correlates with the fall in Scholastic Aptitude Test (SAT) scores.
- So far, the panel concluded, there is no convincing evidence of long-term behavioral effects persisting after marijuana use stops, although it is also not clear that such effects do not occur. In other words, the jury is still out on this one.
- Marijuana and its by-products can remain in the brain and other organs of the body for long periods of time, even months, with unknown but possibly subtle effects.
- Long-term effects of marijuana on the human brain and on behavior are not yet known, but the short-term effects are of sufficient import as to encourage and accelerate intensive research concerning possible long-term consequences.

Clearly, the negative effects of marijuana use on the brain and the rest of the central nervous system, particularly as they affect learning, studying, and neuromuscular coordination skills like driving, ought to be matters of grave concern. This is especially urgent in a society like ours: a society that is knowledge centered and that "runs on wheels."

On the day the National Academy of Sciences released its comprehensive report on the effects of marijuana use, I interviewed the chairman of the panel which prepared it. In the interview, which took place on a local call-in radio program, I asked him what advice he had for his own children about marijuana use—advice resulting from his studies. He advised against its use. I asked him how he would have felt if he had known that the pilot flying the plane which took him back to Boston that day had been smoking marijuana before the flight, or even several days before the flight. He said he would not have wanted to fly on a plane piloted by anyone who smoked marijuana no matter if the smoking had occurred many days before.

What Marijuana Does to the Coping Capability—
Stress, Tensions, and Feeling States

All persons, of whatever age, must learn how to cope. Indeed, it is the inability to cope, to actively and creatively solve personal problems, which impels sizeable numbers of people to use drugs. Young people, in particular, need to learn how to deal with stress and tension because, although these are negative feeling states, they are nevertheless essential to healthy living and to sustaining sound growth to maturity.

Much of our personal growth comes when we find that our current ways of living are not working well for us. At such times, we feel frustration and even pain. Failure at school or at work, disappointment in personal relationships, wanting something we cannot have— all are common experiences for people of all ages. These realities are difficult to cope with. On the other hand, demoralization and retreat from difficulties are also universal. This is where the coping capability comes in. Most of us, in the face of adversity, pull ourselves together and develop as individuals. Many times we grit our teeth, grin, and bear it. If the problem is too tough or too big for us, we look for help. Sometimes we find it in our community: friends, counselors, teachers, and employers. Of course, when the challenges exceed our coping capability, we look for support from those who love us and whom we love. Most often—for teenagers, especially—that means the family, usually the parents. The greatest ally teenagers have in coping with both their drug and their nondrug problems is their family. The greatest threat to their coping capabilities is drug use, especially the use of marijuana and alcohol. Some people—many, perhaps—look to religious faith when their coping machinery breaks down or is overwhelmed. It tells us "who we are," that "we are not alone," and even that "my personal life has meaning beyond whether I feel good or not."

All problems we are likely to encounter in this life have a way of demanding solutions, and if we are strong enough and lucky enough, we manage to find them most of the time. If we cannot, an inner tension, or stress, grabs us. That is when our coping capability must go to work—and fairly quickly. In the typical teenager, the skills needed to handle the uptight feelings are still underdeveloped; the level of his or her coping capability is characteristically low. In the short term, unfortunately, all drugs—including marijuana—have enticing ways of reducing the uncomfortable sensations of stress and tension. What young people often fail to realize is that such reduction drastically curtails the users' learning-to-cope incentive, capability, and flexibility—the very things they are in most immediate need of. This curtailment, in turn, imposes special threats, special barriers, to both the mental and physical development of young people. Without a strong capability for coping, they find that it thwarts their hopes, distorts their vision of themselves, and erodes their chances for a happy and productive future.

Because the adolescent's body and mind are uniquely vulnerable to the effects of all drugs, especially marijuana, the disruptions of the hormone signals from the pituitary gland—a disruption characteristic of marijuana use—are particularly worrisome. These are the signals the body uses to trigger both physical and mental maturity, and disruptions in this message-carrying process at any time during adolescence may produce profound and lifelong effects, a far less likely event in the case of adult use of marijuana or other drugs.

On a psychological level, the ability to identify and manage anxiety—in other words, to cope with it—is one of the most significant functions of adolescent development. Interruptions in the process of acquiring this capability to cope with stress, tension, and other feeling states by reason of short-circuiting the normal anxiety response cycle is likely to have a profoundly negative effect during adolescence and, many times, even later in life. Clinically, when I talk with drug users in their 20s, they often speak about their maturity as having stopped when they started regular drug use. At that point, they feel, they stopped growing up intellectually and socially. They remained "kids" despite their outward appearance of being more grown up and more sophisticated than many of their peers. Thus, a 25-year-old who began regular marijuana use at 15 thinks and acts like a 15-year-old even though he or she may look like a 25-year-old: a case of arrested development induced by drug use. What has been arrested is the capability of the person to cope with the physical and psychological realities of growing up—to meet life honestly on its own terms.

Drug-induced arrested development surfaces in many troublesome forms. Among the most common is the pot smoker's inability or unwillingness to cope with problems in a forthright and self-responsible way. He or she prefers escaping problems to solving problems. For example, many marijuana-using teenagers delude themselves into thinking that their pot smoking is "harmless." Then, when they feel bad or when they are confronted by people who tell them things they do not want to hear, they see this—not as their own personal prob-

lem to be coped with—but as "the other person's problem." They
will not see it as it realistically is: the problem of the teenager himself
or herself and a problem directly traceable to personal marijuana use.
Thus, the intoxicating impact of the drug and the sapping of the
individual's coping capability are cruelest when they cloud the young
user's ability to recognize his own drug dependency and to foresee its
future consequences.

"Cruelest" is the right word because a vicious cycle is set in
motion. For millions, this cycle is continued for years. For many, no
doubt, it will be for a lifetime. Pain and problems lead to marijuana
use. Marijuana use leads to poor adaptive performance—to failure of
coping. This produces more frustration and pain which, in turn, lead
to more marijuana use. As one 20-year-old woman told me recently,
"I was happiest and doing the best when I used the most marijuana,
during my junior and senior years in high school and my freshman
year in college." In exploring this with her, I found that what she
meant was that she felt less frustrated then. When she was drug-free,
she felt more uncomfortable. With some difficulty, I got her to shift
her focus from the question of when she "felt good" to the question
of when she "functioned well" in the sense of confronting and coping
with the problems in her life. Once that refocusing was achieved, it
became clearer to her that she had, during those three drug-using
years, "felt better" but "*functioned* less well." Her grades were
poorer. Her interest in taking on challenging tasks like dating, extracurricular activities, and her family responsibilities all fell during her
pot-smoking years. She was "solving the problem" of her bad feelings
during those years by using drugs. Trapped in self-deception, she had
permitted her drug use to short-circuit the normal, healthy process of
experiencing pain as a stimulus to personal development, to learning.

For this young woman, as for many otherwise intelligent marijuana
users, self-awareness was made more difficult by her belief that she
saw things more clearly and understood them more completely when
she was using marijuana. She believed that now thoroughly discredited argument that drug use "expands" the mind. She did indeed
think differently and feel differently when stoned. But rather than
thinking clearer thoughts, what she was experiencing was a selective
but progressive poisoning of her mental faculties, with the first function knocked out being her ability to grasp realistically her own
diminished capacity for thinking and coping. Even when drug-free, she
had a nostalgic recollection of the dreamy pleasures of intoxication
and, as I saw it, a frightening ambivalence about her drug-free experiences, wondering if her recent struggle to achieve them were worth

the effort it had cost her. From my point of view, it was not hard to wish for her sake that she had never had the drug experience. Without it, her life would have been much simpler, as well as more successful. She saw this point of view as an indication of my being "old-fashioned" and "traditional."

Despite the evidence everywhere, many sophisticated scientists today profess to being confused and in doubt about the precise relationship of marijuana use to the human capability for coping. They note, correctly, that many young people who get into trouble with marijuana had been coping relatively poorly before they used marijuana. They also note that, once drug use began, the coping capability fell even further. For example, kids who use marijuana heavily have higher rates of arrest and lower grades in school *before* they use pot than the kids who go through adolescence without using marijuana. Therefore, some marijuana apologists argue, marijuana use is the *result* of problems, not the *cause* of problems. They thus confuse cause and effect. The error in this assessment, as any teacher or clinician working with teenagers will tell you, is that many of the kids who use pot did not have noticeable problems before their use of the drug. This is true even though, on the average, kids who use marijuana have more problems before use than do kids who do not use pot, and many kids who did have problems before pot use could reasonably have been expected to bounce back—to learn from their problems—except for the fact that pot smoking became a trap for them, undermining their already tenuous capacity for coping. Marijuana, in a few words, makes you stupid, and, what is worse, it makes you not care.

MONITORING THE MARIJUANA MENACE: A CLOSE-UP LOOK AT DAILY USE BY TEENAGERS

Much of the recent, serious national concern about the health threat of marijuana use developed after 1978, having been triggered by the dramatic rise in the percentage of high school students who smoked pot every day of their senior year. This daily use figure stood at six percent in 1975, when the annual survey of high school seniors, called "Monitoring the Future," began. At six percent, it equaled the percentage of the same group of high school seniors who used alcohol on a daily basis.

As Director of the National Institute on Drug Abuse at that time, I was concerned, but not really shocked, by this six percent figure.

However, at the end of the following year, 1976, the percentage of high school seniors using marijuana on a daily basis rose to 8.1 percent. This was cause for more concern: more than a 33 percent rise in one year. In the following year, 1977, the figure hit 9.1 percent, and in 1978 it reached 10.7 percent. Meanwhile, the alcohol use figure stayed level at about six percent. By 1978, the alarm signals were up: daily pot smoking by American high school seniors had almost doubled in three years and stood at nearly twice the rate of daily alcohol use. This shocking rise in the daily use figure was one of the main reasons for my switch from support to determined opposition to marijuana decriminalization or any other policy which appeared to promote or even accept marijuana use.

By zeroing in more closely on this special segment of the nation's high school seniors, we are able to see how these daily smokers of marijuana differ from their peers while, at the same time, providing a somewhat more intimate view of their lifestyles and their drug-using behaviors. Beginning with the basics, daily use of marijuana was twice as common for boys as for girls (13 percent versus seven percent), and it was also twice as common among high school seniors who were not intending to go to college as among those who were college-bound (13 percent versus seven percent).

There were no big differences by region in the country, although there was a higher rate in urban communities than in rural ones. Daily use was also *less* common among blacks than among whites (five percent versus 11 percent). Daily use was not different for upper classes than for lower classes, and there was only a slightly higher rate among students being raised by a single parent compared to those living with both parents.

Daily use of marijuana correlated strongly with levels of scholastic achievement, school attendance, and delinquency. The daily users had lower grades, more truancy, and higher rates of delinquency. Daily use was much less common among students with a religious commitment. It was higher among those who had a paying job, and also among those who spent most of their evenings away from home. In fact, among those high school seniors who were out of their homes with their friends six or seven nights a week, 39 percent were daily users of marijuana—a statistic more highly correlated with daily use than any other. This becomes particularly significant when one realizes that 30 percent of high school seniors spend four or more nights out with their friends each week.

Since this study of marijuana use was initiated in 1975, we have also had opportunities over the intervening years to gather important information about what happened to these youthful users of marijuana *after* they left high school. Those who got married were far more likely to stop daily marijuana use (11 percent versus seven percent). It is not surprising that those living in apartments or rented rooms had higher rates of daily use (12 percent versus 14 percent) after high school, but it is surprising that those living in college dormitories had relatively lower rates: eight percent.

Frequent users of marijuana also have a tendency to use other illicit drugs heavily, as well as tobacco and alcohol. For example, of the daily marijuana smokers, 27 percent were daily alcohol drinkers (versus only seven percent for the whole sample of high school seniors), and 59 percent were daily cigarette smokers (versus 25 percent for the whole sample). In terms of other illicit drugs, the rates of use for the daily marijuana users were five or six times greater than the rates for the study sample as a whole.

This special "six percent segment" of high school seniors provides some illuminating reasons for their daily use of marijuana. Ninety-four percent said they used marijuana "to feel good" or "to get high." The next most frequently cited reason (79 percent) was "to have a good time with friends," followed by the 67 percent who wanted "to relax." Nearly one-half of these daily users said they smoked pot "to avoid boredom." Lesser numbers gave escapist reasons: "to get away from problems"—27 percent; "because of anger or frustration"—23 percent; and "to get through the day"—22 percent. Thirty percent said they used pot to enhance the effects of other drugs they were also taking.

What *consequences* did this group of daily users see resulting from their marijuana habit? Keeping in mind the caveat that individuals or groups who have passed into drug dependence are not likely to be the most sensitive or realistic assessors of the effects of their own drug use (they underreport bad effects of use), such assessments are useful. In addition to shedding light on the drug problem, they serve as a basis for comparisons with more expert and more objective findings—matters explored in earlier pages of this chapter.

Of the high school seniors using marijuana on a daily basis, only eight percent perceived negative effects on their physical health, while 42 percent said it caused them to have less energy. Thirty-one percent said it made them less interested in school and other activities than they were before they began to use the drug. Thirty-four percent said marijuana use hurt their scholastic or work performance, while

38 percent said it hurt their relationships with their parents, and only 10 percent said it adversely affected their friendships. Eleven percent said it caused them to be less stable emotionally, and 28 percent said it made them think less clearly, but only 11 percent thought pot use made their car driving less safe.

Most worrisome, however, was the dogged persistence of the habit of daily marijuana use. Five years after graduating from high school, only 15 percent of this large daily-use group had stopped smoking marijuana completely, and slightly more than one-half (51 percent) were still using the drug daily. This powerfully confirms the fact that marijuana use, like other drug use, is not a habit easily or frequently discarded once it has been acquired.

A DIARY OF A TEENAGE DRUG USER:
A CLOSE-IN LOOK AT HOW AND WHY IT HAPPENS

Unavoidably, theory and statistics make up a large part of this chapter. Sometimes this can leave an unintended and unfortunate impression of a certain remoteness, as if the marijuana problem were merely a matter of conflicting ideas. To counteract any such impression, I am including a personal story of an actual, very much alive marijuana user: excerpts from and commentary about a journal of a teenage crisis, painstakingly and often painfully kept. This diary is, of course, presented for a variety of other reasons also. It captures, enlivens, and reinforces the essence and implications of many things said in these pages, doing it in a way that no other method possibly could. Vividly reflecting the day-to-day feelings of loneliness, hostility, self-anger, and despair suffered by its youthful author, it imparts a reality, an authenticity, that could be imparted in no better way.

As personal, intimate testimony, the diary sustains a commendable warmth and empathy as it brings the spotlight down for a close-in view of what happens to a teenager and his family in a sometimes bitter but always valiant struggle to break free of marijuana dependence. It speaks plainly of endangered dreams, desperate remedies, wracking family tensions, mutual recriminations, and the long, slow, arduous climb up the steep slopes of the mountain called "The Way Things Used To Be." Best and most graphically, of course, it speaks for itself. The author of the diary, Peter Skidmore, was a patient of mine. The reporter who wrote this article, Stephanie Mansfield, is one of the nation's most creative feature writers.

Diary of a Teenage Drug User*

*"How Lonely I Feel . . . So Lost. There
Seems to Be Nothing I Can Hang On To"*

By Stephanie Mansfield

From age 13 to 16, Peter Skidmore got high three or four times a day
and often stayed high for up to four weeks at a time. His teachers
knew, his camp counselor knew, his friends knew. Nobody said anything about it. Like many of his friends, Peter Skidmore sleep-walked
through life, confronting the pain and pleasure of adolescence through
a haze of marijuana smoke.

His parents—intelligent, upper-middle-class people who thought this
sort of nightmare never happened to nice families—finally decided to
do something.

> [January 10, 1981] *Home alone, stoned and quite glad to be at
> home without the 'rents. . . . Call Amy. She's not home. How
> lonely I feel. . . . Afraid, because I was not able to reach someone
> to talk with, to be in touch with the others' lives. And I'm faced
> with my own life, and being the only one in it. By writing in my
> journal I am no longer alone, still lonely, though. . . .*

Peter Skidmore was bored.

He put down the ballpoint pen and closed the blue spiral notebook.
Then he reached for the plastic bong he hid behind his bookcase, the
secret place where he had hidden favorite toys as a kid. He tamped
down the marijuana, lit a match, closed his lips over the plastic mouth-
piece, and inhaled the smoke. He opened the notebook to that day's
entry and picked up the pen.

> *I can't figure out why I get high because I don't really enjoy it. I
> smoke not enough to be escaping life, although to some extent I
> am. . . . I feel so lost in everything. There seems to be nothing I
> can hang on to.*

Of great concern to National Academy of Sciences researchers are
the statistics: One in 14 high school seniors in America uses marijuana
on a near-daily basis. An NAS report released last month found that

---

*"Diary of a Teenage Drug User," *The Washington Post*, Sunday, March 28, 1982.
Reprinted by permission of The Washington Post Company, Washington, D.C.,
Stephanie Mansfield, and the Skidmore family.

marijuana has a broad range of psychological and biological effects, and that the suspected health hazards justify "serious national concern." The major findings concluded that marijuana use impairs motor coordination, interferes with short-term memory, and may produce effects ranging from euphoria to delirium. Dr. Robert L. DuPont, the former director of the National Institute on Drug Abuse who eventually treated Peter Skidmore, says the Washington teenager is typical of adolescent drug abusers. "In some ways it's worse [than heroin]," he says. "It's more insidious. There's a climate of tolerance, of acceptance of marijuana."

What is not typical about Peter Skidmore was his ability to articulate his three-year odyssey in a journal—a sad, revealing diary of a child of the 70s.

Strangers would say Peter Skidmore had it all: good friends, good looks, good grades at a private school, a large house in a quiet Northwest Washington neighborhood. His parents are the kind of people others envy: Bill Skidmore, handsome Ivy League product, successful lawyer with the Commerce Department. Tricia Skidmore: involved, intelligent, soft-spoken, training to be a paralegal.

Tall and slim, with soft blue eyes and blond hair that he used to pull back into a ponytail, Peter Skidmore is the youngest of three children and the only boy. As a child, he was so trouble-free that his mother used to worry. *"We're gonna get it someday,"* she'd say to her husband, half-joking. *"This can't last."*

In the eighth grade at Alice Deal School, 13-year-old Peter Skidmore tried pot for the first time. It was 1978, the peak year of marijuana use among teenagers, when one in nine seniors smoked regularly, according to DuPont.

Peter's best friend had already experimented with drugs. But Peter says he felt naive. He didn't know anything about the drug scene. One night, he went to a dance at St. Albans School and met his friend. They went outside, where a group of boys stood in a tight circle, passing a joint. Peter stood outside the group, uneasy at first. When it was his turn, he took the cigarette, puffing a little too hard, trying to impress the other boys. He didn't feel anything at first. He doesn't remember if he got high.

But if he didn't respond immediately to the drug, he did react to something else: the acceptance from the group. For the first time in his life, he felt he belonged to something. A secret club. After that night, he and the crowd got high often. At first it was weekends and parties, where a joint was always being rolled and bong hits were a rite of teenage passage.

"It just made some things more fun," he recalls. "We used to go out and play Putt Putt golf at 2 in the morning in the freezing rain. No one's going to have fun doing that unless you're high."

Peter worried about getting caught. He squirted Visine in his eyes to clear the redness, chewed gum and sucked on Lifesavers and breath mints to disguise the smell. Still, his parents suspected he had tried marijuana. When they asked him, Peter said yes. They asked him to stop. His father wasn't worried at the time. He thought it was a phase, that pot was pretty harmless. His mother, though, was becoming more and more anxious. She had been reading articles about the harmful effects of marijuana on teenagers, especially on their emotional development. Her husband downplayed it. Don't worry, he'd tell her. _Relax._

By the ninth grade, Peter was stopping off at his best friend's house on the way to school. The two would share a joint before setting off on their bikes. But the drug never interfered with his grades. In fact, Peter was convinced it helped his concentration. Especially in math. When he was stoned, he could really zero in on one problem.

In 1980, Bill and Tricia Skidmore decided to send their son to a private school. They chose Sandy Spring Friends School, a small, relatively progressive oasis of Quaker ideals in suburban Maryland. Peter Skidmore got high three or four times a day. Once before breakfast, once at the break between second and third period, once at lunch, and once again when he got home.

"It kept me company," he says now. "Whenever I needed a break from home, or whenever I was sad or lonely, I'd go down to this bridge in Rock Creek Park near the house and get high."

At school, he'd walk outside to a clearing in the woods, where boys would gather to joke and pass a joint or two. Peter says he never had to buy any marijuana. His friends supplied it. Some grew it in their backyards.

His interest in outside activities began to dwindle. He lived in a state of suspended animation, hardly speaking to his parents. He was irritable. He lied constantly. Bill Skidmore still thought it might be normal. Teenagers always went through a period of estrangement from their parents.

But something else was happening to Peter Skidmore. His memory was becoming hazy. He had a hard time recalling simple things he had done or said. He was exhausted all the time. Since his mother worked three days a week, he was home alone during many afternoons—time he spent smoking pot in his bedroom and writing in his journal.

Bored and listless, he would barely get his homework done before falling asleep. Often, he would spend an entire Sunday in bed.

"I'm sure the teachers knew," he says. "There were a lot of people who smoked pot there. I used to get high a lot because classes were a drag. If I had a test I was worried about, I'd get high so I wouldn't have to think about it. Sometimes, I would fall asleep at my desk."

One night, at a Capital Centre rock concert, he passed out. He says now someone had crushed Quaaludes and mixed them with the marijuana he was smoking. He woke up 45 minutes later in the nurse's station. "I was still dizzy, but I ran back to my seat. It never hit me for a while how dangerous it was."

> [February 18, 1981] *Life gets depressing. I notice myself getting sucked into smoking . . . my partying is not so often, but it is a problem. My whole life seems to be in a different perspective because of pot. I find it hard to imagine doing anything I enjoy without thinking of partying too. Today, I avoided depression and got high. I feel unhealthy. . . . My lifestyle has me trapped in the world of smoke. Why? Why everything?*

His parents found drug paraphernalia in his room and took it away. The pipes, the bongs, the rolling papers, the little glass vials of grass. Tricia called Peter's best friend's mother to tell her what was up. "I expected some resentment," she says now. "We talked over the whole pot issue. She said, in effect, that she still trusted it would pass."

> [February 23, 1981] *Life has become so routine that I am somewhat apathetic. I go to school not caring and come home the same. I don't do homework. Don't do anything. It amazes me how I can do nothing for periods of five or so hours. I'm not excited about anything, barely enjoy dreaming about the future. Have no hopes, no desires. Nothing seems to matter.*

He underlined the last sentence.

Peter Skidmore's drug problem was putting a strain on his parents' marriage. The arguments, the confrontations were taking their toll. Tricia Skidmore had had a malignant tumor taken from her leg a year earlier, which added to the tension.

> [March 27, 1981] *Today was another one of those parents-versus-me days which has brought our relationship down to its lowest yet. Dad thinks that the problem with us "------- kids these days" is that we've never been told what not to do. He said we're immature ------s who think we can do whatever we want and not care about anything. He and Mom are eternally and without cease in anger toward me for treating them so badly and Dad [says] I'm not fit to be a [camp] counselor because I'm a drugged, immature person.*

Peter had spent summers at Catoctin Quaker Camp as a camper. That year, he had planned to return as a counselor. It was the one thing he was living for. It became the one thing his parents could take away.

At about this time, Tricia Skidmore read an article about a drug program that helped teenagers on marijuana. "I was determined, while we still had control, to do something," she says. "I was afraid we would lose it."

[April 12, 1981] *Things have been so ----ed up. School, home, parents, the drug situation, me. I feel that I have lost all touch with life. I can't figure anything out. Mom and Dad are ruining everything I had hoped for. Can that possibly be better for my emotional state? My health, yes, but I think I'm going crazy. Aunt Alice said this weekend, "I think the whole world's going crazy."*

The family consulted a psychiatrist who referred them to Dr. Robert L. DuPont, White House drug abuse adviser under Presidents Nixon and Ford. DuPont had, in recent years, changed his stance on the issue of marijuana. Once in favor of decriminalization, the 46-year-old psychiatrist had become increasingly concerned about teenagers' emotional addiction to pot. He began lecturing at high schools, and last year started a Washington drug abuse clinic.

The drug program was to last 12 weeks and cost about $800, with individual therapy, weekly urinalysis, and group sessions. The Skidmores gave their son an ultimatum: Give up pot or leave the house.

Peter Skidmore enrolled as the program's first patient.

[April 14, 1981] *Today was my first appointment with Ron Levin, drug counselor. He's showing me that relationships based on pot are very superficial and that all the friendships I have now are pretty much based on pot. . . . One thing I did not like too much was that he feels pot smokers are not worthy friends because the deeper feelings, problems, never surface. I'm psyched to make progress. He is really convincing (even if it may be brainwashing) [me] that it is absolutely necessary that life be potless. He's being hard on me and giving me a lot of ----."*

Ron Levin, a 31-year-old social worker, remembers the night Peter Skidmore came in for treatment. "He was hesitant, like most of them are. He didn't know what he was getting into." The first thing Levin told him was to get off drugs immediately. The second order was to find new friends.

"I am going to be on your --- if you continue to hang out with dope fiends," Levin told his patient. Peter agreed to stop smoking pot for the duration of the program, but he resisted giving up his friends. They were his only identity. But he soon discovered that when he stopped smoking pot, he no longer spent as much time with them.

[April 19, 1981] *Four days of completely unstoned, straight, clean fun and happiness. Life is wonderful again. I feel myself growing and experiencing again.*

He experienced withdrawal symptoms, which Levin compares to quitting cigarettes: light-headedness, disorientation, irritability, insomnia. Levin prodded, forcing Peter to "get in touch with his emotions." Often, Peter would cry during these early sessions. After one month, several other boys had joined the program. One weekend, Levin took them hiking—just to show them that it was possible to have fun without drugs.

There were topics of discussion each week: the latest medical research on marijuana, how to deal with peer pressure, immediate versus delayed gratification, love, anger, success, positive addictions.

Generally, the peer pressure Peter Skidmore had experienced at school reversed itself. There was strong support from members of the group to remain drug free.

"It was a lot easier than I expected," he says. "I think when I was getting high I was emotionally addicted to it, but once I stopped, I picked up pretty fast how to deal with the problems. I really started getting into the drug-free life, and it was frustrating when I couldn't convince my friends of the same thing. I felt a lot better about everything I was doing. My parents and I still don't get along that well. I just couldn't admit that I had done something wrong. I think that was the hardest part of the whole program. I always had to retaliate. It had been a long battle and I didn't want to give up."

Summer came and Peter returned to camp. His family picked him up on Mondays and drove him to the sessions with Levin. One night they found a small vial of white powder in his pack. It was cocaine. Peter insisted he was only bringing it back to camp for a friend. The next Sunday, Bill Skidmore drove to the mountains for a confrontation with his son over the cocaine. They sat under a tree as Peter confided in his father for the first time: how he felt about drugs, how he had just broken up with a girl friend, his pain and loneliness.

"I feel so bad about what I've done to you," Peter said.

When they stood up to leave, they put their arms around each other and sobbed. "Peter and I have never been real close," says Bill

Skidmore. But if the emotional exchange broke down any barriers, it was only a temporary detente.

During the first week of August, Peter attended his last session with Levin. Before the individual meeting, the social worker met with Peter and his parents. It was the culmination of the 12-week session. They sat on the hard chrome and leather chairs, staring at the white walls. Levin asked Peter how he felt. Suddenly, the boy exploded with a torrent of complaints.

"You're not supporting me. Where do you ever help me? Where have you been when I needed you?" he cried. "You don't listen to my dreams enough. You don't take an interest in my life."

Tricia Skidmore sat silent, her face ashen. Bill Skidmore wrung his hands, staring at the floor. When he could stand it no longer, he burst into tears.

"You're giving me a bum rap," he shouted at his son, reeling off a list of projects the two had become involved in. At the end of the session, the family had come together, exhausted, and determined to heal the wounds. Bill and Tricia Skidmore went home and wrote their son long, "reaching out" letters.

That night, back at camp, Peter got stoned.

Monday night, Bong hits. Tuesday, ditto. Wednesday, ditto. Monday night was the last drug session, hopefully. . . . I feel pretty ------. My problem with the parents is that I have been subconsciously unable or unwilling to accept or return their love. I've been afraid to, in some respects.

Ron Levin says Peter got high that night to test himself. To see what would happen. It's not unusual, Levin says.

But Peter found more and more excuses to get high. "I got back to the whole drug scene," he says. "By September, I was starting to feel bad about it."

When Peter returned from camp, his parents knew he was using drugs again. There were harsh words, bitter exchanges, more threats and confrontations. Tricia Skidmore looks back on that time as a "nightmare." "It was worse than the cancer," she says.

[September 14, 1981] My pot smoking hasn't diminished since camp and is really a concern now. The relationship with the parents just isn't as wonderful as I thought it was. I'm not getting any of the things which I should do, done. I always get too mellow and stoned, and I feel guilty. My whole life just seems to be banking downhill once again. Nothing seems wonderful anymore.

"I realized I needed help," Peter says now, "but I couldn't ask my parents." One night, as the family was finishing dinner, Peter broke down and cried. For the first time in his life, he was able to ask for help.

The family called Ron Levin. He accepted Peter into the program for another 12 weeks. "The first night was really amazing," Peter says. "There were a whole new group of people, and I had been through it all once before. Everything I had accomplished during the first program came back to me. It was a lot easier that time. I was learning from the group, but I was also able to help them. I was giving *them* encouragement."

One group member Peter couldn't help was a boy who smoked pot two weeks before the end of the program, lied about it, and then ran away from home.

But Peter now understands the emotional risk of giving up drugs.

"Every time I felt I was being real successful, people would notice less. If you don't have a problem, then you're normal and nobody congratulates you for not getting high. That was hard."

Levin agrees.

"I think smoking dope was Peter's way of getting more attention from his parents. I think he was asking, as most kids do, for them to define his parameters, what he could do and what he couldn't do. I think it was peer pressure. I think he really wanted to be needed, as do most of the kids."

"The kids will lie and manipulate and cheat and steal and totally cut themselves off from their parents," Levin adds. "It's what teenagers do normally, but it's really accentuated with dope. You learn that you don't have to deal with stress, you don't have to make any decisions, you don't have to deal with the normal daily activities of just getting along with parents, and you get into this pattern. The more you're away, the more you *want* to be away."

So far, the marijuana program has treated 13 teenage boys. According to Levin, eight of the 13 are now drug free.

"I've learned to enjoy things without it," Peter says. He plays on a frisbee team and recently has taken up ballroom dancing. "I don't think pot should be part of my life. I think it's really dangerous. It stunts your emotional growth. I think a lot of parents are overwhelmed by it. They have no idea how to deal with it. I wonder about all my friends who get high so much. I can't imagine them ever making much out of their lives. I worry about them."

It's been easier since he changed schools. He didn't go back to Sandy Spring this year. He enrolled in School Without Walls, an alternative Washington high school that permits students to take courses at different institutions. He's taking college courses in math at

George Washington University. Next fall, the 17-year-old is enrolling in a small liberal arts college away from home. He is worried about falling into his old patterns. He knows that alcohol and other drugs will be readily available. But he hopes he's learned how to face life without them.

"I feel as if I've grown up," he says. "I had a lot of fun getting high, but I think there's probably a lot that I missed." What he regrets most are the lost years with his parents. "They have told me, literally, that it's been a delight to have me around this year," he says, smiling impishly. "That's nice to hear."

But Peter Skidmore's odyssey isn't over. A week after the program ended last December, a girl he had been dating for several months broke up with him. On New Year's Eve, his parents went out. He was alone and depressed. He knew if he stayed home, he'd "go crazy." He called a few friends and wound up at a party with old friends from Sandy Spring. He was offered a joint. At first, he refused. But then, after a few drinks, he decided to get high.

[January 1, 1982] *I got high for the first time since September and at the time went through so much self-anger because I failed. Because I was escaping, everything bothering me. For every reason, I was bummed about it. Today I feel sure it will not happen again. My worst feelings about it are that I was so stupid to do it after so long. I can no longer say, "since September." Now, it's "yesterday."*

SAVE THE YOUNG—THEY'RE OUR BEST BET

Obviously, the disturbing realities of marijuana use and its pernicious and pervasive effects should be—and are gradually becoming—matters of grave national concern. Whatever you may think about the use of marijuana by adults (I strongly oppose anyone using marijuana), nearly everyone agrees that the young and the very young should not use it. Even the marijuana lobby agrees with this. Most of us agree, too, that there are many sound and urgent reasons to prevent the spread of the marijuana epidemic among the young. Here, at the close of this chapter, I would like to advance two closely related concepts which, if translated into action, may contribute to the goal of stopping the marijuana problem before it begins: (1) the longer a family can *delay* the possible start of marijuana use by its young, the less likely the start-up is to happen, and (2) the more strongly a family *discourages* its youth from experimenting with marijuana (or any other drug), the less likely are its youth to head down the "nowhere" road to drug dependence.

Because marijuana use, and use of other drugs as well, usually starts between the ages of 12 and 20, any delay in drug experimentation reduces the likelihood that the young person will ever start drug use. Research has also shown that the later the person starts using any drug, the less likely that person is to become dependent on it. Although most young people will now concede that frequent use of marijuana *is* hazardous, they often ask me, "Is it so bad, really, to smoke pot just *once*?" Large numbers of America's youth obviously are fascinated by the possibilities of experimentation. "Come on," they insist, "what is wrong with just *trying* it?"

These are seductive questions. I answer by saying that *nobody starts out intending to become dependent on any drug.* I have never known anybody who started using heroin for the purpose of becoming a heroin addict. I have never known anybody who started drinking in order to become an alcoholic. People do not start using drugs to become dependent on them. They start out using a drug, especially marijuana, in a casual way, seeking pleasure and relaxation, usually with peer encouragement and support. One of the great dangers of the casual acceptance of drug experimentation, however, is that a high percentage of the people who begin experimenting will move on to dependence. Neither they nor anyone else can predict with accuracy who will stop use of the drug, who will use it only occasionally for long periods, and who will become dependent.

Only one thing is certain: *chronic dependence is a risk that all experimenters run.* One of the most shocking statistics is this: Half of the people in America who have *ever* at some time in their lives smoked a pack of cigarettes are currently addicted to smoking cigarettes. As a related statistic, I cite this one: One in three Americans who try one marijuana cigarette go on to daily marijuana use. You talk about *risks*! When somebody asks, "Is there anything wrong with smoking a couple of joints of marijuana?" the answer must be an emphatic "YES!" If we are serious about trying to prevent drug abuse and reduce drug problems, in general we are going to have to be much tougher about experimentation—especially with marijuana—than we have been in the past.

Several years ago Senator Charles McC. Mathias, Jr., of my home state of Maryland, held U.S. Senate hearings on the health effects of marijuana use. He assembled experts from all points of the marijuana compass, from the vigorously anti-pot (such as me) to the positively pro-pot members of the board of the marijuana lobby, NORML. He posed two questions to all witnesses: (1) Should children use marijuana? and (2) Is marijuana a health hazard?

Every single witness answered those questions the same way. All said children, at least through age 18, should not smoke marijuana, and all agreed that marijuana was a health hazard.

There was much argument about the legal status of marijuana and how bad marijuana was when compared to other poisons, but on those two points there was unanimous agreement. All effective prevention efforts can be securely based on the answers to those two fundamental questions.

MARIJUANA: THE DUMB HIGH—SUMMING UP

If, in reading this chapter, you have come to understand

- the special role of marijuana in *drug dependence*;
- the pervasiveness of certain marijuana *myths*;
- the disturbing *scope* of the marijuana problem;
- the insidious *appeal* of marijuana for the young;
- the *trends* in marijuana use;
- the *dangers* in marijuana's unique chemistry;
- the increasing *potency* of THC in marijuana;
- the *residual effects* of marijuana on the brain, lungs, liver, and reproductive organs;
- the *cancer potential* contained in marijuana smoke;
- the destructive *impact* of marijuana on memory, learning, motivation, and motor coordination during the formative years of adolescence;
- the *restrictions* imposed by marijuana on the adolescent's ability to cope;
- the potential for *anxiety mismanagement* resulting from marijuana use; and
- the *high risk involved in experimenting* with marijuana,

then—with no great leap in logic—you can readily understand why marijuana so well deserves to be named . . . "The Dumb High."

CHAPTER
FOUR

Alcohol:
Everybody Does It—
Or So It Seems

SEVERAL YEARS AGO I was the guest speaker at a luncheon with the editors of *The New York Times*. They had invited me to talk about heroin addiction, but the conversation turned to America's most often used mind-altering drug, alcohol. As many of the editors sipped sherry or nursed a cocktail (I did not see anyone drinking a martini, and I surely didn't see anyone drinking three martinis at that lunch), I asked them to estimate the percentage of American adults who have as much as one drink of alcohol in the form of beer, wine, or distilled liquor each day. In other words, I asked them to estimate the percentage of American adults who are daily alcohol drinkers. Their estimates ranged from 60 percent to 90 percent. There was surprise, if not disbelief, when I told them the correct number was seven percent and that about 40 percent of American adults are nondrinkers. The seven percent of adults who are daily alcohol drinkers consume about one-half of all the alcohol drunk in this country. My point? Most drinkers *think* "Everybody's Doing It." They are *not*. Whether my remarks had any impact on the behavior of my listeners I have no way of knowing. But a *New York Times* editor told me recently that his colleagues have stopped serving alcohol at those informal luncheons.

ALCOHOL: AMERICA'S FAVORITE INTOXICATING DRUG

Many Americans, especially in the upper social classes, think of alcohol as a normal, if not an essential, part of social life. Alcohol advertisements drive the message home: "If it's time to relax, if you're feeling fine, then it's time to sip a glass of booze!" Most of us see alcohol around us frequently. We have abundant evidence that people who use alcohol are "normal" people. In fact, alcohol is the only drug for which there is some scientific evidence that having a little may improve the health of the user. Yet few families live without the sickening evidence of the hazards inherent in alcohol use. My best friend in high school died in an automobile accident after he had been drinking. Each generation of my family has had tragic casualties from alcohol use.

In 1970, when I first began to treat heroin addicts in Washington, D.C., I was invited to visit the famous hostess, Perle Mesta, then an older woman living elegantly in a large hotel apartment. Our conversation turned to marijuana. She asked me about its effects. Seeking, I now think, to shock her, I compared kids' use of marijuana to adults' use of alcohol. What I remember as if it were yesterday was her energetic response: "Of course. And that's exactly why I'm against it!" She then proceeded to tell me of all the fine careers she had seen ruined by alcohol over the years and of her own approach to alcohol at her parties. She served no guest more than one drink before dinner and, she said, she filled wine glasses only once. No one who came to dinner with Perle Mesta had more than one cocktail and one glass of wine. She considered that to be not only her contribution to preventing alcoholism but her secret to having a successful dinner party. I left her apartment that day doubting that I had educated her, but knowing that she had educated me.

The Scope of Alcohol Use

Alcohol use is the most ordinary and most complex of all American drug problems. Few Americans have to read a government report to believe that alcohol accounts for about 240,000 deaths per year (15 percent of *all deaths* annually in the United States) and costs more than $48 billion in health costs and lost productivity. That comes to just over $200 per year for every man, woman, and child. Alcohol is the most widely used drug in the world. About 95 million American adults—60 percent of Americans over the age of 18—drink alcohol, and an additional 48 million—30 percent—have tried it, but do not currently drink. This leaves only about 18 million Americans 18 and older—10 percent—who have never used the drug, alcohol. Thus, while it is not true, as many drinkers believe, that "everybody drinks," 90 percent of Americans over the age of 18 have had a drink of alcohol at some point in their lives and about 60 percent are regular drinkers. Among Americans from 12 to 17 years of age, all of whom are under the legal drinking age, 65 percent have used alcohol at least once and 26 percent are regular alcohol drinkers. Small wonder that our national and personal attitudes toward alcohol are the most ambivalent, and that the image of "universality" and "normality" of drinking makes alcohol the most difficult drug about which to think clearly.

The scope of alcohol use in this country is further emphasized by information gathered in *Alcohol and Health* (1981), the most recent such report issued by the U.S. Department of Health and Human Services. It points out the following:

- During the 1970s, per-capita consumption of alcohol in America continued to rise, although the rate of rise, compared to that of earlier decades, slowed. By 1978, the most recent year for which statistics were available, the average American consumed 2.7 gallons of pure alcohol per year, or about two drinks per day. However, since 40 percent of adults do not drink at all, the remaining 60 percent drank an average of three drinks per day. Even more disturbing, the top 11 percent of drinkers drank an average of about nine drinks per day.
- Beer accounts for 49 percent of all alcohol consumed, wine for 12 percent, and distilled spirits such as whiskey and vodka for 39 percent. In recent years, American drinking preferences shifted strongly from distilled spirits to beer and wine.
- In the heavy-drinking category, males outnumber females (14 percent of American men compared to four percent of American women are heavy drinkers). Blacks showed higher levels of nonuse of alcohol, but about equal levels of heavy drinking. Hispanics had higher rates of heavy drinking for both men and women than other Americans. Heavy drinking peaks between ages 21 and 34 for men and between 35 and 49 for women, and then declines in later ages.
- Youthful drinking has shown little change in recent years, but is disturbingly high: approximately 15 percent of the young in grades 10 through 12 reported themselves to be heavy drinkers.

The "Special" Nature of Alcohol

Alcohol is a unique drug in a number of important ways. It is special because of its chemistry, its history of use in this country, its caloric but nonnutritional inputs, and the economic pressures which support its manufacture, sale, and use.

Alcohol's "Special" Nature—Chemically. The chemical composition of alcohol—$C_2H_6O_2$ or ethanol—makes it chemically the simplest of psychoactive drugs. Also, alcohol is unique because it is the only nonmedical drug in common use which is taken *only* by mouth: it is never "shot," "smoked," or "snorted." Alcohol is the only drug which has a large number of regular users who do not become physically dependent on it. In this regard, it contrasts sharply with tobacco, our other legal but nonintoxicating drug, which—after a few years of use—practically forces smokers either to quit altogether or to use it all day, every day.

The principal psychoactive ingredient in beer, wine, and distilled liquor, ethyl alcohol or ethanol, is a substance produced by fermenting sugar with yeast spores or bacteria. There are many kinds of alcohols, but the only one used in alcoholic beverages is ethanol: a colorless, inflammable liquid which produces an intoxicating effect when used as a drug. In this capacity, ethanol can produce feelings of elation, well-being, sedation, intoxication, or unconsciousness—depending upon the quantity, manner, and circumstances in which it is imbibed. Thus it fits perfectly the definition of a *drug* as specified in Chapter 2.

Variations in the manufacture of different alcoholic drinks are achieved by using different sources of sugar for fermentation. Beer, for instance, is made from malted or "germinated" barley; wine is fermented from grapes or berries; whiskey is made from grains like corn or rye, usually; and rum has molasses as its base. Because the yeast and bacteria which convert sugar to alcohol are killed by the rising alcohol content as the fermentation progresses, there is a biological ceiling for alcohol content: roughly five percent for beer and 12 percent for wine. However, with the development of the distillation process (which began in Europe in the 17th century), the alcohol content of beverage alcohol was raised—potentially to almost pure ethanol. Thus, distillation—by raising the "strength" of alcohol to vastly higher levels—made possible the making of "hard" liquors: whiskey, gin, and vodka.

Alcohol's "Special" Nature—Nutritionally. Alcohol is the only drug which contains calories. In the liver, the metabolism or burning of alcohol produces water and carbon dioxide and releases about 200 calories per ounce of pure alcohol. A typical drink contains about one-half ounce of pure alcohol (the approximate amount contained in 12 ounces of beer, five ounces of wine, or 1½ ounces of whiskey or gin), or about 100 calories. Since a great many alcoholic beverages are mixed with other calorie-containing substances, most drinks consumed in the United States today have between 100 and 150 calories. Fully eight percent of all the calories consumed in America today are imbibed in the form of alcoholic beverages: one in every 12 calories consumed by Americans comes from ethyl alcohol.

Although many of the negative health effects of alcohol use result from the problems of intoxication and dependence, there are—in addition—a wide range of *nutritional* problems which are not so readily recognized. One of the functions of the stomach is to store food and water, often swallowed over a very short period of time, for more gradual release into the small intestine for absorption into the bloodstream and metabolic processing in the body. Alcohol is unusual in this respect because, being a simple chemical that is easily dissolved in either fat or water, it "short-circuits" this mechanism for gradual release and is partially absorbed into the bloodstream directly through the stomach wall without having to pass out of the stomach and into the intestines. Water is virtually the only other common substance which is handled by the body in this way. This makes alcohol more quickly available to the blood and the brain than if it were required to pass out of the stomach before absorption, as are other foods. Because it is rapidly and completely absorbed into the bloodstream, the effects of drinking alcohol begin within a few minutes after the drink has been taken. Even so, the absorption of alcohol is still far slower than is the absorption of drugs taken intravenously or by smoking.

It is especially important to note that if the drinker's stomach has food in it when the alcohol is swallowed, some of the alcohol is absorbed by the food and then released into the bloodstream more slowly. The speed of absorption is a significant factor because the brain adjusts relatively slowly to alcohol and also because the liver "burns" the alcohol relatively slowly. Thus, if alcohol is taken into the bloodstream more slowly, the liver and the brain have a better chance of handling the dose without problems arising either in terms of metabolism or behavior. Conversely, if a given dose of alcohol is drunk on an empty stomach, it hits the liver and the brain faster and harder and is therefore more likely to produce health hazards. When people drink alcohol to get high, or intoxicated, this overwhelming of the body's protective mechanisms is exactly the desired effect. If alcohol is drunk slowly, in small quantities, after eating food, there is relatively little high and relatively little altered thinking or acting. By contrast, if alcohol is drunk rapidly, in large quantities and on an empty stomach, the behavioral toxicity is increased, and a high is produced.

Alcohol's "Special" Nature—Historically. Alcohol is special, too, because it has a long national and international history. For thousands of years, in virtually all societies which used grain for food, people learned to ferment the grain starch and sugar to make beer and wine. The simplicity of the process of fermentation and the ubiquity of grains made alcohol the "world's drug" throughout the ages. Despite this historical preeminence, however, and despite the fact that alcohol has long been the most commonly used drug in America, the people of the United States have held mixed feelings about the drinking of alcohol. Through the years since the founding of our nation, some have been "for" it and others "against" it. The balance of these forces has ebbed and flowed over our country's history. There have been "whiskey rebellions" and Carrie Nation crusades. There seem always to have been pro-alcohol forces and anti-alcohol forces. Wherever and whenever alcohol has been a question, we have been a nation of fence-straddlers. Tightrope walkers.

Our historic ambivalence toward alcohol is illustrated in a story told by Professor Robert Saunders, Dean of the College of Education at Memphis State University. According to the tale (Professor Saunders does not remember the source), a Tennessee lawmaker received a letter from a farmer-constituent who wanted to know where he stood on "the whiskey question." This was the legislator's remarkable response:

Dear Friend:

I had not intended to discuss the controversial subject at this particular time.

However, I want you to know that I do not shun a controversy. On the contrary, I will take a stand on any issue at any time, regardless of how fraught with controversy it may be. You have asked me how I feel about whiskey. Here's how I stand on the question:

If, when you say whiskey, you mean the Devil's brew, the poison scourge, the bloody monster that defiles innocence, dethrones reason, destroys the home, creates misery and poverty—yes, literally takes the bread from the mouths of little children; if you mean the drink that topples the Christian man and woman from the pinnacle of the righteous, gracious living into the bottomless pit of degradation, despair, shame, and helplessness, then certainly I am against it with all my power.

But if, when you say whiskey, you mean the oil of conversation, the philosophic wine, the ale that is consumed when good fellows get together, that puts a song in their hearts and laughter on their lips and the warm glow of contentment in their eyes; if you mean Christmas cheer; if you mean the stimulating drink that puts the spring in an old gentleman's step on a frosty morning; if you mean that drink, the sale of which pours into our treasury untold millions of dollars which are used to provide tender care for our crippled children, our blind, our deaf, our dumb, pitiful, aged and infirm, to build highways, hospitals, and schools, then certainly I am in favor of it.

This is my stand, and I will not compromise.

In 1919, the "Temperance" or anti-alcohol forces, which had been steadily building strength in this country since the middle of the 19th century, succeeded in enacting national prohibition of alcohol into the federal law of the land. They could hardly have imagined that just 14 years later a reform president, Franklin Roosevelt, would make repeal of Prohibition a major first act of his administration. This, of course, humiliated the temperance forces and led to a discrediting of the abstinence of the "no alcohol at all" movement. This twist of fate was more remarkable because the temperance forces throughout the last half of the 19th century were the reform forces in American politics. The same political alliances which made heroin and cocaine illegal, which got dangerous and fraudulent patent medicines out of our lives, and which cleaned up the nation's food supply were at work supporting the elimination of alcohol from American life. Initially, these reformers were successful at local and state levels. Only in the zeal for national reform in the early decades of the 20th century was prohibition of alcohol made a national law. By that time, most states had already gone "dry." Nor was the temperance movement limited to the United States. Canada and the Scandinavian countries went right along with us. While there was always a tension between those who sought the total elimination of drinking and those who promoted moderate drinking, it was the former which came to dominate the American temperance movement.

Over the last 50 years or so, since the repeal of Prohibition, a new attitude toward drinking alcohol has emerged. In one of the most unusual of alliances, in the 1940s and 1950s the alcohol industry and the newly developed Alcoholics Anonymous made common cause around the peculiar concept that there were two separate kinds of drinkers of alcohol: *social drinkers* and *alcoholics*. The former were "like you and me"—people who drank alcohol for pleasure and who did not have "problems" with alcohol. Alcoholics, by contrast, were far fewer in number, and they had a "disease"—presumably genetically determined—which prevented them from drinking sensibly: they lost control of their drinking. They were "problem drinkers." After the political disaster of the repeal of Prohibition, this bizarre compromise was as strong a position as could be adopted by the survivors of the old temperance movement. Today we see this convenient classification of drinkers sustained by the alcohol industry and echoed by many recovering alcoholics. We also see it played out dramatically in the suddenly militant efforts to get drunk drivers off the highways.

Alcohol's "Special" Nature—Economically.   Alcohol shares with tobacco the deep penetration of our nation's economic life. Alcohol, it is loudly and proudly proclaimed, brings wealth into the public coffers in the form of taxes and also provides many jobs for many people. Understandably, therefore, any attempt to reduce alcohol consumption raises howls of protest from people with perfectly legitimate economic interests in promoting the sale and use of the drug. The economic, as well as the legal, aspects of alcohol have been further complicated by the fact that our nation went from wide-open legal use of alcohol to its complete prohibition in 1919 and then *back* again to a somewhat more restrained legal availability in 1933. This 14-year span, the importance of which is often underestimated, cast a long shadow over our national alcohol policy—especially as it affects the prevalence and economics of alcohol use. Almost any attempt to limit the consumption of beer, wine, or liquor is stubbornly resisted by powerful and vocal special-interest groups which often conceal their true motivations by mocking the attempt as "Neo-Prohibitionism."

Despite its unique chemical, nutritional, historical, and economic nature, alcohol is still a typical drug in that it is a self-reinforcing substance—a psychoactive substance—that makes users feel good and want more on a purely biological basis.

IF ALCOHOL IS SO "NORMAL," WHY IS IT SO DEADLY? OR—THE CONSEQUENCES OF ALCOHOL USE

The ultimate optimist might—if he or she looked hard and long—find a bit of good news about alcohol drinking and health. Some studies, it is true, have suggested that people who drink two or fewer drinks per day have higher levels of high-density lipoproteins in their blood, and this may help reduce very slightly their risk of heart attacks. Experts emphasize, however, that when a person consumes more than two drinks per day, the effect of drinking on mortality is progressively and strongly negative. Probably, you are already beginning to suspect why this is so. Let us consider briefly some of the more life-consuming consequences of drinking alcohol.

The Effects of Alcohol on the Liver

Keeping in mind the crucial role of the liver in metabolizing alcohol, we can see that it can quickly and easily become overworked. When the liver is forced to metabolize excessive amounts of alcohol, it also produces fat which soon begins to build up. When the drinker has downed even a few drinks, fat accumulates in the liver. If heavy drinking continues, the fat buildup continues, producing a fat-laden, enlarged liver. In about 15 percent of heavy drinkers, this fatty buildup leads eventually to scarring and the destruction of healthy liver cells, thus producing a small, rock-hard liver. This deterioration is called cirrhosis of the liver, a disease which is often fatal. Virtually all cirrhosis of the liver in the United States is caused by heavy drinking of alcohol; as a cause of death, it is in sixth place overall in the United States today. Although cirrhosis deaths have been decreasing slightly since 1973, the decline has been offset by an increase in other forms of alcohol-related deaths, especially highway accidents, particularly among the young.

The Effects of Alcohol on the Brain

Once in the bloodstream and past the liver, alcohol has powerful effects on most of the other organs of the body, including the brain, lungs, heart, kidneys, and pancreas. In the brain, alcohol begins by depressing the highest brain functions first, those of the frontal lobes having to do with the individual's maintenance of values and self-awareness. With higher intakes of alcohol, the drinker's judgment, decision making, and reaction time are all affected adversely. Indeed, almost all of the user's *cognitive functions* and *neuromuscular coordination*, as we analyzed them in Chapter 3, are seriously impaired by the drinking of alcohol, just as they are by the smoking of marijuana.

In still larger dosages, alcohol depresses the more primitive brain functions, including—ultimately, if the quantity is large enough—the breathing center, thereby causing breathing to stop. Fortunately for many users of alcohol, before this fatal level of anesthesia is reached, the vomiting center of the brain is activated, and—reinforced by the stomach irritation also produced by overdrinking—causes the user to vomit. The lives of many who overdose on alcohol are thus saved.

Many experts have pointed out a new threat posed by the combined use of alcohol and marijuana. Since marijuana suppresses the brain's vomiting center, it is possible that people stoned on marijuana may, when also drinking large amounts of alcohol, not vomit before they pass out. This can cause a raised risk of deaths due to alcohol overdose. This raises the increasingly frequent problem of the poorly understood interactive effects of multiple drug use, which has become increasingly common during the last two decades.

The effects of alcohol on the brain are not all temporary, by any means, any more than are the effects on the liver. There is, in fact, evidence that *irreversible brain damage* from heavy drinking may begin even before the onset of cirrhosis. As a clinician I have been impressed by the fact that many people who manage to recover from as many as 20 years of heroin addiction seem, amazingly enough, to have normal brain function. This is decidedly not the case for the alcoholic. The brain function of alcoholics who have been addicted for 20 years is often noticeably and permanently impaired.

One brain-based effect of alcohol consumption is decreased ability to drive safely. While it is now well known that drinking and driving in combination are dangerous, I remember from my own youth, before such studies were widely reported, that many teenage drivers really believed they were safer drivers when they drove under the influence of alcohol. That may sound bizarre. It is bizarre. But it is also true. The conventional teenage wisdom then was that driving after drinking made one more relaxed and more likely to feel "one" with the car, and thus a better, more instinctive driver. Further, if one were drunk and did have an accident, he would be less likely to be injured because he would "go with the experience, relaxed, and not fight it." These misguided views were not only widespread 30 years ago, but they are also still typical of many drug user's beliefs about the effects of many drugs, especially the effects of marijuana, on driving. The sober mind is not only always better for driving; it is also better for all types of neuromuscular activities. Any intoxication impairs driving ability.

Recent research adds an important new dimension to this. It has been found that memory is impaired after very modest levels of drinking, even those well under the legal limit. Another study shows that people who drink large amounts of alcohol, say five or six drinks at a time, have mental impairments related to driving which last long after all traces of alcohol are out of their bodies. These studies also show that mental efficiency is reduced during sober periods following bouts of drinking, not only for alcoholics but for social drinkers who drink large quantities of alcohol at one time.

The Effects of Alcohol on the Heart

The drinking of alcohol is closely associated with, and frequently responsible for, a large number of adverse effects on the human cardiovascular system. Increased intakes of alcohol have been found to significantly increase the work load on the heart and to reduce the coronary blood flow to the heart muscle. Heart muscle strength is decreased at blood alcohol levels associated with even mild intoxication; biochemical and microscopic deterioration is seen in the heart muscles of heavy drinkers. All of this naturally decreases cardiac output: the heart just cannot work as smoothly and as efficiently as nature intended. Alcohol consumption also reduces the "flexibility"— the contractability—of the muscles forming the heart walls. Characteristically, too, alcohol can affect the strength and regularity of the heartbeats and can produce hazardous abnormalities in the heart rhythm. Oftentimes, this leads to a condition known as arrhythmia, an uncharacteristic and potentially fatal alteration in the rhythm of the heartbeat.

Alcohol use and blood pressure are closely related, too. Much evidence indicates that, among all races and in both sexes, drinking larger amounts of alcohol is associated with substantially increased rates of high blood pressure. Worse still, patients who are heavy drinkers not infrequently experience heart failure, most often right-sided—a crisis sometimes signaled by an insidious or abrupt shortness of breath or a coughing spasm.

In addition to these dangerously adverse and, at times, fatal effects, indulgence in alcohol over a period of time can—and often does— produce such attendant risks as angina or heart pain, phlebitis, and stroke, as well as other hazards to the heart and blood vessels. Indeed, when almost any other part of the body is affected adversely by regular or heavy ingestion of alcohol, the heart is also affected either directly or indirectly.

The Cancerous Effects of Alcohol on the Body

Heavy drinkers have an increased risk of cancer of the mouth, esophagus, stomach, liver, and bladder. This risk is even greater if they also smoke cigarettes, as many heavy drinkers do. This point deserves special emphasis: the risk of cancers is increased for drinkers, and it is increased for smokers, but for those who are both drinkers and smokers, the extra risk is not merely additive—it appears to be multiplicative. Alcohol also acts as a promoter of cancers in the lungs, the pancreas, the intestines, and the prostate. The use of alcohol causes, in addition, a wide spectrum of other diseases, such as pancreatitis (one of the most painful of all diseases) and painful peripheral nerve damage.

The Effects of Alcohol on Pregnant Mothers and Unborn Infants

Alcohol has a profoundly toxic effect on the unborn human infant. For pregnant and nursing mothers who drink, the alcohol crosses the placenta to reach the unborn baby. Alcohol also enters the mother's breast milk. Thus alcohol, consumed by the mother, reaches the infant both before and after birth. For pregnant women who consume three drinks of alcohol per day, there is a 10 percent chance that their babies will be born with the Fetal Alcohol Syndrome (FAS). The risk rises to 33 percent if the mother imbibes six drinks per day. Experiments with animals suggest that, although lower maternal alcohol consumption rates reduce the risk of FAS, there is no safe maternal level of alcohol intake. Any maternal intake of alcohol, regardless of its size, increases the risk, just as any inhalation of cigarette smoke increases the risk of lung cancer. And, in both cases, of course, the risk rises as the dose increases.

Effects of maternal drinking on children range from mild deficits to full-blown Fetal Alcohol Syndrome, which is characterized by mental retardation, irritability, poor motor development, and growth deficiency before birth and through childhood. FAS children also have a characteristic cluster of facial abnormalities: a short upturned nose, a sunken nasal bridge, a thin upper lip, and retarded growth of the jaws. Children born to alcoholic mothers are at risk for lower birth weight, cardiac defects, and learning deficits and, on the average, have lowered intelligence. In the United States, about one in 600 births today is an FAS infant—each one a victim of an alcohol-drinking mother. To perpetuate this tragedy, even now most pregnant women seem completely unaware of the danger that their drinking imposes upon their unborn children. Drinking of alcohol by prospective fathers can be a problem, too. For one thing, it tends to encourage the mother of the unborn infant to drink. Furthermore, the father's drinking, if chronic and heavy, can reduce male sex hormones, thereby reducing fertility, to say nothing of reducing sexual interest and effectiveness.

The Effects of Alcohol on Nutrition

For the 95 million American adults who drink alcohol, from 10 to 20 percent, or more, of all of their caloric intake comes from alcohol. Because alcohol has virtually no nutritional value and since it displaces more healthful foods in most drinkers' diets, these drinkers are at a substantially greater risk of nutritional deficiencies and attendant disorders, including obesity. The tendency to supplant nutritional food with alcohol is compounded because the drinking of alcohol actually increases the body's need for many nutriments, including the B vitamins, niacin, thiamin, and folic acid, as well as such minerals as potassium, zinc, and magnesium. These nutrient deficiencies come about when excessive intakes of alcohol interact and interfere with the physiological and metabolic processes of digestion. Such deficiencies contribute to anemia, convulsions, and general poor health.

Given this array of profoundly disturbing consequences, can anyone doubt that alcohol is a serious threat to human health and life in our country today? And this is only part of the picture. As the *Journal of the American Medical Association* points out: "One-third of all traffic fatalities are alcohol related; a significant number of industrial accidents, drownings, burns, and falls have been attributed to drinking; and a relatively high involvement of alcohol has been reported in assault, rape, child abuse and neglect, child molestation, and family violence in general." Alcoholics die at 2½ times the rate for nonalcoholics. Overall, alcohol use causes about 240,000 premature deaths each year in the United States. This is about 15 percent of all deaths. Alcohol use as a cause of premature death is surpassed only by the smoking of tobacco. Since drinking and smoking are often linked—that is, smokers are far more likely to be drinkers and vice versa—the consequences of both are further aggravated by the combination and interaction of the use of these two drugs. Though a decision not to drink or smoke will certainly not insure immortality, it will dramatically reduce the risk of having to make a premature call to an undertaker.

FACTORS GOVERNING IRRATIONAL RISK ASSESSMENT OF ALCOHOL

We have examined the paradox of why alcohol is so "normal" and, at the same time, so "deadly." Notice another and quite different paradox: Why do we as a nation and as individuals tolerate with such calm a health risk of such magnitude? A large part of the answer lies in psychological factors which appear to govern risk assessment. Working sometimes singly but more often in combination, these seven factors regulate the priority rating we attribute to health dangers. They anesthetize our susceptibility to shock from many great risks. By looking at these factors as they operate in the assessment so many make when confronted with the death-dealing consequences of alcohol use, we can better understand why the immensity of the risk is so often shrugged off or so vehemently denied.

The Big Event Versus Small, Scattered Events

Most of us assess the risk of alcohol use in terms of one "big event" (seven persons killed in a three-car collision caused by an alcohol-sodden driver) and ignore the small, separate events spread out over time and space. During bad years, for example, crashes of commercial aircraft kill a few hundred people in the United States. Yet airplane crashes are big, scary news. Twenty-five million Americans are so afraid to fly that they stay out of airplanes. The media, however, cover only single *big* disasters as major news. When was the last time you saw a front-page headline about an airplane crash? Today, maybe, or last week, or last year? Whenever it was, you are likely to remember it. How many people were killed? Ninety-one! When was the last time you saw a newspaper headline—on any page of any newspaper—announcing the sad, everyday fact that, "Today 660 Americans Died Because of the Use of Alcohol"? Think about that number for a moment: over 600 Americans die every day because of alcohol use.

Who Controls the Risk?

The second factor explaining the typical unconcern over alcohol's deadly effect is whether or not the individual at risk thinks he or she controls the risk. If drinkers feel they control the risk (and they usually feel that they do), they will—and do—take enormous chances. If someone else controls the risk, virtually no risk (however small) is acceptable. Think about the contrast between the risk of death from smoking cigarettes (320,000 deaths per year) and the risk of death from nuclear power plants. How many people fear nuclear power plants, even though no one, worker or neighbor, has been killed by radiation from the more than 70 operating plants in the United States during more than 20 years of commercial operation? When was the last time you saw a political demonstration about nuclear power? Last week? When was the last time you saw pickets outside the plant of the "Lucky Lucre Tobacco Company" denouncing the manufacture and sale of cigarettes? Or when was the last time you watched a movie about pregnant mothers who, because of their alcohol drinking, posed terrible dangers to the unborn of future generations? Did you ever see pickets protesting the fact that about 15 children per day, in this country alone, are born handicapped for life by their mothers' fondness for alcohol? Or a documentary depicting in detail the brutal beatings and sexual molestations visited upon thousands and thousands of young and innocent children by drunken fathers?

Familiar Risk Versus Unfamiliar Risk

The third psychological factor influencing the way we assess a health risk—an alcohol-induced cardiovascular shutdown or a cardiac arrest, for instance—is whether we view the risk as familiar or unfamiliar. If the risk is familiar, it is usually downplayed, often ignored. Only when a risk is strikingly unfamiliar does anyone pay much attention to it. The more familiar the hazards of alcohol use, the less attention we are likely to give them. After all, "drinking is such a 'friendly, fun thing,' how could anything so familiar possibly be dangerous? Our neighborhood is full of people I see drinking all the time."

Again, contrast the risk of alcohol consumption with the risk of flying in a commercial airplane. People fearful of flying do not fly, so—for them—flight is unfamiliar. In fact, the basic principle underlying successful treatment of phobias (excessive fear reactions which cripple tens of millions of Americans) is repeated exposure to the feared situation. The only way to overcome fear of flying is to get into an airplane again and again until the fear reaction literally withers away. Much the same conditioning characterizes alcohol use. So many people have drunk so much alcohol that they no longer fear it—even though they may have cirrhosis of the liver or cancer of the bladder and are only a nudge away from death's trapdoor. Drinking alcohol is so familiar that virtually no one fears it, even though one out of every seven Americans who die each day die for reasons directly attributable to alcohol use.

Risk for Pleasure or Risk for Need?

The fourth factor which shapes the way we assess the magnitude of a risk is whether we associate the risk with pleasure or with need. And, naturally, for most users of alcohol, pleasure is the goal, while for the many components of the alcohol industry, need (if not greed) is the basis for turning a blind eye to the health threat of alcohol. Contrasting with the widespread nonreaction to the health threat of alcohol (a drug perceived by drinkers to be pleasurable and important) is the public reaction to the health threat of food additives or preservatives. Many Americans perceive these additives as being unnecessary, and they are widely feared. We tend not to fear what we like or need. We fear excessively what we consider to be unnecessary or unpleasant.

Public and Personal Denial

Denial of drug use and its consequences comprises another factor which powerfully inhibits appropriate concern for the risk in all drug problems, including alcohol. Denial means, as you will recall from Chapter 2, that the drug user almost invariably denies the consequences, and even the extent, of his drug or alcohol use. He does this because he likes the feelings produced by his drug use and drinking, and he does not want to give them up. Out of considerations of love or guilt or even simple laziness, the user's family and friends also frequently deny the extent and consequences of the drinker's use of alcohol and other drugs. After all, it takes work and courage to deal with the conflict which will almost surely be precipitated by an honest confrontation with a drug- or alcohol-abusing but often well-meaning family member or friend.

Another aspect of denial which makes a proper risk assessment difficult is that the consequences of alcohol use (and other drug use)—particularly such physical consequences as cancer, brain damage, and cirrhosis of the liver—take years to emerge and develop fully. Moreover, their occurrence is, for any particular person, unpredictable and uncertain. Almost always the drug or alcohol user rationalizes: "It won't happen to me." Even more frequently, the alcohol user says, "Alcohol really doesn't bother me. But if I ever do have a problem because of my drinking, I'll just quit." And, alas, those around the drinker often appear to share the same type of destructive denial.

"All My Friends Drink—So Why Shouldn't I?"

A final factor influencing the size of the risk people are willing to take with alcohol arises from the socializing lure of "downing a few" with friends and business associates. Most drug users, including drinkers of alcohol, tend to mingle and mix with people who use drugs as they do. This makes it easy for them to blind themselves to the actual quantities they consume. I talked recently with a businessman who told me he drank "about a pint of vodka a day." His wife, who had carefully monitored his consumption for a week, told me that he drank more nearly *one quart* of vodka per day: an almost universal type of underestimation engaged in by users. The man considered his heavy, daily consumption of vodka as "ordinary social drinking" because, he insisted, most of his business associates drank similarly. His father and his brother, he said, drank as much as he did. "After all," the self-deluded rationale goes, "if everybody else is drinking as much as I am and is still perpendicular—as I am—where's the *risk*?"

The seven psychological factors I have described demonstrate the easily understood, even if not rationally arrived at, reasons for the lack of concern about alcohol problems in our society. The human psychological deck of cards is stacked in favor of those who want us to drink alcohol, just as it is, for example, stacked against those who want us to use electricity generated by nuclear power. If, however, we can manage to see clearly beyond the hazy fumes arising from these prevalent types of risky miscalculations, the jolting fact that meets our eyes is that alcohol is a leading cause of preventable illness, death, and social cost to this nation.

THE "SOCIAL DRINKER" VERSUS THE ALCOHOLIC OR—"IS THERE REALLY SUCH AN ANIMAL?"

One out of every 10 adults who drink alcoholic beverages is an alcoholic or an alcohol abuser. This adds up to about 10 million serious problem drinkers in this country. Millions upon millions of dollars are wasted each year because of alcoholism. About 50 percent of the alcoholics in America are unemployed, and those who do have jobs lose between two and three times more work days per year than the nonalcoholic worker does. Alcoholic workers are involved in almost three times the number of accidents that other employees are. They are an almost constant threat to the safety of those around them, and they reduce the efficiency and morale of their co-workers.

"Alcoholism" and "Alcohol" Defined

The National Council on Alcoholism defines this addiction as "a chronic, progressive, and potentially fatal disease. It is characterized by tolerance and physical dependency or pathologic organ changes,

or both—all the direct or indirect consequences of the alcohol ingested." Others have defined alcoholism more loosely by saying that
it includes the behaviors of virtually anyone who has any problem
because of his or her drinking—hence the more general terms "problem drinking" and "alcohol abuse." Most people who give the matter
thought understand "alcohol abuse" and even "problem drinking" to
involve excessive, continuous, or binge drinking, or drinking by a
person who has lost control of his or her drinking behavior.

What, then, is an alcoholic? Contrary to the popularly held image,
alcoholics are not necessarily skid row bums. In fact, only about five
percent of all alcoholics fall into this stereotype. In outward appearance, at least, many alcoholics look like anyone else who lives among
us. For quite a long time, usually, he or she is able to live and work,
but not as effectively as if alcoholism had not fastened its grip. You
find alcoholics among your co-workers, your friends, the housewives
and househusbands in your neighborhood, and possibly even in your
own family. In this country, there are about three male alcoholics to
every female alcoholic.

The "Social Drinker" and the
"Alcoholic": Some Distinctions

The term "social drinker" is even more elusive. Actually, it is not
definable scientifically: the separation of the social drinker from the
alcoholic is an arbitrary one, born primarily of compromise and conve-
nience. Comfortable and convenient though the social-drinker/alco-
holic classification may be, its flaws are glaring. Whether one looks at
the amount of alcohol consumed or at the problems produced by
drinking, the scientific data show no clear-cut boundary line between
the social drinker, or "safe" drinker, and the alcoholic. The consumption and problem curves, as the scientists say, are not "bimodal"—
they describe one population of drinkers, not two distinct groups—
one healthy and one sick. There are, to be sure, people who have
numerous problems and who drink enormous quantities of alcohol,
and there are many people who drink moderately and have no
problems whatsoever with their drinking. But the boundaries between
the extremes are filled with people "in the middle."

The implications of this reality are only beginning to dawn. For
example, it is now widely agreed within the scientific community that
the only way to reduce the number of "heavy" or "problem" drinkers
is to reduce overall, per capita alcohol consumption. This can be seen
in studies comparing the drinking of alcohol in one country with the
drinking of alcohol in another: the levels of alcohol consumption are

directly proportional to the levels of alcohol problems. In a given population, there is no way to reduce problems caused by alcohol without reducing overall alcohol consumption.

Looking at alcohol and health, we must come to a similar conclusion. Those who talk of the benign or even the desirable health effects of alcohol focus *only* on those who drink minimally. When we consider the effects of alcohol drinking, we should, as a practical matter, consider *all* the effects of *all* the drinkers because they are all parts of one whole. When that is done—and it seldom is done by the industry supporters who insist on separating the people with problems from those without problems—the true nature of the effects of alcohol on our lives becomes apparent. It is not a pretty picture.

An additional complication for the separation of the social drinker from the alcoholic is that social drinking is the soil from which alcoholism grows: without social drinking there is no alcoholism. Put another way, only by drinking alcohol can you become an alcoholic. Another consequent flaw is that the social drinker, without realizing what is happening, can very quickly or quite gradually over a long period of time become an alcoholic. Basically, the difference between the social drinker and the alcoholic is that the social drinker stands a couple of short, uncertain steps away from dependence and has been a little bit luckier—so far. Realistically, whatever difference does exist is a matter of degree and of time.

Alcohol and the Drug Dependence Syndrome

Even a brief second look at the Drug Dependence Syndrome will readily remind us why this is so. Alcohol is a drug—a fact with which few any longer disagree. Being a drug, its use often causes the user to move through the same stages of the dependence process which is characteristic of all drugs. The Drug Dependence Syndrome—the deteriorative patterns of drug use—follows the four-stage sequence outlined in Chapter 2:

Stage One:
First or
Experimental Use

      Stage Two:
      Occasional Use

            Stage Three:
            Regular Use

                  Stage Four:
                  Dependence—in this
                  instance, "alcoholism"

The person, therefore, who refers to his or her regular or heavy use of alcohol as "only social drinking" stands perilously close to dependence—to becoming an alcoholic.

The Phases of Alcoholism. "But," you may ask, "how can I personally know when a social drinker is becoming an alcoholic? How can I tell?" The short answer: you can't. But you can *observe*, continuing to keep in mind that the prospective alcoholic is moving through a process: a sequence of deteriorative phases. In the beginning phase, certain visible clues may emerge: frequent drinking, possibly to cope with stress or a particular worry; promises (almost always broken) to "quit" or "cut down"; increased tolerance to the drug; and minor personality changes, especially irritability.

In the middle phase, the drinker often tries to conceal his drinking behavior. Typically, too, he starts drinking earlier in the day. By now, signs of his approaching alcoholism are growing more and more apparent, especially at home and on weekends when the pressures to perform are less. Regardless of how much booze he imbibes, he finds it harder and harder to get the euphoric "kick" or "high" he wants. So he drinks more—and daily; he needs it.

In the final phase of alcoholism, the alcoholic lives only to drink. Neglecting his health, he undergoes physical changes and severe personality deterioration. He feels—by turns—sad, isolated, lonely, guilty, and depressed. Irritable and tense, he sees his bottle as his only true friend. Eventually his health, aggravated by physical debility brought on by a combination of excessive alcohol and by malnutrition, hits the pits. Usually, near the end: *delirium tremens* (the DTs—the alcohol withdrawal syndrome), pancreatitis, problems with the esophagus and stomach, liver failure, brain damage, and . . . finally . . . death.

Is Alcoholism Inheritable—a Genetic Susceptibility? A person who has an alcoholic parent or sibling is four or five times more likely to be an alcoholic than is a person without such an alcoholic relative. Roughly one-half of hospitalized alcoholics have such familial alcoholism. Compared to nonfamilial alcoholism, these people have an earlier onset of alcoholism and more severe symptoms. Further, studies have shown that identical twins are more similar in their drinking habits than are fraternal twins. Children born to nonalcoholic parents, but raised by alcoholic adoptive parents, did not have an increased rate of alcoholism. By contrast, children born to alcoholic parents but raised by nonalcoholic adoptive parents were four or five times more likely to be alcoholic than the biological children of the nonalcoholics.

Whether this increased rate of alcoholism is genetic or reflects some intrauterine experience (such as heavy maternal drinking) remains unclear, but most experts now believe that the vulnerability to alcoholism is genetic. This has important implications for children of alcoholics and for alcoholic parents. Such children are at an elevated risk, and this is something which must be taken into careful consideration, discussed openly by both parents and children, and watched closely for possible negative developments as these at-risk youngsters go through their teenage and young-adult years. A new self-help group, spun off from Alcoholics Anonymous, attempts to work with and meet the needs of these youths. It is called COA, or Children of Alcoholics.

Having said this—and it *is* important—it is essential that I point out that many alcoholics do not have alcoholic parents or siblings. Additionally, what is inherited is not "alcoholism" but a *susceptibility* to it. Many children grow up without becoming alcoholic even when born to alcoholic parents, and many children born to nonalcoholics do become alcoholics. Thus, if one has alcoholism in his or her family, special and continuing concern is essential. If one does not have alcoholic relatives, concern is still warranted because no one can safely consider himself or herself genetically immune.

BUT . . . on the Other Hand . . . You Don't Have to Be an Alcoholic to Have Serious Drinking Problems. What alcoholism is and who "catches" it—important as those concerns are—are only a part of the alcoholism problem that plagues the nation as a whole. A great many of the most serious alcohol-related problems occur among people who do not drink in the alcoholic fashion I have been describing. A recent example was the tragic death of screen star Natalie Wood. From press accounts, it appeared that she had had several drinks while on a sailboat with her husband and a business associate. When the two men quarreled, she apparently decided to leave the main boat and step down into a smaller craft for a solitary spin around the harbor, as she reportedly often did. In the act of stepping down, however, she apparently slipped, hit her head, fell into the water, and drowned. The presumption was that, in the first place, without the alcohol in her brain she might not have fallen and, in the second place, even if she had fallen, she might have been able to save herself. Again from press accounts, it appeared that Natalie Wood was neither an alcoholic nor a problem drinker except in this one tragic and fatal instance. In those fateful moments immediately before her death, she did indeed have a problem with her drinking.

Obviously, social drinkers can find themselves in real trouble, even if they are not alcoholic and may never become one. A host of studies and surveys have shown that large numbers of social drinkers do, in fact, have serious health problems because of alcohol use. These difficulties include excessively high rates of heart disorders, high blood pressure, and injuries resulting from motor vehicle accidents and accidents occurring when drinkers try to operate industrial machinery and power tools while under the influence of alcohol. The point is that people do not have to be alcoholics to have serious problems from drinking. This conclusion was strongly emphasized recently in a report from the National Academy of Sciences. The panel's chairman, Mark H. Moore of Harvard University, put it this way: "There is a piece of the alcohol problem that lies *outside* the area of heavy drinking." He stressed the significant fact that many alcohol problems—drunk driving, domestic violence, teenage auto accidents, and stress-related drinking that leads to job loss—all result from "ill-timed periods of alcohol use," not from chronic heavy drinking.

The current crusade against drunk drivers on highways will, one day, lead to the recognition of another significant conclusion included in the Academy's report: There is no safe level for alcohol in the brains of automobile drivers, and many of the dangerous drunk drivers are "social drinkers," not "alcoholics." When that realization sinks in, the true national education about the dangers and destructive effects of alcohol will have begun. We will then conclude that our goal is not only to get drunk drivers off our highways but to get *anyone* with any alcohol in his or her brain out from behind the steering wheel of an automobile. In sum, a drinker of alcohol does not have to be "dependent" on alcohol to have serious problems arising both directly and indirectly from alcohol use.

FACTORS PROMOTING MODERATION IN ALCOHOL CONSUMPTION

There has been much speculation as to why alcohol, of all commonly used drugs, is the most likely to be used regularly without causing complete dependence. Why, people ask, are there so many "social drinkers" in comparison to the number of "alcoholics?" Part of the answer is to be found in the fact that as many as 30 percent of "normal social drinkers" will—at some time during their drinking careers—experience significant bouts of alcoholism or serious alcohol-caused problems. Another part of the answer lies in the fact that a large number of social drinkers refrain from regressing to dependence because of what might usefully be thought of as "enforced" moderation.

Alcohol drinking is the most socialized of all drug-using behavior in the world, and many informal, complex, and often effective *social controls* help to keep alcohol drinking moderate. In most social circles, for example, drinking by adults is accepted, but drunkenness is strongly discouraged. Alcohol users in those circumstances do not want to become drunk, and when they begin to feel "tipsy," they stop drinking. These and similar social controls motivate moderation for many drinkers and help keep down the number of alcoholics. Moreover, few people want—if they can possibly avoid it—to be socially stigmatized by the opprobrium accorded a "drunk," a "sot," or a "lush."

In addition to the moderation enforced by social restriction, there are two *biological factors* which, for many alcohol users, promote moderation. A first biological plus for moderation is the *route of administration*. As I have pointed out, because alcohol is taken only by mouth, this oral route of administration ensures the slowest rate of buildup of the drug in the bloodstream and, of course, in the brain, the latter being the target organ for the intoxicating effect sought by the user. This means that the concentration of the drug in the brain rises and falls more slowly for alcohol than for drugs taken in other ways. Any brain-targeted drug delivery which is slower tends to be less reinforcing and, therefore, less addicting. To some extent, this helps to keep down the number of alcoholics in the drinking population.

A second biological plus for moderation in alcohol has to do with *caloric content*, the fact that alcohol contains calories. Although, as we have seen, these calories have no real nutritional value, a great many people nevertheless closely associate drinking with eating. Eating food both before and along with drinking helps some drinkers keep their alcohol consumption at moderate levels. This, clearly, is another plus. Increasingly, drinkers of alcoholic beverages are actively concerned with the actual caloric content of what they drink. Thus, they moderate their drinking in order to limit their caloric intake. This is one of the primary attractions of "light" or so-called "lite" beer.

Paradoxically, neither social controls nor biological factors work well to limit cigarette smoking, even though smoking—like drinking—is legal and has been common for many generations. Unlike alcohol, however, tobacco is not intoxicating, so it has no internal "off" switch equivalent to the onset of drunkenness with which to warn the tobacco user to stop before he or she smokes enough to become addicted or dependent. In contrast to alcohol, both tobacco and marijuana smoking promptly deliver a drug—nicotine and THC, respectively—to the brain of the smoker. In the smoker's case, the route of administration of the drug is via the lungs, and when tobacco or pot is smoked, it produces a sharp burst of nicotine or of THC which hits the brain just a few seconds after each puff is taken. This fast drug delivery makes tobacco and marijuana smoking more reinforcing and therefore more addicting than alcohol is. This is, then, another plus for the biological factors which tend to moderate the consumption of alcohol.

ALCOHOL AND TEENAGERS: ESTABLISHING THE GROUND RULES

As we have seen, for both teenagers and adults the health hazards from even moderate drinking of alcohol are enormous: enormous to the drinkers and to those around them. Even if a single drop of the fermented grape or distilled corn never slides down your throat, you can be killed by alcohol in the brain of a careening car driver. All of these health hazards are particularly severe for younger drinkers because they are more likely to drink excessively. One recent study, for example, found that 41 percent of all high school seniors down *five or more drinks* in rapid succession—that is, drink to drunkenness—at least once every two weeks. That, appropriately, is called binge drinking. It will help you as a reader, I believe, to better understand the personalized approach to the prevention of alcohol use by teenagers if we take a moment at this point to review together the role and significance of alcohol in the GATEWAY concept in particular and—in general—its illegality and its destructive impact upon teenagers.

The casual acceptance of the normality of teenage drinking was emphasized for me recently when I was the host of a talk show on the local NBC radio station in Washington, D.C. My guest was a nationally recognized sports-medicine physician who had just been featured in an extensive interview published in *U.S. News and World Report.* We were talking, on the air, about tension among athletes. He said that high school sports are highly competitive, so he tells student athletes to "let the tension off" by "going out and getting drunk from time to time." In so saying, this physician was obviously and shamelessly ignoring the health, safety, and legal implications of the advice he was so casually giving. I can understand (though not easily) how this doctor could say such a thing, because teenage drinking is so "normal," so "ordinary," that scarcely anyone gives it a second thought. What I cannot understand—nor condone—is his apparent willingness to encourage thousands upon thousands of young students and promising young athletes to engage in such chancey and potentially self-destructive behavior.

A Personalized Approach to the Prevention of Alcohol Use by Teenagers

Get Tough on Teenage Drinking.   We start at the point where drinking begins—typically, in the United States, between the ages of 12 and 16. Of course, all drug use, especially alcohol use, is legally prohibited for ages under at least 18. Parents, teachers, law-enforcement officials, and youth peer groups themselves need to get tough on underage, youthful drinking. No drinking under legal age is acceptable. It is all illegal and it is unhealthy. For many American teenagers today, this comes as a rude and unwelcome shock. They consider alcohol a normal rite of passage into early and middle adolescence. Nevertheless, we need an all-out, family-based effort to stop teenage alcohol use. The most important means to achieve this goal is the *re-education* of parents and teachers who, along with our youth, have come to accept teenage drinking as both inevitable and normal.

Demolish the Myth That Alcohol Use Is a "Right."   The casual assumption of the normality of drinking by teenagers is seductive. Here I need only point out that—by any definition whatsoever—teenage alcohol use is definitely *not* a civil right; it is a criminal law violation. That such a baseless and fractious "civil-rights" argument can maintain even the appearance of legitimacy is a manifestation of the confusion of our values on this issue which has occurred and—to a great extent—handicapped our society during the last two decades.

Help Teenagers Through Their Eight Most Critical Years.   In these pages I have emphasized that virtually all nonmedical drug use begins between the ages of 12 and 20. If we can help a growing adolescent get through these eight critical years without drinking alcohol, not only will we be able to drastically reduce the likelihood that this young person will use other drugs, but we will also reduce the possibility that he or she will ever drink alcohol. And, should this person choose to drink as an adult, we will reduce the likelihood that such drinking will be excessive. Once a socially active young person has reached the age of 20 or thereabouts and has been telling friends, especially at parties, that he or she does not drink alcohol and has learned to have fun and to relax without alcohol-induced intoxication, the temptation to drink alcohol falls sharply. This is especially true when the young person has reasons not to drink: reasons of personal values, health, or religion. The widespread acceptance of alcohol use in America today, however, makes this awareness and the personal convictions needed to avoid drinking alcohol difficult—more difficult than for them to avoid other drugs, including marijuana and tobacco.

Recently, in talking about making decisions about drug use, I spent some time discussing each of the several commonly used drugs. One woman in the audience spoke up, identifying herself as a Mormon. She said, "I find this so confusing, trying to sort out the conflicting claims about so many different drugs. For me, the issue is simple. I made one decision at one time in my life about all these drugs: not to use any of them—ever. That way, I don't have to worry about each new headline or each new expert I might run into." She made a good point. The most crucial drug in making that "one decision" is alcohol, and the critical time to make it is adolescence.

Don't Even IMPLY That Alcohol Use by Kids Is Okay!   A short time ago I reviewed a pamphlet for teenagers about alcohol. Published by a prestigious organization, it was entitled "A Message to Teenagers: How to Tell When Your Drinking Is Becoming a Problem." Inside, with attractive graphics, were 12 questions, three of which asked:

   "Do you drink because you have a problem?"
   "Do you ever have loss of memory due to your drinking?"
   "Do you think it is cool to be able to hold your liquor?"

The teen reader is advised that alcoholism is a disease which can hit the young and that "If you can answer yes to any of the 12 questions, maybe it's time you took a serious look at what your drinking might be doing to you."

I find appalling the approach suggested by this pamphlet. As they have stated it, the formulators of that approach imply that teenagers customarily are inbibing considerable, if not quite yet staggering, amounts of alcohol. None of the questions is so worded as to warn off the nonusing teenager. None asks: "Is *any* use of alcohol by young people okay?" Nowhere in this pamphlet is there any hint that so-called social drinking ("safe" or "responsible" drinking) may in any way lead to alcoholism. Nowhere is the law about the drinking age even alluded to. I have to ask: Isn't this whole approach, in fact, like waiting for the Drug Dependence Syndrome to develop before sounding the first warning bell?

I understand that a publication of a prestigious organization like this one does not want to scare off kids it might be able to help, and maybe that is why the pamphlet ends with this invitation: "And, if you do need help or if you'd just like to talk to someone about your drinking, call us. We're in the phone book." My concern, however, is that many teenage drinkers and those on the verge of becoming teenage drinkers will read this pamphlet and conclude that underage, illegal drinking—being so widespread—is apparently okay even though, if any of them have one or more of those 12 "problems," maybe it's time they took "a serious look" at their drinking. When it comes to teens and drinking, that approach strikes me as being much too little . . . *and* far too late.

A PERSONALIZED ALCOHOL-USE POLICY FOR ADULTS: HOW MUCH IS TOO MUCH?

THIS Much Is Too Much: The "Four-by-Four" Solution

In developing a personal policy for the use of alcohol *by adults*, we need to deal directly with sensible and workable limitations on the kind of drinking they actually do. For adult members of the family, we need to set unmistakably clear guidelines about "If," "When," and "How Much" to drink. Although there are no completely satisfactory "rules" in the strict sense of that term, I have found that many families have responded favorably and have attested to the help given them by these basic guidelines:

Four Definite "Don'ts"

1. *Don't drink if you're underage.* It's dangerous, illegal, and should be avoided.
2. *Don't drink if you have a history of excessive or "problem" drinking or any kind of drug dependence.* It's dangerous. Avoid it.
3. *Don't drink if you are a pregnant or nursing mother.* It is dangerous to the unborn or nursing child and should be avoided.
4. *Don't drink if you are using any other drugs which reduce alertness:*

painkillers, sleeping pills, antihistamines, prescription tranquilizers, or any illegal "substances." Drinking in combination with these or any other drugs is dangerous and should be avoided.

Four Protective Boundaries—If You Choose to Drink

1. *Drinking more than two or three drinks during any 24-hour period is potentially dangerous and should be avoided.* One "drink" equals 12 ounces of beer or five ounces of wine or 1½ ounces of distilled spirits.
2. *Daily drinking is dangerous and should be avoided.* Do not drink on more than four days per week. Drinking more frequently than that is potentially habit forming, dangerous, and should be avoided.
3. *Any drinking within six hours prior to driving a motor vehicle or going to work is dangerous and should be avoided.* This "boundary" applies likewise to operating any other complex piece of machinery and to other activities requiring mental alertness.
4. *If you choose to drink, find yourself an "alcohol monitor."* Identify a person who knows you well and who either does not drink at all or drinks less than you do. Ask this person to monitor the amounts of alcohol you drink and your drinking-related behavior, and if he or she sees that you have a problem, pledge that you will stop drinking.

This Four-by-Four Solution is not likely to be supported by many sophisticated alcohol experts or by the alcohol industry. They urge far more "flexible" guidelines. I urge the Four-by-Four Solution for its simplicity, directness, and proved practical worth. It is simple for the potential drinker, for his or her family, and for others in the drinker's life. Without such simple directness, the Drug Dependence Syndrome makes personal and social control of alcohol drinking difficult or—in far too many cases—impossible. And, above all, I know that it *works*. As a clinician and a physician, I have watched these recommended "Don'ts" and "Boundaries" evolve over a substantial period of time. Most of the reasonable people I have encountered and worked with in recent years have concluded, as I have, that the drinking of alcohol should be limited to people over the legal drinking age who are not pregnant or nursing and who do not have a history of drug or alcohol problems. And, again like me, they have also concluded, almost unanimously, that drinking should not occur on more than four days in any one week, that alcohol intake should never exceed two or three drinks in any 24-hour period, and that alcohol should never be mixed with other drugs, with driving, or with work. As a result of this extensive effort and collaboration, I know—beyond any reasonable doubt—that the guidelines I have laid out here are *functional* and, if widely adopted and conscientiously followed, will deal straightforwardly and effectively with many of the major problems among drinkers: alcoholism, Fetal Alcoholism Syndrome (FAS), teenage drinking, spree drinking, drunken driving, and the multiplicative effects of mixed drugs. If these constraints were to be widely supported, the individual drinker would be less likely to have serious physical, legal, or social problems with his or her drinking.

I am far less concerned about the criticisms of so-called sophisticates or the adverse reactions of the alcohol industry to these guidelines than I am about two other groups whose opinions are of more immediate concern to me in writing this book. People who do not drink at all, roughly 40 percent of American adults, are likely to find them a bit startling and probably disappointing because they permit, or even encourage, a level of drinking which seems, at first glance, to be staggeringly high. The second group about whose reactions I am considerably concerned are the 11 percent of American adults who are heavy drinkers. This group will, I little doubt, find my recommended limitations positively antediluvian, the stuff that marching militant females with parasols protested about at the turn of the century. To both groups I say this: What I am trying to establish here is an acceptable middle-ground position that can reasonably and safely apply to everyone. The fact that light drinkers and nondrinkers may find my recommended levels too high simply reflects the moderation, the desirable moderation, they practice. Similarly, the fact that heavy drinkers may initially find the guidelines repressive or too restrictive reflects the reality of the unhealthy and excessive extent of the drinking they consider "normal." In particular sum, note that what I intend is *a family-based alcohol policy.* It is a policy which can, if implemented broadly and with good judgment, reduce both alcohol consumption and alcohol problems. Its goals can, I believe, be achieved without creating a "new Prohibition," without unduly or unfairly impinging upon the right of adults to drink alcohol moderately, and without stigmatizing drinkers.

Develop a Strong Program to Educate the Public About the Dangers of Alcohol

Why haven't the alcohol industries or, for that matter, agencies of the government adopted a similar set of simple warnings or restrictions for drinking alcohol? Why are such limits not taught to our children, advertised in the media, and printed on alcohol-containing products?

One of the major reasons, certainly, is economics. Most of the alcohol consumed in this country is consumed in violation of these guidelines. If such guidelines were widely communicated and widely adopted, the total national consumption of alcohol would fall by more than 50 percent. That, admittedly, would hurt some people and some businesses financially, but it would also save both drinkers and non-drinkers—to say nothing of the tax-paying public—enormous sums of money by reducing the social costs of drinking and alcohol-related deaths. Most directly, however, it would give to all a clear signal that heavy drinking is dangerous. An awareness of such simple restraints and boundary lines would, moreover, help drinkers and nondrinkers alike to know when drinking has become excessive so that they can take appropriate actions or preventive measures early in the drug-taking process—preferably well *before* dependency sets in. Unfortunately, there are many people and numerous groups who for a variety of reasons—many of them having to do with economics—do not want to know that. And they do not want others to know it.

What societal losses, other than reduced profits for distillers and breweries and related industries, would be suffered if these guidelines were adopted? Or, to put the question in a more specific frame, what benefit does the drinker derive from drinking dangerously? Or, for that matter, from drinking alcohol at all? The answer is that, once hooked, most drinkers like their habit and will not readily give it up.

There is excellent evidence, however, based on the nation's experience with cigarette smoking over the last two decades, that tough-minded public education about drug dangers does change behavior—not for everyone, of course, but for a significantly large number of people. For instance, as a result of a campaign to educate the public about the dangers of tobacco, we now have more than 35 million *former* smokers. Happily, we also have several million young people who otherwise would have become cigarette smokers but decided not to because of increased public education developed about the subject since the U.S. Surgeon General's first report on *Smoking and Health* in 1964. That type of educational program worked, and is now working, with admirable effectiveness. We need to apply these same effective principles to reduce alcohol use in this country. We can do it—and we must.

The effort to reduce alcohol use through an educational program will not, as I am fully aware, be all smooth sailing. In addition to the economic obstructions, there is the roadblock placed by the drinkers themselves—for the most part, unintentionally. As our understanding of the Drug Dependence Syndrome has shown us, despite such semantic antics with weasel words like "social," "moderate," or "safe," the so-called safe use of alcohol is *not* safe for many drinkers. A large segment of the alcohol-using population, perhaps as many as 30 percent of all drinkers who begin "social drinking," cannot, in fact, restrict their intake within the limits set by these guidelines. These vulnerable imbibers *cannot be identified in advance* by any biological or psychological traits. Many of these drinkers, most of whom are otherwise physically and psychologically healthy, can expect to lose control and go over the line into serious alcohol problems of all kinds, including—but not limited to—outright alcoholism. However, if understood and supported by a public educated as to the jeopardizing nature of this drug, the guidelines I have laid out will help people with alcohol problems to identify those problems earlier and to seek the assistance needed to surmount them—an assistance to be described later in Chapter 7.

Print the Truth on the Liquor Bottle and the Beer Can

The third component of the strong, personalized, alcohol use policy I am advocating can best be described as "truth in packaging" and is aimed principally at the brewers of beer, the vintners, and the distillers of alcoholic beverages. Appropriately consumer oriented, this component can also serve a valuable function in programs designed to educate the public as to the problems and potential dangers of alcohol use and misuse. It should be a continuing concern that adults of legal drinking age know what is in the drink they are drinking, and this can—in no small part—be ensured by (1) printing the actual *alcoholic content* on each bottle or can, (2) listing all the *actual ingredients* on the bottle or can, and (3) printing *warnings and danger signs* on each alcohol container.

The greatest failure of health organizations and the alcohol industries, in my view, is their failure to give the consumer of alcohol some pertinent and much-needed information. They could start with this basic fact, one that is generally overlooked or ignored by the alcohol industry: all alcoholic beverages necessarily contain the same toxic agent—alcohol. Thus, all forms of drinking can be equated in terms of the amount of alcohol each drink contains. In more or less standard terms, one beer contains the same amount of alcohol as five ounces of wine, or the same amount of alcohol as contained in a cocktail having one and one-half ounces of distilled spirits, such as vodka or whiskey. Although distilled liquor and wine have the alcohol content printed on the label of the container, beer usually does not. Furthermore, no alcoholic beverage of any kind has its actual ingredients, including potentially unhealthy additives, listed on the label, even though almost all other calorie-laden foods do. This is particularly important for people who may be allergic to one of more of the ingredients in a particular beverage. Without ingredient labeling, there is no way for the allergic person to know what he or she is drinking.

No container of any alcoholic beverage carries printed warnings about the negative health effects of drinking, nor does it identify or describe the warning signs and possible dangers of excessive drinking of this drug. The alcohol consumer, therefore, cannot know what substances have been added, substances to which he or she may be allergic. Furthermore, there is no information on the label which informs consumers about the likely consequences of their use of the drug. Why is this necessary data not shown on the whiskey bottle or the beer can? Why is alcohol treated neither like a "drug" nor a "food"? Fundamentally and plainly, the answer is that the alcohol industry does not want to "scare" consumers for fear they might drink less. Far sadder and more unfortunate in a democratic society is the fact that the liquor lobby has for many years succeeded in preventing the government's regulators from carrying out their responsibility for protecting the public's health by applying normal safety rules to alcohol use. Recently, when the administration was seeking ways to raise federal tax revenue, a variety of "nuisance" and "sin" taxes were considered. Taxes on alcohol, not increased at the federal level for 20 years, were quietly dropped from the tax-raising proposals after the liquor industry did its job on the Congress and the Executive branch of the government.

GETTING FROM ABSTINENT TEENHOOD TO DRINKING ADULTHOOD—CAN IT BE DONE?

Since this book is being written primarily for parents and their teenagers, the possible move from no drinking to self-controlled consumption of alcohol by adults is of more than passing concern. Repeatedly, as you have seen, I have strongly advised against underage drinking. I have also outlined the Four-by-Four Solution to excessive adult drinking. Recognizing the reality that most Americans will continue to drink, how is the teenager to get from an abstinent teenhood to a drinking adulthood? Some have urged parents to teach and support "responsible drinking" at an early age, say 15 or 16. Aside from the obvious illegality of underage drinking, training a youngster to "handle" alcohol at that age is, in my professional opinion, both unwise and inadvisable.

A patient of mine recently told me of a neighboring family who had instructed their 15-year-old son to limit his drinking to "no more than three beers at parties." Fairly soon thereafter, I saw this family because their own 15-year-old son was having real problems, not only with alcohol but also with PCP and cocaine. In our talks together, the young man told me that his friend, a lawyer's son, also drank heavily and used lots of other drugs, too. These two adolescents obviously were already deep into the drug scene. Without laboring my disapproval of the ill-advised approach taken by such permissive families, I ask myself, "How can families teach responsible drinking when and if it becomes desirable to do so?" My answer, evolved over much time and trial-and-error effort is: *Wait until the child attains the legal drinking age.* When that age is reached, then—at that time—help him or her learn how to use alcohol within clearly understood boundaries, if he or she decides to drink. At that time also reinforce for your child the potential dangers of drinking, how to spot them, and what to do about them if they should occur. If this education goes on in the open and when the child is mature, it is not unlikely to be a fairly successful, positive experience for both the parents and the children.

There can be no question that this "when and how to drink" policy raises some troublesome family issues. This, for instance, is one which is often confusing: What is the family to do about giving children, including teenagers, small quantities of wine or champagne at times of celebration, such as a wedding or a New Year's Eve party? This kind of family-centered, modest use of alcohol is no more likely to be a problem for the child or teenager than is the use of wine for a church communion service. It is, in my view, reasonable to share with teenagers, and even younger children, small portions of wine on special occasions. It is not reasonable, or wise, in my view, for children to consume large quantities of alcohol on such occasions or for wine drinking to be a routine part of a child's life. These distinctions can be difficult for families where wine drinking is an everyday occurrence. They are not likely to be a problem in families where alcohol is used—in modest portions—primarily for special occasions.

This point, I think, is well illustrated by an experience which involved a family with whom I had been working. The father, who had taken a tough but not harsh antidrug stand, told me that the best friend of his 15-year-old daughter came to him and told him in confidence that the daughter believed her father would "kill" her if she ever even tried beer or marijuana. The father, surprised—appalled, really—by this information, sat down for a talk with his daughter. He said to her, "Listen, I would not kill you if you tried marijuana or beer. *Nothing* you could do would lead me to hurt you, let alone kill you. I do not want you to use alcohol and drugs because I love you. If I found that you had used drugs or alcohol, I would simply do whatever was necessary to get you to stop. I'm not sure what that would be, but I assume it would be both nonviolent and effective." This reassured the girl.

Three years later, this same father told me his daughter had traveled with the family to a neighboring state where the legal drinking age was 18. She asked to have a glass of wine with the family at dinner. The father, who did not drink and who had emphasized that family decisions to drink alcohol were limited at least by the legal drinking age, agreed. The daughter, joining her moderate-drinking mother, had the glass of wine. Everyone enjoyed the meal. This girl was learning to drink alcohol responsibly, within the framework of family values and the laws of the community. This I consider a successful outcome for both the father and the daughter.

In any event, unless parents use alcohol excessively and permit their children to use it excessively, the alcohol problem for teenagers in America today is *not* the alcohol they drink in face-to-face settings with their families. The alcohol problem for teenagers is drinking alcohol *outside* adult supervision in peer and party settings. Because it is not reasonable, my experience tells me, to expect teenagers to learn how to become moderate or responsible drinkers in unsupervised peer-group settings, I definitely do not encourage it.

Overriding this central concern is the additional fact that many of the young people attending such "drinking" parties are likely to be under the legal age and will, nevertheless, tend to ignore the restriction that such drinking is illegal in all parts of the United States. This adds one more reason why I invariably discourage this type of approach to learning how and when to drink. However families elect to work out their own unique response to issues of this kind—and I do recognize the variety of possible solutions—I strongly urge that the problem of drinking in general, and of teenage drinking in particular, be discussed fully and frankly by all adolescent and adult members of the family and that the resulting decisions should be firmly rooted in family values and clearly defined, ongoing guidelines for the teenagers.

DRINKING MORE AND FEELING IT LESS?
MAYBE WE'RE JUST GETTING "LITE-HEADED"!

Those who call every attempt to reduce alcohol consumption "neo-Prohibitionism" and see Americans' use of alcohol as inevitably rising can learn a lesson from the folks who make Alka-Seltzer. After years of marketing their product to treat hangovers, in 1984 they turned their advertising campaign around because, as *The Wall Street Journal* reported, "Americans are drinking less, and they are becoming increasingly antagonistic toward those who drink to excess." The new theme for Alka-Seltzer: get that plop plop, fizz fizz to relieve "the symptoms of stress that come with success." The agency handling the Alka-Seltzer advertising account noted that in 1983 the male population between ages 18 and 24 shrank for the first time in many years. This is the group which drinks the most beer; so, not surprisingly, after a decade of spectacular growth, beer sales trailed off in 1983. Liquor sales have been flat or falling for a decade, and American wine consumption, which had risen sharply in the 1970s, showed only tiny gains in 1983. These trends, tied to the fitness and self-improvement movements, produced a fall in per-capita alcohol consumption which the alcohol industry itself related to the country's greater concern for health. In addition to this concern for health and also society's decreasing tolerance for excessive drinking, other important factors contributed to the decline in alcohol consumption, probably the most noteworthy being the raised legal drinking age and the explosive growth of community groups campaigning against drunk driving.

The alcohol industry is beginning to take a page from the experience book of the tobacco industry, which for two decades has faced similar health-related pressures aimed principally at a reduction in the smoking of cigarettes. Just as the tobacco companies have recognized that the nicotine and tar in cigarettes comprise their greatest threat to America's health, the alcohol industry is now aware that the greatest menace it contributes to the nation's health is alcohol itself. The makers of beer and other alcoholic beverages, taking a significant step to change this dangerous and negative image, are moving toward "lighter" products, those with less alcohol.

Brewers and distillers, always with a quick eye for big bucks, have not failed to notice that tobacco companies benefitted financially from the shift to low-tar and low-nicotine cigarettes. Apparently, they also see in the experience of the tobacco industry a shrewd and potent marketing strategy: Even though the number of Americans who had

successfully quit smoking increased dramatically, the declining percentage of the population who continued to smoke cigarettes actually
smoked so many *more* of the new, weaker cigarettes that the total
per-capita cigarette consumption—and the overall income of the tobacco industry—actually rose in recent years.

This profit picture was also helped by rising prices for tobacco, and
rising taxes also increased the government's revenue from smokers. It
is not hard to foresee a similar pattern and market strategy developing in the alcohol industry: lighter beverages, more nondrinkers, but
more drinkers who—continuing to drink—are drinking *more gallons*
of beverages, each containing less alcohol, each generating increased
sales and income—all this with rising profits in the industry and rising
tax revenues from alcohol sales.

Meanwhile, Americans are already beginning to get the message.
Alcohol-free wines and beers are being mass-marketed for the first
time in many years. Brewers of "light" beers incessantly flood the ad
slots flickering across our television screens, acting out the nutritional
glories of their bibulous product with seemingly endless casts of occu-
pationally heroic "good guys" drinking it more and feeling it less.
Ah . . . great is the Gusto! Especially when brewed as "Just the Rite
Lite."

SUMMING UP

Before leaving this chapter, look again at these salient facts:

- Alcohol is a drug which produces predictable and regular stages in
  its use.
- Alcohol is a common GATEWAY into all nonmedical or recreational drug-taking.
- Alcohol is a leading cause of potentially preventable illness and
  death in our society.
- With alcohol, as with any other drug, *nonuse* is preferable to use.
- If alcohol is to be used, it should be used only by adults, and use
  should be moderate with explicit social and legal controls.
- Once alcohol use has reached the dependence stage, to stop drinking almost always requires the active supervision of someone who is
  not a user and who is sensitive to the signs of danger.
- The denial of drug use is such a universal characteristic of the
  drinker's own psychology that he or she will not detect or admit
  problems until the end stages of the dependence process.

- The Four-by-Four Alcohol Guidelines:

  Don't drink if you are underage, if you are a pregnant or nursing mother, if you are using any medicine which decreases your alertness, or if you have a history of problems with alcohol or any other drug.

  If you must drink alcohol, drink no more than two or three drinks in any 24-hour period, drink on no more than four days a week, don't drink within six hours of driving a car or going to work, and do use a personal alcohol monitor.

CHAPTER FIVE

Cocaine:
Deadly Nose Candy

COCAINE IS FOR THE 1980s what marijuana was for the 1970s: a mass-appeal, chic drug with an undeserved reputation as "safe," or almost safe. Cocaine also shares with alcohol, especially with champagne, the image as the party drug of the rich, a way to reward yourself extravagantly. Like marijuana in the early 1970s, cocaine has become a naughty, exciting drug which new users share with innocent excitement, having discovered that "It's fun, and there's really no problem with it. Try some, you'll like it."

Consider the contrast between marijuana in the early 1970s and cocaine in the early 1980s. Pot was the drug of the dropout kid. Coke—short for cocaine—is the drug of the hot-shot executive. Or so it appears. Why the one image 10 years ago and the other today? The Baby Boom Generation—those born between 1946 and about 1965—are the drug epidemic generation. The modal member of the group was born in 1955. In 1974, he was 19 and just right for the pot-smoking image of the 70s. In 1984, he was 29 and just as right for the contemporary cocaine image. As we will see, the coke of that "image" is no more appropriate than the pot of the earlier time. But the image itself, real and powerful, persists and is reinforced many times over in the media.

A LOOK BACK AT COCAINE:
ITS ORIGINS—AND SOME HISTORY

South American Primitive

Cocaine in its natural state is found in the leaves of the South American bush, *Erythroxylum coca*. Although the Indians in the Andes Mountains on the west coast of South America did not have a written history, archeological evidence shows that the coca plant was used for its psychoactive properties prior to the arrival of Europeans in the New World. Several important principles underlying the way traditional cultures handled dependence-producing drugs are illustrated by the Inca experience with coca leaves. There the use of the drug was limited to religious and ceremonial events, and access to it was controlled by the authorities: priests and nobles. The masses did not use it for recreation. These limitations were similar to those imposed by other primitive cultures for the handling of dependence-producing drugs such as alcohol, opium, and marijuana. In no case was the use of psychoactive drugs freely permissive or to be determined by the individual drug user. Those primitive cultures clearly recognized a danger we described in Chapter 2: the use of psychoactive drugs distorts the user's judgment, and there is little chance that he will be able to limit his own use of the drug without strong social control supplied by nonusers. There is no evidence, certainly, of abuse of coca by the Incas in the pre-Columbian era, probably because of tight social controls over the use of the drug. This control was made easier by the low-potency form in which the drug was used. The coca leaves themselves contain less than one percent cocaine, in dramatic contrast to the pure drug which modern technology can produce. The chewing or oral route of administration helped reduce Incan dependence on coca by reducing the peaking of drug levels hitting the brain—an important part of the reason why the effects of drinking a drug like alcohol are comparatively more easily controlled than the effects of drugs taken into the body by intravenous injection or the inhaling of smoke.

This stable situation of socially controlled use of the coca leaf in the pre-Columbian Andes was disrupted when the Europeans arrived. On his exploratory voyage of 1499, Amerigo Vespucci observed Indians chewing the coca leaf in what is now northern Venezuela. He was the first European to describe the practice to the rest of the world. The Europeans lost little time in overturning the old cultural order in South America, and thereby destroyed the social controls over coca leaf chewing. Moreover, they soon discovered that they could pay the tin miners in Bolivia and other Indian laborers in coca leaves rather than in money and thus reduce their costs of mining the metal. This pattern of foreign conquest, followed by disruption of well-establshed cultural controls over the use of locally available psychoactive drugs, has been repeated in many other parts of the world. Similar problems occurred in the Near and Far East with the use of opium. The introduction of alcohol to the American Indians was a particularly tragic example of the combination of social breakdown by conquest and the introduction of a dependence-producing drug.

Following the destabilization of the Incas' initial, pre-Columbian, socially controlled use, the practice of coca leaf chewing expanded to become virtually universal among the Indians of the Andes Mountains. The low potency of the leaf itself, the relatively inefficient oral route of administration, and the fact that the leaves rapidly lost their cocaine content shortly after harvest—all acted to keep coca leaf chewing localized to the Indians living near the growing sites in the Andes of South America.

The European Fascination with Cocaine

The coca situation remained relatively stable, with the chewing of the coca leaf being limited almost exclusively to the Indians in the Andes until the middle of the 19th century. At about that time, the search for new medicines prompted European chemists to identify and extract the active chemicals from many plants and traditional plant remedies from around the world, including the South American coca leaf. Medicine's long linkage with botany, which flourished most dramatically in the Middle Ages, promoted a search for new therapeutic agents as they existed in native cultures in order to identify and purify the effective ingredients by modern chemistry. During much of the 19th century, there was almost no awareness of the dependence-producing potentials of some of the resultant drugs. In the mid-19th century, the hypodermic needle was invented. This invention permitted a far more efficient method of drug administration and, in turn, made self-administration of dependence-producing drugs much more difficult to control. These changes—identification of new drugs, chemical purification of the active chemicals, and more efficient administration—created an impact similar to that created by the development of the distillation process for alcohol in Europe in the 17th century and the introduction of the tobacco cigarette in the early 20th century: the marked increase in the potency of a dependence-producing drug created havoc with the social-control processes. Thus, with naive recklessness, the Europeans in the late 19th century broke the bonds which had restrained cocaine use throughout the preceding centuries. Thus was the stage set for the first worldwide explosion of cocaine use. The genie was out of the bottle—or the bush.

Early in the European rush to cocaine, an Italian neurologist, Dr. Paola Montegazza, tried the newly purified cocaine himself and wrote in Olympian prose:

I sneered at the poor mortals condemned to live in this valley of tears while I, carried on the winds of two leaves of coca, went flying through the spaces of 77,438 worlds, each more splendid than the one before. God is unjust because he made man incapable of sustaining the effect of coca all life long. I would rather have a life span of 10 years with coca than one of 1,000,000 [and here he inserted another line of zeros] centuries without coca.

Dr. Montegazza, one might say, was one of the first in a long line of modern gurus to extol the shaky glories of turning on and tuning out.

Dr. Sigmund Freud Meets Cocaine—And Blunders a Bit.
Another enthusiast for cocaine use was Sigmund Freud. In 1884, Freud was a struggling 28-year-old neurologist in Vienna, Austria. He had read in a Detroit medical journal of the near-magical powers of cocaine. With youthful enthusiasm he proceeded to write medical articles on the uses of cocaine as a curative for conditions ranging from depression to morphine addiction. Freud also promoted cocaine use for digestive disorders and asthma, as well as for its beneficial effects on creativity. He gave some pure cocaine to a friend who was addicted to morphine; he recommended cocaine use for his fiancee when she felt gloomy; and he used it himself to deal with his own depressed moods. On one occasion, very early in the game, Freud declared: "I discovered in myself and in other observers who were capable of judging such things that even repeated doses of cocaine produced no compulsive desire to use the stimulant further; on the contrary one feels a certain unmotivated aversion to the substance." And, he euphorically exclaimed, "Inebriate hospitals can be entirely dispensed with," and "For humans the toxic dose is very high, and there seems to be no lethal dose."

Soon, of course, Freud discovered the darker side of cocaine magic: the cocaine craving and the postcocaine depression which were far worse than the problem for which the drug was taken in the first place. His addicted friend deteriorated mentally, became chronically paranoid, and nearly died from cocaine use as his dependency on the drug quickly eclipsed his morphine problems. Indeed, Freud's friend rapidly went from being the first morphine addict in Europe to be cured by cocaine to the first cocaine addict in Europe.

More specifically, this man, treated with cocaine by Freud, also experienced the unusual tactile hallucinations of animals crawling under his skin, thinking them to be "cocaine bugs," a symptom later seen commonly in chronic, high-dose cocaine users. In severe cases, sufferers even today become so distressed by this symptom that they literally scratch sores in their skin in a delusional attempt to dig out the bugs.

In one of life's ironic twists, Freud missed—but barely—the one really important medical use for cocaine: as a local anesthetic useful in surgery. Before leaving Vienna for a holiday, he gave some of the drug to an ophthalmologist colleague to experiment with in eye surgery. When Freud returned, the ophthalmologist friend had discovered that a solution of cocaine applied directly to the eye was a near-perfect anesthetic for eye operations—a discovery which brought him great and lasting renown.

One of Freud's many critics at that time flailed him for his advocacy of cocaine and accused him of having unleashed the "Third Scourge on Humanity," the other two being alcohol and morphine. Freud, meanwhile, having missed an opportunity for fame by discovering cocaine's use in eye surgery, had to face the embarrassment of his mistaken and overzealous promotion of cocaine, an embarrassment which was to be lifelong. He was forced to move on to new areas of interest, including the development of psychoanalysis and his own historical fate as one of the giants of 20th-century thought.

Meanwhile, in the final decades of the 19th century, cocaine was widely used as a patent medicine and even as a component of an apparently magical wine called Vin Mariani. The latter was a favorite of kings, presidents, authors, and popes: perhaps the "media stars" of that era, who were playing a role which cocaine-using sports and music celebrities are playing in our era 100 years later.

The American Flirtation with Cocaine

First Fling: Patent Medicines, Cough Syrup—and "The Real Thing." In a drugstore in Atlanta, Georgia, in 1886, cocaine was introduced into a popular new drink, Coca-Cola, by the company which brought us the world's first mass-consumed "soft drink." That first Coke was sold more as medicine than as fun. The claims made for the drink then, like the claims made for the first breakfast cereals originating during the same era, pointed to the power of the product to overcome fatigue, pains, and upset stomachs. This comparatively free-wheeling era also saw heroin introduced in the form of a cough syrup and a concoction for soothing colicky babies.

For a time, Coca-Cola continued its interesting cocaine connection. In 1903, however, cocaine was removed from the product and replaced by caffeine, an alternative but far less-reinforcing stimulant.

But the unmistakable name stuck, and the coca taste apparently remains to this day, for Coca-Cola is still flavored by the leaves from the same bush that produces cocaine. When I visited Peru and Bolivia several years ago to study the cocaine problem there, I was surprised to learn that tons of coca leaves are still exported to the United States. When it gets here, the cocaine, I was told, is extracted, legally, for medicinal use in surgery, especially in throat surgery, and the flavor is extracted to make Coca-Cola. The dose of cocaine in Coca-Cola in those early days was probably small and, as will be seen later in this chapter, 90 percent of cocaine taken orally is destroyed in the body before it gets to the brain. Thus, it is doubtful that early Coca-Cola was an intoxicating product.

This story is not intended to criticize modern Coca-Cola. I drink Coca-Cola, and the college from which I graduated, Emory University in Atlanta, is often called "Coca-Cola U" because of the close association over many decades between that company and the university. I remember as an undergraduate visiting the Emory library and seeing the pictures of the coca leaves used in the manufacture of the early Coke, along with the assorted paraphernalia of coca leaf use from the Andes. That was 30 years ago, between the nation's second and third enthrallments with cocaine, when no one was embarrassed by such a connection. The coca was then long out of the cola.

In the first decades of the 20th century, when the muckraking journalists and the populist reformers reached the peak of their power, the American public reacted strongly against the earlier wide-open, "let the buyer beware" era of foods and medicines. Prompted by the public outcry, in 1906 Congress passed the Pure Food and Drug Act, thereby removing such drugs as cocaine from food and patent medicines. Subsequently, in 1914, Congress enacted the Harrison Narcotics Act prohibiting heroin and cocaine, and the Volstead Act prohibiting alcohol, in 1919. With those bold reforms, America's first fickle flirtation with cocaine came to a close. It was not mourned. Dr. Sigmund Freud and the manufacturers of Coca-Cola had been embarrassed by their misguided use of cocaine. Individuals, families, and communities seemed to believe they were all well rid of the drug which, except for increasingly rare medical use, had become illegal in this country and throughout the rest of the world.

Second Dance: Jazz It Up—It's Still Gotta Thrill. America's second spin with cocaine came in the 1920s. Cocaine, along with bootlegged booze, put a lot of the roar into those Roaring Twenties. In those hectic years, in contrast to the country's earlier love affair with this drug, cocaine use was illegal, and instead of being used to cure upset stomachs and middle-aged blahs, it was used for illicit fun. Instead of the typical cocaine user being a postmenopausal rural woman, as had been the case in the 1890s, the typical cocaine user in the 1920s was an urban young man, sometimes a restless, raccoon-coated young man in a noisy, honking convertible. Cocaine use was considered bohemian and was often associated with blacks and with jazz music. It was an era in which cocaine use was often intravenous, and when cocaine was—for the first time—tied closely to the use of intravenously injected heroin in what became known as the "speed-ball." Songwriter Cole Porter immortalized it all with this line: "I get no kick from cocaine; mere alcohol doesn't thrill me at all." The cocaine image was thought of, as it is today, as simultaneously a part of the lifestyle of the predatory, criminal underworld and of the fast-track, unconventional, wealthy thrill-seekers. During this fateful de-cade, cocaine use never reached the masses. Harsh antidrug laws were in place and were being enforced with progressively greater severity. Cocaine's popularity ended abruptly, as did a vast number of other things, with the resounding economic crash of 1929.

Third Time Around: Dancing . . . Peak to Peak. The irony of the cocaine story in the 1980s is that this is the third time around for cocaine in America. This is the third time Americans have undertaken a disastrous flirtation with this drug. Now, apparently forgetting those earlier unhappy experiences, a whole new generation of Americans is discovering cocaine and repeating the same old tragedies: the lost hopes, the broken lives, the deaths. In 1982, more than 22 million Americans had used cocaine at least once, and more than four million had used the drug during the month before the survey. This amorous, but by no means coy, embracing began in the early 1970s. Cocaine inherited the increasingly tarnished mantle of marijuana. Cocaine, a stimulant producing intense, brief euphoria, seemed at first sight the "ultimate safe high."

Its use, as in the 1920s, was associated with the risk-takers, those modern princes who seem to fly above the rules and laws which bog down ordinary people. The media played a powerful and invidious role in this glamorization of cocaine. A barrage of accounts of the rich and famous caught using cocaine filled our television screens and the front pages of our newspapers. Stories about the fabulous wealth to be made in the cocaine trade lured many greedy people from all walks of life—from the dropout kid down the street to desperate, failed tycoons. The key to this current cocaine epidemic was its penetration of the unprecedented mass-drug market of the last 20 years. This time, unlike the 1920s, the cocaine market was not limited to offbeat jazz musicians, unconventional collegians, and high-kicking flappers. The 1980s cocaine market was those tens of millions of young Americans who, during the raucous 60s and 70s, had grown up using illegal drugs, especially the 55 million who had used marijuana. Cocaine became the snow cap on the modern drug-epidemic mountain.

Cocaine's image fit America in the 1980s as neatly as marijuana's image fit us in the 1960s. The early pot smoker of popular culture was a long-haired, middle-class kid, sitting cross-legged in a park at sunset and heeding the admonition of Timothy Leary to "Turn on, Tune in, Drop out." The popular image of the 1980s cocaine user is the elegantly dressed, sophisticated young executive at an exclusive New York disco, celebrating his latest "big deal" as he rockets to success. Both images are stereotypes of the aging, drug abuse epidemic population of the post–World War II Baby Boom.

THE CURRENT COCAINE SCENE

Who's Using It? How Much? And Where?

We have no data on the numbers of people involved in those earlier cocaine cycles in American history. Surely the numbers were large at the turn of the century and small in the 1920s. In 1972, before the current illicit drug boom peaked, but after it had begun in the mid-1960s, cocaine had been used at least once by two percent of 12- to 17-year-olds, by 9.9 percent of 18- to 25-year-olds, and by two percent of Americans over the age of 25. The comparable figures for 1982, the most recent national data available, were seven percent, 29 percent, and nine percent, respectively. The rises in just 10 years amount to over 300 percent for youth, over 200 percent for young adults, and over 400 percent for older adults. Of course, using 1962 as a base (if such data were available), before the illicit drug epidemic began, would undoubtedly reveal far larger percentage increases in cocaine use.

Among American high school seniors, a group for which we have annual surveys from 1975 through 1983, the percentage having used cocaine at least once rose from nine percent to 16 percent, and the percentage using cocaine during the preceding month rose from two percent to five percent. On the other hand, the figures for 1980 to

1983 show a leveling off of cocaine use rates in this age group. In fact, lifetime use by high school seniors peaked at 17 percent in 1981. Use within the last month by high school seniors peaked that same year at six percent (a figure also reached in 1979).

National surveys show that cocaine is most likely to be used by high school students who are already heavy users of alcohol and marijuana and that, compared to those drugs, the initiation of cocaine use is relatively late. In addition, the use rates of cocaine differ dramatically from the use rates of marijuana and alcohol. There are only small numbers of high school students who use cocaine at a very high frequency, including daily use. While 5.5 percent of high school seniors used alcohol daily in 1983, and an identical 5.5 percent used marijuana daily, only 0.2 percent reported daily use of cocaine. This 1983 daily cocaine use figure was down slightly from its peak in 1981 at 0.3 percent. Among Americans aged 18 to 25, the highest drug-using segment of our population, 7.1 percent used cocaine one or more times in the month prior to the last national survey in 1982.

The 1982 survey of American households found that 22.1 million Americans 12 years of age and older had used cocaine at least once, 17.4 million had used it within the last year, and 4.2 million had used it within the last month. Since we know that the millions of Americans who do not live in traditional households have higher use rates for cocaine and other drugs, and since we also know that all illicit drug use is underreported in survey data, this can be taken as a minimum estimate of the size of the contemporary American cocaine problem.

As cocaine use has risen in the United States, so have problems caused by cocaine. The Centers for Disease Control (CDC) reported in 1982 that the number of cocaine-related deaths rose fourfold from 1976 to 1981 to more than 300 a year and that the rate of hospital emergency room visits caused by cocaine rose sixfold in the same period. The CDC also reported that, among those seeking treatment at an emergency room for a cocaine-related problem, the percentage of cocaine users injecting and smoking the drug (as opposed to snorting it into the nose) rose during those years. In 1977, 24 percent of users reported injecting cocaine, while in 1980 the figure was 31 percent.

All surveys of American cocaine use show that it is typically episodic or what is described as "spree" use, with the percentage of cocaine users demonstrating patterns of daily or near-daily use being relatively small when compared to the percentage of users of alcohol, marijuana, and other drugs when daily use is reported. Even among those who do use cocaine regularly over the course of months or years, there is a tendency to spree use, with cocaine runs or almost continuous use lasting for hours or days, interspersed with episodes of crashing: intervals during which the user abstains from the use of cocaine.

There's No Biz Like "Snow" Biz:
The Economics of Cocaine

Cocaine is not cheap. A single use of the drug typically costs from $5 to $20 for a high lasting about 30 minutes. Frequent compulsive use of the drug is enormously expensive, and even occasional use of it is not affordable by many. This cost barrier to compulsive cocaine use is different from the cost barrier to alcohol use, where the frequent, high-dose intake of the drug is affordable by the large majority of the American population, including teenagers. Marijuana, like alcohol, offers no insurmountable cost barrier to heavy use. A big marijuana habit, like a heavy alcohol habit, might cost $10 a day. By way of contrast, compulsive use of cocaine, extending to several hundred dollars or even to thousands of dollars a day, is not uncommon. Regular cocaine users, when asked how much cocaine they use, frequently comment, "I use cocaine until it is gone," which translates into "until my money is gone." This pattern of cost-limiting the amount of the drug to be used is similar to that followed in compulsive gambling but is different from the pattern of alcohol and marijuana use. It is not different from the considerably less common pattern governing heroin use, which is also usually money limited.

Why are the "economics" of alcohol and marijuana use different from those of heroin and cocaine in this regard? For one thing, the inflation in the cost of heroin and cocaine, created by relatively effective American prohibition of these drugs, drives their cost up to between 50 and 200 times the cost of the same drug if it were sold openly the way aspirin is now sold in this country. Heroin, for example, which could be easily retailed for one cent per milligram, costs the illicit user in the United States today about $2.00 for that quantity. With a typical daily heroin habit being about 50 milligrams, the cost is boosted from a hypothetical legalized price of 50 cents a day to a prohibition or illicit price of $100 a day. The economics of cocaine are similar. Alcohol, while taxed more heavily than aspirin, is sold at about two times the ordinary retail markup because about half the cost is tax. A big alcohol habit of 10 ounces of pure alcohol per day can easily be met by buying two bottles of fortified wine for less than $6.00 per day. Marijuana prohibition is relatively less effective than prohibition of cocaine and heroin in the United States. This helps to raise the price to perhaps five times the potential open-market price. Five or six marijuana "joints" a day cost from $5 to $20.

There is another, but not easily understood, factor that works hard and painfully to produce Big Bucks for the illicit drug trade. It's a phenomenon called *tolerance*. Tolerance means that as a person (or a laboratory animal) uses more and more of a drug over time, each dose produces a smaller and smaller effect. Cocaine and heroin are short-acting drugs frequently taken by smoking or by the intravenous route. Tolerance develops rapidly, and users typically escalate the amount of the drug used over time. Frequent drinkers of alcohol have a much smaller reaction to a single drink than occasional drinkers have. Some drugs produce more tolerance than others. Cocaine and heroin are unusually effective in producing tolerance following heavy, frequent use. While heroin habits of 600 milligrams per day (10 times the heavy use-rate among chronic abusers) are not uncommon when the drug is cheap, an alcohol habit of 20 bottles of fortified wine a day (10 times a big habit) is unthinkable. Further contributing to the high consumption of such high-priced drugs as cocaine and heroin are the rapid peaking of blood levels and the short duration of action of these drugs. It is a never-ending circle: more and more drug use means more and more money means more and more profits for the pockets of the purveyors of these poisonous potions, adding further to their incentives to provide users with more and more drugs.

Finally, enormous economic benefits (for all the wrong people) are generated by the supposed glamour, glitz, and grandeur evoked by the current cocaine scene. Probably the single most striking aspect of that scene is the emergence of cocaine as the champagne of illicit drugs, its image as the party drug of the rich and famous. There are at least two reasons for this perception. First, cocaine is a stimulant, and that makes it distinctive and different from the other more commonly used drugs like alcohol and marijuana, for example. Second, cocaine is expensive, at least when used with any frequency. And high cost, as they say, is the ultimate "touch of class."

Let's look, for a moment, at the way wealth "grows" in the drug world. Like everything these days, the price of illicit drugs is inflated in value—and going up. The escalation of the value of cocaine in the illicit market is readily apparent from the fact that cocaine sells for about $50 an ounce for pure medicinal purposes. That same ounce, adulterated many times over, will bring about $1,500 to $2,500 when sold to cocaine users in the United States. We can see the inflation of the drug's value perhaps even more clearly by tracing its progression from the time it leaves the South American farmer and moves to the eventual U.S. consumer.

Drugs are often measured, even by high school dropout junkies, in metric weights of grams and kilograms. One kilogram, or one kilo, is equal to 2.2 pounds. One ounce equals 28 grams. On the slopes of the Andes, it takes about 500 kilos of coca leaves to produce 2.5 kilos of coca paste. This quantity of leaves sells for about $1,200, whereas 2.5 kilos of coca paste sells for about $5,000 once it enters the illicit traffic. That 2.5 kilos of paste, in turn, produces one kilo of cocaine base worth $11,000, which is then refined into one kilo of pure cocaine worth $20,000 in Colombia. That same kilo smuggled into the United States sells for $60,000. When cut initially to 50 percent purity, its value goes to $120,000. At the street level where it is sold to American cocaine users, that kilo is an average of 12 percent pure and brings $500,000. Thus, an ounce of cocaine worth about $50 in a pharmacy sells for $14,000 in the illicit market. That is a 30,000 percent markup!

The total U.S. cocaine market, supplying 22 million cocaine users, is estimated to be 40 tons of cocaine a year. The U.S. cocaine market, estimated at more than $25 billion a year, is now three times as big as the total U.S. recording and movie industries put together.

Such figures can be misread and often are. Many people, not all of whom are basically criminal, read these numbers and are excited by the lure of huge, easy profits. They drift, or leap, into the cocaine traffic. I have met many drug traffickers in my professional life, most of them either seeking treatment for their cocaine habits or serving long prison sentences, both being occupational hazards that make other serious job risks, such as black lung disease for coal miners, seem trivial. I understate the case when I say that traffic in cocaine is terribly risky and almost certain to be disastrous. While cocaine traffickers, like gamblers, often have large sums of cash pass through their hands, the money doesn't stick. Those I have known never have anything. They are constantly being arrested or ripped off by other traffickers. They never know which of their "friends," to save his own neck, has become an informer for the police, and they never know which of their customers is an undercover agent.

The high level of paranoia caused by the trafficking itself is compounded by the fact that most dealers also are cocaine users. They often self-administer large amounts of cocaine because it is so easily available. This consumes their profits and, in addition, frequently produces intense problems, of which severe paranoia is but one. I have been amazed by the contrast between the media's image of the fabulous wealth of cocaine traffickers and the actual reality I have seen personally. They are among the most unhappy, haunted, sick people I have worked with. Almost invariably broke—and broken—human beings.

The money factor in cocaine trafficking should also be looked at from the typical user's point of view. One "line" of cocaine used for one snort of the drug contains about 10 milligrams of pure cocaine and has about eight times that quantity of dilutants. One gram of diluted street cocaine, selling for about $150, has about 30 such "lines." In one evening, the cocaine user may consume a few lines costing roughly $10 a line, or several grams costing $500 or more. These numbers are slippery, of course. The costs to the user are highly varied. The street market is constantly changing the value of cocaine and other illicit products, thus producing far larger and sharper swings than occur in legal commerce. Rises and falls of 200 percent or more can occur from week to week. In addition, the cocaine user never knows the true potency of the product he is using. When he buys a "gram of cocaine," he is buying a gram of white powder which may be nearly pure cocaine (a distinctly rare occurrence), or he may be getting no cocaine at all for his money. It is standard practice to substitute far cheaper, bitter-tasting substances, as well as synthetic local anesthetics and stimulants, for cocaine. More will be said later about this "cutting" procedure.

Making It Big: Rock Stars, Supersports—
And Shattered Images

While rock stars and sports heroes are comparatively rare in the population, they cast a large shadow because of the attention we pay to them. They are "special" people. Successful musicians and sports figures are young men and women who, typically, come from relatively obscure—and often impoverished—backgrounds into sudden wealth. The typical lifestyle of both professional sports stars and musicians uniquely combines rootlessness and deprivation with sudden and lavish access to money. Astounding amounts of it. This combination makes these young people uniquely vulnerable to all drug habits, especially the habit associated with high living in America in the 1980s: cocaine use.

There is still another reason why these special people are particularly attracted to cocaine. They become rapidly addicted to applause and to excitement. They get high on it. They require more and more of it. Having worked with several stars, I have become acutely aware

of their distress when the roar of the crowd subsides and the spot-
lights go out. After leaving a stadium where 50,000 or 100,000
people have been screaming their names, they walk out alone into a
less frenzied, less enchanted, community. Wearied and emptied after
giving their all in a dramatic performance on the stage or in the sports
arena, they often find themselves in a hotel room, in a strange city,
alone. This is a jarring, unnerving experience for a great many of
these young stars. Old friends, family, and traditional values are out
of place in this new world of wealth and glamour. Large quantities of
leisure, money, sex, drugs, and all sorts of high living are easily
available. New friends spring up everywhere—varying from the hang-
ers-on and adoring groupies to the big-ego businessman to the wily
agent to the equally lost colleague or competitor. One feels special,
even chosen. All the earlier periods of struggle and obscurity seem
like nothing more than a waiting period for the current entitlement to
success. In all the din and confusion, the one thing clear is that the
applause of the crowd is the key to all this success. But, when the
key is lost and the doors no longer swing invitingly open, shadows and
unnameable terrors can descend.

The cocaine high (to be discussed later) has many similarities to the
intoxicating high of applause and excitement. Many of these painfully
vulnerable stars seek to recreate, sustain, and control this intensely
exciting experience through their use of cocaine. Of course, because
of their living outside of the ordinary bounds of family control over
pleasure-producing behaviors including drug use, and because of their
easy access to large amounts of money, the restraining forces affecting most young people do not apply to stars. This sets up a vicious
pattern of cocaine and other drug dependence.

Such a pattern would remain a relatively infrequent and highly
personal tragedy if it were not for the flood of attention given to
young stars and their drug habits. Unfortunately, these celebrities
have lost themselves in a "land of the spree and the home of the
rave." The repetition in the media of arrests of the heroes of America's young people not only adds to the glamour of drug use in
general, and cocaine use in particular, but it also creates an image of
the desirability and even the normality of cocaine and other illicit drug
use.

After years of relative neglect of this issue, there are recent, and
hopeful, signs that the music and the sports industries are beginning
to wake up to the negative effect exerted by these obsessively publi-
cized events, not only on the lives of some of the most talented stars
in their fields but also on the public acceptance of the sports and

music industries on which they all depend. Recent headlines have contrasted dramatically with those of 10 years ago, showing a modest increase in the commitment of both the music industry and the sports industry to promoting drug-free lifestyles among their stars and in their public messages. They are now, belatedly, handing out increasingly severe penalties to people who violate the drug laws.

I hasten to correct a possible wrong impression. If one asks, "What drug is the sports star most likely to be arrested for possessing?" the answer is "cocaine." However, if the question is "Who is the *typical American user of cocaine* in the 1980s?" the answer is *not* a rock star or a professional athlete. The typical modern cocaine user is a young man or, less often, a young woman aged 18 to 35 who used marijuana and other illicit drugs heavily during the teenage years and who later developed a taste for cocaine. The typical cocaine user remains a heavy consumer of other drugs, especially depressant drugs such as alcohol and, less often, opiates including heroin and such synthetic opiates as Dilaudid. He or she is more likely to be pathetic and grubby than to be sophisticated. The cocaine user who achieved success in middle age, the successful businessman or the rich and bored housewife, is—like the addicted rock star—a distinct rarity in America today. The media image is, as I have emphasized, in stark contrast with this reality. The pathetic, unemployed youth strung out on cocaine will not make the evening news or a television documentary. Cocaine use is today predominantly a part of the polydrug scene for the aging Baby Boom Generation.

Cocaine in the Executive Suite and in Other Workplaces

No examination of the current cocaine scene in America would be complete without at least a fleeting look at how this drug has infiltrated the country's corporate and industrial enterprises. Cocaine use, by the young and not quite so young has, for the first time, brought high-cost, compulsive drug use into the corporate executive suite and the workplace on a large scale. Alcoholism has been a common problem among top executives for generations, but, however deadly excessive use of alcohol is, it is not expensive. Booze is relatively cheap. Heroin addiction, the only other truly expensive American drug habit, has been for decades limited to lower economic levels.

But, with the infiltration of cocaine, the corporate/industrial picture has changed drastically. Now cocaine habits of $2,000 a week and more are showing up in men and women with personal access to the highest levels of corporate life. As one Washington, D.C. attorney said about his clients: "They are just waking up to the threat posed by cocaine users. Not only are these people desperate for cash and involved in theft of money and property, but they are also involved in selling company secrets and vital information. That is far more menacing than the simple theft of a few thousand dollars worth of electric typewriters, or a few missing pocketbooks. In one case a multinational corporation found itself in serious tax trouble when its records were sold by a money-hungry employee." Trade secrets, highly prized technologies, and long-term corporate strategies are immensely valuable commodities which can be sold for money to buy cocaine. And this is being done on a far, far larger scale than you may have imagined.

Drug use which requires lots of money—and that mostly means cocaine and heroin habits—changes personal values fast. People I have worked with, and who were previously reasonably honest, rather quickly became thieves once they got hooked on either cocaine or heroin.

The connection of cocaine to depressant drugs, especially the ultimate downer heroin, has recently added to this threat as the two high-cost, compulsive habits have often been combined in people who were previously practically immune to this type of drug dependence and the thefts and the peccadilloes required to support it. The next time you read about drug abuse in the workplace, remember that the problem is not limited to the laborer who drives the forklift off the ramp because he is stoned on marijuana, or to the secretary who missed work because of her alcohol problem.

. . . And, Meanwhile, in Other Countries

In describing the current cocaine scene, we should be aware of what is happening in other countries. Europe, and to a lesser extent the more developed nations of Asia and Latin America, are following the American pattern. There is a trendy use of cocaine both among the local jet setters and the down and out, heavy drug users. Even more disturbing has been the explosive rise in cocaine problems in the countries producing cocaine for export, notably Bolivia, Peru, and Colombia. In these nations, cocaine problems are most common among urban, unemployed young men (who are numerous in these generally depressed economies). Rather than snorting cocaine, as is common in the United States, a large proportion of these Latin youths are smoking *coca paste*, the first-line product produced after cocaine has been extracted locally from the coca leaf. The smoking route of administration, like the smoking route employed in the United States that is called "freebasing," produces an intense cocaine effect with an intense dependence. Coca-paste smoking has become epidemic, producing horrifying stories and dismal treatment outcomes. To cite one example, for those compulsive coca paste smokers who have failed repeatedly to respond to more traditional treatments, some Peruvian neurologists are resorting to lobotomy, the surgical cutting of part of the brain. The considerable extent of the cocaine problem in that part of the world is suggested by this recent sampling of the 3,000,000 people who reside in Lima, Peru: an estimated 160,000 chewed coca leaves, 39,000 smoked coca paste, and 21,000 sniffed cocaine.

WHAT COCAINE IS

The Process of Making Cocaine

The source of cocaine is the plant *Erythroxylum coca*, an evergreen bush growing on the slopes of the Andes Mountains in South America, principally in Bolivia and Peru. Unlike the other major drug-producing plants, marijuana and opium (which are easily grown in all parts of the world), coca grows best between the elevations of 1,500 and 6,000 feet, and the coca plant must be three or four years old before the leaves can be harvested for processing to make cocaine. Plants continue to produce for about 20 years. Once the coca plant is mature, the leaves are harvested several times a year by stripping off some of them just as tea leaves are taken from the tea plants at similar elevations in the mountains of Africa and Asia.

When the leaves of the coca bush are soaked with kerosene, sulfuric acid, and an alkali, a crude paste known as coca base or coca paste is created. This is a mixture of coca alkyloids and oil having a cocaine content of up to 70 percent. When hydrochloric acid is added, the cocaine salt is produced with a purity of about 90 percent. Then, in the form of white flakes or rocks, it is crushed to produce a snowy white powder. This appearance leads to cocaine's street name, "snow." Because the coca leaves are bulky and difficult to transport, the cocaine is quickly extracted from them, and they are reduced to the form of coca paste near the Peruvian and Bolivian growing sites. Before extraction, the coca leaves themselves contain nearly 20 alkyloids, of which cocaine is the principal component.

Botanists have suggested that the coca shrub's biological advantage in producing cocaine comes from the bitter taste of the chemical, making it less attractive to foraging animals. One can speculate that the percentage of cocaine in the coca leaf would have to be, by evolutionary selection, carefully kept high enough to make the leaf taste bad, but low enough to prevent blood levels of cocaine (following even massive leaf eating) from rising to a level that would produce intense drug dependence. This fine-line "target" has been hit well enough in nature to keep the plant competitive in the Andes environment. It may also give us a clue as to why the South American Indians had a relatively easy time controlling coca use levels, and the consequences of such use, as long as use was restricted to chewing the coca leaves.

What would have happened to the social control processes if the coca leaf produced 10 percent cocaine? What would the foraging habits have been of wild herbivores in the Andes if the coca leaves produced 10 percent cocaine? Similarly, what would have happened if the Indians 500 years ago had known how to purify the cocaine above the leaves' one percent cocaine content, or if the foraging animals had been able to purify or inject the cocaine? In recent years, we have had a chance to find out more about the unfortunate impact of purified cocaine on the local Andes populations. Additionally, modern laboratory experiments tell us all we need to know about the behavior of animals when exposed to pure cocaine by the intravenous route, as will be described shortly.

Smuggling the Cocaine to Market

After being processed into coca paste in or near the Andes Mountain growing sites, the crude drug product is transported into the worldwide, illicit drug-trafficking networks, principally via highly organized criminal networks in the neighboring country of Colombia, where it is often manufactured into pure cocaine. Cocaine then travels by a variety of routes through the Caribbean and Mexico to the United States, as well as to worldwide distribution throughout Latin America and Europe.

Why, you may wonder, is cocaine so carefully purified from the one percent state existing in the crude, natural coca leaves, to the nearly 100 percent pure cocaine in illicit-drug laboratories, only to be diluted subsequently to about 12 percent purity for sale to American drug users? The answer, in one word, is *smuggling*. The law enforcement effort to stop cocaine trafficking is now focused on the high-level criminal traffickers at the points of entry into the United States.

Traffickers, responding to this reality, concentrate or compress their product into the smallest possible volume to make smuggling easier and detection by the law more difficult. It is hard to detect cocaine when it is in its pure form, when it can be concealed virtually anywhere. This same accordion effect has major implications for efforts to dry up the supply of cocaine. Namely, it is easier to find cocaine and punish sellers when the volume is large: where it is grown at one percent purity and where it is ultimately sold at roughly 12 percent purity. Once the cocaine is marketed to the ultimate consumer, the product is again diluted, near the site of use, to inflate profits.

For years the coca bushes must remain rooted in the soil, exposed to the sunlight. These bushes are almost as easy to spot in Peru and Bolivia as a wheat field is in Kansas. They cannot be easily concealed. They could be easily destroyed if the political will could be mustered. I had the experience several years ago of visiting the countries involved in coca trade in South America, including Colombia, Ecuador, Bolivia, and Peru. A relatively small amount of coca leaf is cultivated for legitimate medicinal cocaine. The vast majority of the coca cultivation is dedicated from the start to illicit cocaine traffic. Both Peru and Bolivia have international treaty obligations to stop all illicit cultivation of coca bushes. Despite this, I was disheartened to see large sections of the Andean forests being cleared by the most modern equipment as coca bushes were openly planted for illicit cultivation. Because it takes several years of growth to allow the plants to reach maturity, it is quite easy to identify coca cultivation in Latin America before the first harvest is made. The failure of the countries involved, as well as of the international community, to stop this cocaine traffic at its source, where it is most easily stopped, represents one of many widely shared tragedies of international drug abuse prevention.

"Cutting" the Product

Once the cocaine has been purified and enters the illicit market, it travels to the United States and other cocaine-consuming countries, going through a complex distribution system that includes a dramatic dilution of the drug. This dilution procedure adds a variety of inexpensive agents to "cut" the product. These include amphetamines, ephedrine, procaine, xylocaine, and lidocaine. These chemicals are synthetic stimulants, many of which are used medically as local anesthetics. In addition, a variety of inert filler substances are often added to illicit cocaine to increase its volume. These additives include sugars of various kinds. Quinine is commonly added to illicit cocaine because its bitter taste (like cocaine itself) leads the cocaine customer to believe he or she has a purer product than is actually the case.

GETTING COCAINE INTO THE BODY: FOUR ROADS TO EUPHORIA

Since, earlier in this chapter, I have alluded to some of the means by which cocaine is taken into the human body, it is useful now to be more specific about them. We are about to see what happens when cocaine is *snorted*, when it is *injected* intravenously, when it is *eaten*, and when it is *smoked*. These are the so-called "routes of administration." We will consider, too, why users commonly pick one or another of these routes for getting the coke to their brains.

What Happens When Cocaine Is Eaten?

Cocaine can be *eaten* or *taken orally*. However, only about 10 percent of the cocaine enters the bloodstream after oral administration, and the drug's effect is spread out over several hours. Thus, oral administration is doubly inefficient: the high is blunted by the very gradual rise and fall of the cocaine level in the blood, and 90 percent of the ingested cocaine is destroyed by digestion before it enters the bloodstream. Thus, for purely practical reasons, cocaine is seldom used orally. It is too expensive to "waste" in this way.

What Happens When Cocaine Is Snorted or Sniffed?

The second and most common route of cocaine administration in the United States is to *sniff* or *snort* the white powder into the nose. For the taking of many of the illicit drugs used in the world, certain highly personalized, ritualized procedures have been developed. This is the ritual for snorting or sniffing cocaine. The powder is measured out with a coke spoon into small piles on a glass, often a mirror, and divided (with a razor blade or other sharp instrument) into "lines." Each line is a single dose of the drug. A tube is then used to sniff the cocaine up into the user's nose. The initial effects are quick because the cocaine passes rapidly into the bloodstream and thence to the brain. However, further absorption is then slowed because the cocaine also constricts the small blood vessels in the lining of the nose at the site of administration. Measurable levels of cocaine are found in the blood within about 10 minutes after nasal use, with the peak occurring at about 60 minutes. As is often the case with drug effects, the user's sense of peak drug-induced euphoria occurs earlier than the peak blood level: peak euphoria occurs in about 20 minutes after sniffing even though peak blood level occurs after 60 minutes. Subsequent to sniffing, about 60 percent of the cocaine taken into the nose eventually enters the bloodstream.

What Happens When Cocaine Is Injected Intravenously?

The third route of administration is to *inject* the cocaine intravenously. Following injection, 100 percent of the drug (and 100 percent of the cutting dilutants) reaches the bloodstream—and very quickly. The peak mental effect, the "rush," occurs in about 30 seconds after injection. Economics push the cocaine user toward the intravenous injection route. Besides, it is easy and 100 percent effective in delivering an intense, almost instantaneous high. Many cocaine users do not inject because they associate intravenous drug practices with "junkies" and "addicts." Of course, injection has some unique health hazards, including hepatitis, Acquired Immune Deficiency Syndrome (AIDS), and other needle-borne infections, to say nothing of the whole range of adverse effects resulting from the injection of the often toxic dilutants used in cutting street cocaine. All of these dangers notwithstanding, increasing numbers of the nation's millions of cocaine users, seeking the most potent and efficient high, are being lured into intravenously injected cocaine use.

What Happens When Cocaine Is Smoked?

The fourth route of administration is *smoking*. Cocaine can be smoked in two ways. The first of these is to burn the primitive coca paste, thus producing a smoke with high-cocaine content which is then inhaled. This is the pattern of smoking in South America, where coca paste is far more common and much cheaper than cocaine. In the United States, the reverse is true, but coca paste is now becoming more available here also.

The second type of smoking is called "freebasing." Ordinary street cocaine containing its many dilutants and impurities is dissolved in water to which is added a strong alkali. A highly flammable solvent is then used to extract the purified cocaine from the mixture. These caustic and highly flammable chemicals have caused serious and even fatal accidents. Once the purified "freebase" has been extracted, it is burned and the smoke inhaled. To smoke freebase, the purified powder is either sprinkled on a cigarette or burned in a special freebase pipe. The freebase extraction process has become so popular with the cocaine-smoking public that a minor industry has developed to provide the necessary implements. Some freebasers no longer bother extracting the alkaloid with a solvent. They just add a chemical that releases the purified cocaine and inhale the material.

Freebasing produces an intense two- to five-minute "super high." Smoking coca paste and freebasing both involve the absorption of cocaine across a membrane in the respiratory tract, just as snorting cocaine into the nose does. However, in smoking, the total membrane area exposed to the drug is thousands of times larger than when the nose is used. Thus, in contrast to the nasal route, where absorption of the cocaine is slowed by the constriction of blood vessels soon after the drug gets to them, the huge inner surfaces of the lungs promote far more rapid and complete drug absorption.

On the other hand, the *toxic, local effects* of the cocaine, rather than being limited to the relatively small area of the nasal mucous membrane as occurs when the drug is snorted, are also spread over the entire lung lining when cocaine is smoked.

From some who have used cocaine both by injection and by smoking, I have heard that the rush is similar. Despite the relative inefficiency of smoking, some people simply do not want to inject drugs. Moreover, because marijuana smoking has become so common and so apparently "normal" in the lives of so many illicit-drug users, they are strongly attracted to smoking cocaine. What should give pause, of course, is the fact that all the negative effects of cocaine use are more frequent and more intense among those who either inject or smoke the drug. There is a tendency in all drug use for the more intense and more potent techniques of use to displace the milder methods.

Freebasing, in addition to its problems arising from danger of burns and the possible trouble and mess of a difficult extraction, has a serious economic drawback. Because burning destroys between 10 percent and 80 percent of the cocaine, smoking is relatively wasteful and inefficient. This factor, and the terribly short period of the high which follows smoking, combine to make freebasing especially expensive. In short, the cocaine smoker does not get as much for his money. The smoking route of administration would no doubt be more popular if it were not for this factor. Freebasing is especially popular with cocaine users who are used to smoking marijuana and tobacco, who are unwilling to use the intravenous route of administration, and who are willing to pay truly astronomical sums of money for a very short, but very intense, cocaine high.

HOW COCAINE DOES ITS WORK

Neurotransmitters, Synapses, and Responses

Unlike most other drugs, particularly alcohol and marijuana, where the mechanisms by which the drug works remain mysterious, we have a good understanding of the way cocaine works. Normally, nerve cells communicate messages to each other by sending a signal from one cell to another across a tiny gap known as the synapse. The sending nerve cell releases into the synapse neurotransmitter chemicals which, on reaching the receiving cell, trigger a response in that cell. After the nerve discharge has occurred, the neurotransmitters are taken back into the sending cell for reuse in sending the next message. When cocaine is taken into the body, the drug enters the synapse, the space between two nerve cells, and blocks this "re-uptake" of neurotransmitters, particularly in those parts of the brain associated with reward or pleasure. These brain areas are in the deep or midbrain. They are called the *ventral tegmentum* and the *nucleus accumbens*. The principal neurotransmitters involved are norepinephrine, serotonin, and dopamine.

In addition to blocking re-uptake, cocaine promotes release of neurotransmitters from the sending neuron. When these chemicals are not taken up and therefore remain in the synapse, there tends to be a high firing rate which produces excitement and euphoria. It is not hard to understand why the cocaine state is associated with euphoria, and it is not difficult to understand why the postcocaine state is associated with lethargy and depression: at the end of a run of cocaine use, the neurotransmitters involved in pleasure are depleted. It takes many hours, sometimes even days or weeks, for the nerve cells to recover their precocaine neurotransmitter reserves.

Newton's Third Law (for every action there is an equal and opposite reaction) seems to apply to many drug effects, including those produced by cocaine. The more intense the euphoria of the cocaine high, the lower the postcocaine depression. This alternating flooding/depletion process can be explained biologically. The acute cocaine high comes from the spilled neurotransmitters flooding the synapse in the brain's pleasure centers. The subsequent acute depression and fatigue come from the depletion of these same vital neurotransmitters.

In my clinical experience, I have observed a pathetic twist to this: The more enthusiastic the cocaine user is at the outset of the cocaine use, the more horrible the deterioration at the end stages of his or her dependence.

Overstimulation, Adaptation, and Paranoia

The more chronic problems resulting from cocaine use are not quite so easily understood. The long-term hyperstimulation of plea-sure-producing nerve centers seems to make them resistant to normal stimulation. When cocaine is taken into the system over an extended period of time, the more ordinary pleasures of life, from food to sex to achievement, pale into insignificance when compared to the intense high produced by the drug. The brain's pleasure centers, having been repeatedly overstimulated by chronic cocaine use, become resistant to *any* stimulation—a process known in biology as adaptation, or homeo-stasis—as the organism attempts to moderate the effects of an ex-treme stimulation.

The cocaine user who began his drug use feeling that life with his new friend, cocaine, was as exciting as the Italian neurologist Montegazza described it to be over 100 years ago, progresses inev-itably (if he continues to use cocaine at high doses) to experiencing life as empty and gray and—if paranoia develops—as positively hostile.

To compound this irony at yet one more level, as the cocaine user gets deeper and deeper into his cocaine use to pursue pleasure, with chronic use he *looks* more and more miserable and unhappy. While he can often inspire novices to try the drug when he is in his initial, honeymoon stages of cocaine use, at the end stages no one would follow his lead because his mind, his body, and his life are so discern-ibly and unmistakably ruined. In laboratories, when monkeys are given free access to cocaine, it takes them five days or less to die. During that time, they look anything but happy as they waste away, scratch their skin for "bugs" that are not there, and suffer tremors and seizures. It would be hard for a fair-minded observer to conclude they were seeking, much less finding, pleasure.

WHAT COCAINE DOES: THE EFFECTS IT CREATES

Physiological and Psychological Effects

Cocaine produces a wide variety of physical and psychological effects, both locally where it first touches the body and, later, in parts of the body far removed from its point of entry. Locally, as we now know, cocaine constricts the blood vessels and produces complete but temporary local anesthesia. We need to remember that when it is snorted, it produces these effects on the linings of the nose. When it is smoked, the lungs are similarly affected. Recently, a heavy user, who smoked cocaine, described his first experience with it in these words: "I inhaled deeply, the way I do cigarettes or marijuana. I felt I'd been hit in the chest by a hammer. I was in shock, I couldn't feel myself breathing, my throat and lungs went numb. I was scared to death."

The moment cocaine enters the bloodstream and passes swiftly to all parts of the body, it produces a profound effect on the heart, rapidly increasing the heart rate and raising the blood pressure. Cocaine also raises the body temperature, dilates the pupils of the eyes, and can affect the vision. Some experienced eye doctors report that they can detect cocaine crystals in the retinas of long-term, high-dose cocaine users. The cocaine users whose vision is affected report seeing flashes like small stars darting back and forth.

Cocaine is often taken initially as an aphrodisiac, but regular and persistent users frequently report decreased interest in sex, and male users often report impotence.

Cocaine can cause death in several ways. It can produce a fatal disturbance in the heart rhythm (arrhythmia); it can cause fatal epileptic seizures; and, because it characteristically causes severe depression and paranoia, it can produce suicide and homicide. These fatal and near-fatal episodes are, of course, more likely to occur among chronic high-dose users, but they can also occur unpredictably among low-dose, infrequent users.

In addition to the almost universally and invariably unpleasant runny nose, scarring, and tissue death which result from snorting and sniffing cocaine, there is the danger of a more serious problem: perforation of the septum between the left and right nasal passages. In recent years, in the United States, this problem of septal perforation has, in fact, led to a dramatic rise in the need for plastic surgeons to repair such defects. When cocaine is smoked, serious lung pathology can develop, including a bloody cough and serious lung disease as the blood-vessel-constricting effects are repeated and prolonged. Clinicians now call this syndrome "cocaine lung."

When cocaine is injected, a variety of complications can develop— complications which are secondary to use of the intravenous route of drug administration. The dilutants in the cocaine can produce severe problems. These range from blocking the arteries in the lungs to producing pulmonary hypertension or heart and brain impairments, which—when combined with a sudden, high-dose shock—can bring on collapse and death. Sterile practices are virtually never followed in the drugged state, so serious and potentially fatal serum hepatitis and Acquired Immune Deficiency Syndrome (AIDS) can occur. In addition, the use of the intravenous route of administration for cocaine users has become a common entry into intravenous use of other drugs, including heroin. In sum, intensified cocaine use, with its rapid escalation of amounts of the drug used, often leads to loss of control over use, and this, in turn, almost inevitably generates severe physical and mental consequences.

Reinforcement—Cocaine's Relentless Effects

Whatever its other effects, the illicit use of cocaine has one target and *only* one: the effect on the brain. This is the central stimulant or excitory effect which produces the cocaine high. One of the best ways to study the reinforcing properties of any drug is to give small doses of it to laboratory animals to measure how much work the animals will do to get them. Such studies have been carried out with many drugs.

Cocaine has proved to be the most potent reinforcer of them all. In one study, for example, monkeys pressed a lever an average of 12,800 times to obtain a single dose of cocaine. Even when they were starving, the monkeys preferred cocaine to eating food. Male monkeys preferred to press the bar and get cocaine rather than have sex with a receptive female monkey placed in their cages. Monkeys worked for cocaine even when it was paired with severe electric shocks that were administered every time they succeeded in getting the cocaine. Monkeys hate to get electrical shocks. If given free access to the cocaine, the monkeys continued to self-administer it until they had convulsions and died. Laboratory monkeys given free access to intravenously administered cocaine rapidly developed severe symptoms, including hyperactivity, tactile hallucinations (cocaine "bugs"), staggering, severe weight loss, shakes, and convulsions. If they had free access to that drug, there was no possibility of the monkeys' exerting personal control over their cocaine craving. Only death could end their unrelenting struggle for it.

Several lessons about drug reinforcement can be learned from this animal model, and they need to be emphasized. There are no social or psychological characteristics of monkeys which produced in them the intense cocaine craving they exhibited. It was more intense than the craving for any other commonly used drug and clearly more powerful than the attraction of such natural pleasures as food and sex. It overrode strong punishments: electrical shocks. It was not possible for the monkeys to control their own demand for and use of cocaine prior to their demise.

Cocaine Addiction and the Drug Dependence Syndrome

One of the most curious arguments about cocaine use in America in the 1980s has been whether cocaine is addictive. The modern concept of addiction was developed to deal with the problems of addiction to such drugs as morphine and heroin. It is now well known in the United States that heroin was introduced as a nonaddictive cure for morphine addiction in the late 19th century. During that same misguided era, cocaine was often prescribed to help overcome morphine and alcohol addiction. The humiliation of medical science produced by the unexpected problems of heroin and other drug dependence led, in the middle of the 20th century, to an impressive clarification of the biological process of dependence on drugs like morphine, called opiates or opioids. This biological state of dependence on opiates was called addiction. The hallmarks of the addictive process were that the test drug—heroin, for example—could substitute for morphine (or other opiate) to prevent withdrawal, and that abrupt withdrawal of the test drug produced "classical withdrawal symptoms of the morphine type," including sweating, aches, and pains, as well as diarrhea and vomiting. Heroin and methadone, for example, can easily and completely substitute for morphine in such tests. Cocaine cannot. Animals addicted to morphine in laboratory studies, when they are switched from morphine to cocaine, experience withdrawal symptoms. Thus, using this model, it was concluded that cocaine was not addictive. Marijuana, incidentally, was also non-addictive in this sense. Since the 1940s, no new drug has been marketed with this opioid type of dependence without first having been identified as addicting.

This substantial scientific achievement has had one terribly negative effect: we have *overlearned* the lesson. A mistaken assumption has been widely created that drugs which do not produce dependence of this type are not addicting in the sense that they cannot produce severe, physically based drug dependence. This distinction (which required some new, semantically agile, but not truly scientific terms) led to separation of addictive from nonaddictive drugs, of hard drugs from soft drugs, and of physical dependence from psychological dependence. In all cases, the nonaddictive or "soft" drugs, which produced only psychological dependence were thought of as safe or at least safer. This is wrong. Many drugs, most notably cocaine, which fit the pattern of the nonaddicting, soft drugs which produce a psychological dependence, are highly reinforcing and dependence-producing. As I pointed out in Chapter 2, the critical question is "Does the drug produce pleasure?" or "Is the drug use self-reinforcing?" If the answers to both of these questions is "yes," then the drug is indeed addicting in the most meaningful sense of the word. The most important way the term *addiction* can be used in drug abuse prevention is to know whether the substance produces reinforcement and whether, when the drug is withdrawn, there is craving. On both these counts, cocaine is not only addictive, but it is *more addictive than heroin*.

Many modern apologists for cocaine have repeated the message of the 100-year-old, now discredited quotation from Sigmund Freud: "I discovered in myself and in other observers who were capable of judging such things that even repeated doses of cocaine produced no compulsive desire to use the stimulant further; on the contrary one feels a certain unmotivated aversion to the substance." What the apologists have conveniently forgotten is that Freud had made *the* classic mistake: he had misjudged the fundamental nature of the Drug Dependence Syndrome. He had been wrong in his assessment of cocaine's addictive potential. He observed only that in the *earliest stages* of cocaine use, which I have called the Experimentation and Occasional Use Stages, is there indeed no addiction. The novice user of any of the dependence-producing drugs easily concludes, as Freud did, that there is "no compulsive desire to use," and that there is even an "unmotivated aversion to the substance." Tens of millions of American teenagers have conducted the same misguided experiment themselves during the last two decades and reached the same conclusion Freud reached. And they have been just as tragically wrong as Freud was. When one separates the early stages of infrequent use of any drug from the later stages of frequent, dependent use, one necessarily misses the true nature of the syndrome, or the process of dependence.

The same sort of mental sleight of hand can be shown in separating cigarette smokers who get heart attacks and have lung cancer from those who do not. The latter group one could call "safe" smokers, and the former could be called "sick" smokers—those with a mysterious "disease." Since there are more of the latter than of the former, one might conclude that it is the illness of this group of cigarette smokers that is responsible for their problems—not their smoking. One can do the same with speeding drivers: separate those who speed and do not get killed from those who speed and are killed. The former are "social speeders," and the latter are "diseased." In these other areas, most of us now know that when we are trying to determine the risk of smoking or speeding, we must count *all* smokers and *all* speeders, not separate them into groups that are convenient for our purpose. In the drug field, however, many people—including more than a few experts and many millions of kids—have persisted in making this fundamental and tragic error of logic.

Cocaine's Cozy Cousin: ''Speed'' on the Fast Track

Another curious aspect of modern cocaine usage deserves to be highlighted. In the 1930s, a class of drugs called stimulants was first synthesized. Of these stimulants, amphetamine is the best-known example. Because of their stimulative effects, mimicking the body's alarm or sympathetic nervous system, they were appropriately called "speed" by drug users. Initially, these drugs were incorporated into medical practice as "safe and nonaddictive" treatments for many conditions, such as obesity and depression. This pattern, as you can see, is the old familiar one: A new drug is introduced as curative and safe. Then, in subsequent decades, the effectiveness of the drug is questioned, and its dependence-producing liability is recognized. Today, virtually the only legitimate uses for amphetamine and other drugs of this class are the paradoxical calming effect they have on hyperactive children and their effectiveness in the treatment of a rare sleep disorder, narcolepsy. Shortly after the stimulants became available for use in medical practice, they were picked up by drug abusers, first for oral use and later for intravenous injection. Amphetamine, taken intravenously, was common in Japan, Sweden, and the United States after World War II. Fortunately, this highly specific, short-lived drug epidemic was controlled fairly well through strict law enforcement.

Speed became popular by the intravenous route again in the early stages of the U.S. drug epidemic which began in the 1960s. The doses used were tremendous. The horrible consequences, from dependence to paranoia to death, were unmistakable. The sick, emaciated, paranoid, helpless "speed freak" became as characteristic of that era as the marijuana burn-out became 10 years later. This sad situation led, eventually, to imposition of strict controls over stimulant drugs worldwide and to the warning from the street-drug users themselves: "Speed Kills." After a peak on the West Coast in the late 1960s, intravenous amphetamine use dropped sharply but has not disappeared.

It is ironic and scientifically inappropriate that cocaine shares with amphetamines virtually all of the latter's toxic effects, and yet cocaine use, including intravenous injection, retains the glamour long since lost by speed. Studies using pure cocaine and pure amphetamine for intravenous use have shown that, when injected, even the most experienced intravenous cocaine user cannot distinguish cocaine from amphetamine. I wonder how long it will take for cocaine use to develop the same grubby image now attached by street users to amphetamines, and how long it will take for the drug users themselves to conclude that "Coke kills"? Maybe the day is not as far off as it seems. A high school girl recently told me that the most common graffiti in her suburban school's restrooms are dismal reports of cocaine problems. Someone, for instance, had scribbled "Cocaine" in bright red script on one wall. Later, someone else had marked over it in black with derogatory comments, including "Cocaine sucks" and "Cocaine is a bad trip." The recent leveling off of cocaine use rates, after rocket-like rises through the late 1970s, may reflect this late-developing awareness.

THE COCAINE STATE: GETTING HIGH . . . AND FALLING LOW

Feeling States and Consequent Vulnerability

How does it *feel* to take cocaine? By this time, you have probably formed a few general impressions, so let us take some time here to enlarge upon them and try to pull the picture into sharper focus. When cocaine is used, there is a sudden, specific, jolting impact on the central nervous system. This produces feeling states of euphoria and heightened alertness. There is a subjective sense of a diminished fatigue, making the cocaine state in some ways similar to the effect of coffee or amphetamine use. In contrast to the feelings produced by coffee, of course, those produced by cocaine are far more pervasive and intense, and, in contrast to amphetamines, they tend to be of relatively short duration. There are also the feeling states attendant upon other physical effects of cocaine: a rise in the body temperature, a rise in the pulse rate, an increase in the respiratory rate, etc.

The psychological states produced by cocaine use depend, as those of all psychoactive drugs do, on a complex interaction of the individual and the drug itself. The controlling variables include the amount of drug taken, the user's past history with the drug, the physical and psychological state of the user at the time he uses the drug, his expectations for the use, and many other factors. Working in combination, these variables make the drug effect far less predictable than a simple reading of a table of drug effects would lead you to believe. Alcohol is a good example of the varied, unpredictable effects which may be generated by a drug. Alcohol provides all too familiar evidence that the same drug produces many different effects in different people, and even on the same person at different times.

After a single use, the cocaine high lasts from 10 to 30 minutes. The most common reaction when it passes is to want more cocaine. A typical pattern involves use of the drug three or four times in the course of several hours. At the conclusion of such a run, the user generally feels tired, irritable, and depressed. These negative feelings can last for many hours and—along with the stuffy, runny nose—are often the most noticeable effects of cocaine use. Irritability and an unpleasant personality are common in the postcocaine state. The sad fact is, of course, that the "cure" for this dismal feeling is further use of cocaine, which is precisely the vicious cycle that cocaine users get into. Often, this cycle is interrupted only by the availability of money to support the cocaine habit.

VULNERABILITIES AND PREDISPOSITIONS
OR—FALLING INTO THE COCAINE DEPENDENCE TRAP

As is characteristic of all drug use, the cocaine user frequently progresses through stages beginning with experimentation and ending with dependence. As is the case with users of other drugs, however, the cocaine user does not inevitably progress through all four stages of the syndrome. Some people start and quickly stop cocaine use. Others use the drug in an apparently moderate and controlled fashion for short or long periods. Still others progress rapidly from experimentation to high-dose, compulsive cocaine use. While controversy on the subject continues in the scientific community, it seems clear that the psychological and physical characteristics of the user which predisposes to dependence have more to do with the willingness to use the drug heavily than with some deep, mysterious personal vulnerability or invulnerability to dependence itself.

Scientific studies of laboratory animals exposed to cocaine and other drugs tend to confirm this: Experiments with the self-administering of drugs clearly demonstrate that there are substantial differences between one animal and another in their willingness to use various drugs. Some of these differences seem to be genetically determined, others characterize whole species, and still other differences seem to relate to the specific drugs (no animals can be induced to self-administer LSD, for example). However, when given the drugs repeatedly (whether they take them voluntarily or involuntarily), the animals become dependent on the same drugs which produce human drug dependence. They then seek to self-administer the drug.

Psychological and physical factors do indeed seem to be key determinants. Thus, people who are already heavy drug users, people who are risk takers, and people who hold values permissive of drug use are more vulnerable to cocaine dependence. People with a family or personal history of drug dependence also seem more vulnerable to using cocaine heavily enough to produce dependence. It is also true that those who have large amounts of money or in some other way have easy access to a supply of cocaine are more vulnerable to progression from experimentation to dependence. Cocaine dealers, physicians, and others working with cocaine professionally are particularly vulnerable to trying the drug and, having tried it, to escalate its use to the point of severe dependence.

Victims of the Cocaine State

The victims are legion. One cocaine user I saw in treatment said he had used marijuana heavily since his teenage years and then began to use cocaine in his early 20s. He snorted the drug occasionally with few problems until several of his friends became cocaine dealers, and he suddenly found that cocaine was everywhere. That triggered an explosive rise in his levels of cocaine use and a rapid loss of control over it. His cocaine use, which had initially generated relatively few problems, abruptly produced a severe disruption in his work life and in his marriage which, in turn, forced him into treatment. Another patient entered treatment only after he was fired from a job for stealing to pay off his cocaine debts. In his teenage years he, too, began illicit drug use with marijuana and then added cocaine in his early 20s. The pattern of his cocaine use was destabilized when he began to shoot the drug intravenously. He promptly lost control of his cocaine use, and his life fell into complete disarray. A third pattern I have seen is for a relatively stable cocaine use level to deteriorate following some traumatic life experience, such as loss of a job or a divorce.

From such experiences certain warnings emerge: Anything that makes money or cocaine more available and anything that encourages more cocaine use can trigger a disastrous loss of control over the drug even in those who have controlled their use for relatively long periods of time. Anything that reduces social controls over drug use in general and cocaine use in particular, and anything that upsets one's life in ways that produce emotional turmoil and pain is likely to produce an escalation in cocaine use, with a resultant loss of apparently controlled-use patterns. When cocaine use becomes frequent and involves high doses, self-control is out of the question. And when loss of control has occurred—when the addiction switch is turned on—it is just as impossible for the cocaine user to return to controlled use as it is for a recovered alcoholic ever again to become a "social" drinker. The signals sent out here flash an unmistakable warning: Never fool yourself into thinking anyone can get away with "social coking," at least for long.

Cocaine and the Infrequent User: Where the Honeymoon Ends

Some cocaine users, and some cocaine experts who may read this account, will complain that I have been describing only the experience of the compulsive, high-dose user of the drug. Reacting to the negative portrait I have painted, they will ask, "But what about the *infrequent* user?" As is the case with the use of any dependence-producing drug, people in the early stages of the Drug Dependence Syndrome have few problems and hold the often-mistaken belief that they can control their drug use. Further, numerous people I have spoken with have tried cocaine once or twice and concluded that it "did nothing for me." This reaction will surprise some readers of this chapter, since I have portrayed cocaine as terribly seductive. In answer I cite again the implications of the Drug Dependence Syndrome. Cocaine fits right into the pattern of all dependence-producing drugs.

It takes time to learn to love cocaine. Early users, as we have seen, almost all have the illusion of safe, controlled consumption. Many people are saved from cocaine dependence by lack of contact with the drug and by personal values which discourage them from using it. Unfortunately for those who do try the drug, and for whatever reasons are willing to learn to love it, the consequences are disastrous. I hope the siren call of so-called experts and cocaine users in the honeymoon stage will not obscure the powerful and more relevant testimony of the hooked cocaine addicts. They are as tragically dependent drug users as I have ever seen.

One of my patients, a young bank executive, described his personal use of cocaine and its cost by saying that "running out of coke means running out of money." He buys coke in varying amounts, depending on his money supply. A "quarter" equals a fourth of a gram or about six to eight lines, or single doses, costing about $25. What he called "good" coke costs him as much as $150 a gram. "Good" coke might produce 50 lines, while "bad" coke might make only 30 lines. At times he would buy as much as one-eighth of an ounce, 3½ grams, for $350 or even more. Using one-half of a gram of coke in an hour of snorting it was "nothing," and he could shoot intravenously a similar amount in just 10 minutes.

He described one memorable experience when he went six or seven days without sleep, using cocaine all the time he was not at work. About the fifth day, he asked the buddy he was using cocaine with to tell him "How long has it been since we slept?" The answer: "About five days—I'm not sure." He had no idea how long he had been on this cocaine run. In retrospect, he calculated that he spent $2,000 that week for cocaine. The run ended when he was making a loan to a customer at the bank. He fell asleep while sitting at his desk and talking to the customer. He knew he was falling asleep and that it would jeopardize his job, but he could not resist sleep any longer— once he had run out of coke to keep going.

More typical for this man are coke runs from 2:00 P.M. (bank closing time) until 6:00 A.M. the following day. During such an average run, he uses two to four grams of cocaine costing $300 to $600. Once the coke run ends, he usually sleeps for 12 to 18 hours and then, if he has money, starts the cycle all over again. This same young man explained that high-dose use of coke produces tense, unpleasant feelings that he "needs to level out." He does this with depressant drugs—most often using alcohol—but frequently he also uses Valium and methaqualone. His favorite "downer" is heroin which, combined with cocaine, he calls "the top of the line."

SOME CONSEQUENCES OF COCAINE USE

Around His Neck the Albatross Clings . . . and Clings

The most common comment I have heard from cocaine users is the horrified, and belated, realization they have of their loss of control over their own lives as cocaine takes over. Their ensuing downward spiral parallels the decline of those monkeys, making cocaine in reality the fast track to calamity. Even in the late stages of this process, however, many cocaine users persist in thinking that cocaine use is generally easy to control, and that somehow they will again be able to control their own cocaine use. Rather than correctly seeing their current predicament as the all-but-inevitable result of their cocaine use, they see it as an accident or a slip.

In recent years, anonymous telephone hotlines have been established to provide information to drug users and those concerned about drug use. One, in New York, recently conducted a 30-minute interview of 55 callers concerned about their personal problems with cocaine. The findings illustrate the current consequences of cocaine use in America.

Note that this information is drawn from a sample of people who have recognized their problems with cocaine and who have called for information. As such it is, no doubt, a sample with both higher levels of cocaine use and cocaine problems, and a higher educational level than those of the typical cocaine user in this country. The average age of the callers was 33; 78 percent were male, and 50 percent had incomes of $25,000 or more. They spent an average of $800 a week for cocaine. Fifty-one percent reported that they only snorted the drug. The remainder also smoked it or injected it intravenously. More than one-half of the sample used cocaine at least five days a week.

When asked to describe their feelings on initially using cocaine, they said it made them feel in control, sexually aroused, talkative, energetic, confident, elated, and content. Most were amazed by their rapid progression from this positive feeling state to compulsive use of cocaine characterized by craving for the drug and loss of control over its use despite serious physical and psychological consequences.

In the later stages of their cocaine use, this sample reported the following consequences, which they attributed to their cocaine use: exhaustion, sleep disturbances, headaches, trembling, nausea, irritability, anxiety, confused thoughts, lack of motivation, disruption in work performance, and disturbances of relationships with family and friends. Forty-seven percent reported paranoid thoughts, 20 percent reported panic attacks, 18 percent felt violent, and six of the 55 had injured another person while intoxicated on cocaine. Sixteen percent had hallucinations, and six of the 55 had grand mal epileptic seizures with loss of consciousness.

Significantly, serious physical and mental problems were reported equally by those only snorting the drug. These and similar difficulties were reported by those using cocaine relatively lightly, even those using only one to five grams per week.

Billy Ylvisaker: The Personal Story of a Cocaine User

As accounts of cocaine tragedies have mounted in the popular press and virtually all of the mass media have given significant attention to cocaine, one brief biographical sketch from *Newsweek* will illustrate the current sad state of affairs. As you read this article, recall that most people who begin cocaine use think the drug is harmless and that they can easily control their use of the drug. Also recall those monkeys who were given free access to cocaine and how they chose cocaine over food (when starving), over sex (when it was easily available to them), and even when they had to endure painful electric shocks when they got the drug. Recall also that until those monkeys died of cocaine overdoses, not one of them could stop using the drug.

Throwing It All Away*

By Pete Axthelm

On Saturday night, Billy Ylvisaker danced with his girlfriend at the Cartier Ball, on the splendid grounds of the Palm Beach Polo and Country Club. The party tent was as reasonable a facsimile of the Place Vendome as a few hundred thousand dollars' worth of carpentry could achieve. The fun also felt vaguely sculpted, ordered, man-made. Revelers arrived on time, ate the masterfully catered courses on schedule, left shortly after midnight. After all, there would be polo the next day. Most would watch, some would play.

Billy Ylvisaker played very well Sunday afternoon. His five-goal handicap, on a scale on which 10 is perfection, placed him among the 56 best Americans in the sport. Sunday he looked even better than that, meshing his horsemanship smoothly with the headlong rushes of his team's 10-goal Argentine star Gonzalo Tanoira and the fierce thrusts of his father and teammate, Bill Sr. The Ylvisakers' team lost narrowly, but Billy scored three goals and accepted hugs and congratulations amid the traditional postmatch champagne sipping.

No Dilettante: Billy had other reasons for the broad smile and dancing eyes beneath his tousled blond hair. He had just signed on to play this summer with Tommy Wayman, the Oklahoma-born hero who is one of only two American 10-goalers. There were also plans for a campaign in England, where Billy had already beaten Prince Charles and met the queen. Perhaps most satisfying of all, Billy sold a pony that day for a lot of money. In the delicate pro-amateur balance of high-style international polo, the development and sale of top horses are among the qualities that distinguish the pros. Bill Ylvisaker Sr. happens to be a hugely successful business entrepreneur as well as the

---

*"Throwing It All Away," *Newsweek*, April 11, 1983. Reprinted by permission.

major force behind polo in America. But son Billy was no idle-rich dilettante. Sunday's events confirmed him as a horseman, athlete, pro. He told friends he was planning to do some celebrating.

The party began at sundown at the Players' Club. It ended less than 12 hours later in the bathroom of Billy's home on the ambitious Wellington sports and housing complex that his father has carved out of a vast barren tract west of Palm Beach. Sarah Port, Billy's girlfriend, found his body. He had snorted a large amount of cocaine and injected some intravenously. Friends recalled that he had struggled with a drug problem some years ago, but they thought he had licked it. They were wrong. Billy was 27 when he died last week.

The funeral took place Wednesday in a modest church called St. David's in the Pines. Billy's favorite pony stood under tack outside. His dog Brandy romped nearby. The mourners sat on folding chairs and listened to a service said by Father John Mangrum, known as the "polo priest." Then Bill Ylvisaker Sr. rose and spoke with sad and savage eloquence. "I guess you all know my son died of an overdose of cocaine. What a waste. I can only hope that there will be a lesson in this terrible occurrence for some young people somewhere."

The lesson has been cried out and unheard depressingly often in sports as in life. We have sorrowed for the needle-tracked wizards of the ghetto hoops, the naive and cocky kids who figured that all the big stars dabbled in coke, the faded shells who played too long at a high-stakes game that they hollowly labeled "recreational." But for those of us who knew Billy and his world, his demise is worth crying out once more. This was a high-spirited young man with almost everything. His death is a grim tribute to the lure of white lines and smooth mirrors on the path toward nothingness.

Bill Ylvisaker Sr., a man of sweeping vision and fiery intensity, never dreamt of such a turn to darkness. He is chairman and chief executive officer of Gould Inc., a $2 billion conglomerate. It has more than a hundred subsidiaries worldwide. Palm Beach Polo, which is merely the most opulent sports venue imaginable, is one of the smallest Gould holdings. But it is Bill's best-loved project. His boiling energies have shaped both the place and the entire game of polo.

The Ylvisaker children were hardly spoiled. One daughter is a jewelry designer, another a college student. The eldest, Laurie, is an effective publicity director who has helped spur the expanding interest in polo. Like his father, Billy asked no favors and took pride in toughness and challenges. A poor student, he was struggling at junior college when he decided he would like to play polo at the University of Virginia. The school demanded that he fashion a straight-A semester in JC to earn that. Billy did it.

Achievement: Similarly, he was not satisfied to be one of the wealthy patrons who pay the feed and tack bills for the privilege of riding with the 10-goal stars. His game improved steadily in recent years, and the elite of international polo respected him as a peer and a friend. Under the peculiar code of the polo life, the achievement was considerable.

"A player must be judged by his conduct, on and off the fields," explains Memo Gracida, the second American 10-goaler. "He can lose respect not just by playing poorly or dirty, but by behaving rudely at a party or putting a pony's bandages on sloppily." Tommy Wayman's wife, Rosemary, adds: "Polo is a passport to the whole world, but you have to keep earning it."

By all accounts, Billy Ylvisaker earned it. Perhaps that memory will fortify his father as he reaches down for a toughness that not even more than 100 subsidiaries ever demanded. Maybe, under some striped party tent after the pain is dulled by time, it will even allow Billy's friends to raise stemmed glasses to recall the best and boldest days of his fast, brief life. As the polo goes on this month and for winters and springs to come, there will probably be tournaments or trophies honoring his name or reflecting his image. Billy's father knew a better way, as he said at the funeral. The truest honor would be to remember all that a young man can erase with a jab of a needle into a vein.

Understanding Sudden Cocaine Deaths

Despite the common perception among users that cocaine is a safe drug, there are increasing numbers of cocaine users who die suddenly, apparently from doses of the drug they had used previously without noticeable ill effects. In many cases, sudden death occurs even when the drug is snorted, rather than just being smoked or injected intravenously.

There are at least two likely mechanisms for these cocaine deaths. The first is the powerful and often unpredictable effect of cocaine on the heart. Among all cocaine users there is an increase in heart rate and blood pressure which is more intense the more cocaine is used. However, for some users at some times, cocaine use, even at relatively moderate doses, produces a sudden, extreme increase in the heart rate, leading to the heart literally quivering rather than beating. When this happens, blood is no longer pumped, and the user dies if he does not receive instantaneous medical assistance. This sometimes happens in surgery when cocaine is used as an anesthetic agent, but there it is relatively easily managed and is unlikely to produce death. Some surgeons have stopped using the drug because of this problem. Researchers using cocaine also must be prepared for this problem.

When such an event occurs as part of illicit cocaine use, sudden death is the likely outcome.

Cocaine also reduces the seizure threshold, sometimes producing epileptic seizures. In high doses, and apparently even in low doses through the mechanism of kindling, cocaine can produce sudden death. This process deserves explanation. Cocaine used repeatedly, even at low doses, produces a progressively increasing risk of epileptic seizures, even when the drug is taken by inhaling it up the nose. Because cocaine commonly is taken repeatedly over a relatively short period of time, this process builds through a mechanism known by neurologists as *kindling*. It is well known in neurology that repeated, subseizure stimuli can reduce the brain's resistance to seizures. This, along with the heart rhythm problem, may explain the increasingly common experience of sudden death by cocaine users, even when the dose of cocaine used is not unusual for them. Both mechanisms can produce death without warning.

THE TREATMENT OF COCAINE DEPENDENCE

Overcome the Twin Fallacies of *"Safety" and "Easy Control"*

Treatment of cocaine dependence is just one part of the larger problem of drug dependence treatment which is dealt with in Chapter 7. There are several problems, however, which can be usefully highlighted here. Cocaine treatment is made more difficult precisely because so many cocaine users, even after having terrible problems, believe that they can again control their cocaine use. This is a characteristic that cocaine shares with alcohol and marijuana because those two drugs also are widely thought of as safe and easily controlled. These drugs are not only the GATEWAY into drug dependence, but for many attempting to recover from dependence by entering drug abuse treatment, they are the GATEWAY *back* to drug dependence. Both sad facts are traceable to the same misperception: the images of safety and controllability which these drugs have. Complete and permanent abstinence must be established early and firmly if treatment for cocaine dependence is to be successful. It is, in my experience, vital to engage the user's family in the treatment procedures to reinforce this process. Family members can help the user cope with the family problems which may have served to encourage the cocaine dependence and which are surely the result of that dependence.

Treat with Antidepressant Drugs—But Sparingly

Because depression is such a common part of the postcocaine
state, I have found the use of antidepressant (and non-dependence-
producing) drugs helpful in some cases. These drugs, of which amitriptyline and imipramine are the most commonly prescribed, often
help remove the characteristic depression and insomnia which almost
invariably prove troubling for the recovering cocaine-dependent person.

Use Inpatient Treatment—If and When Needed

Inpatient treatment may be necessary to stop the use of cocaine. It
need not be extended beyond about a month. Usually, such a drug-
free period is necessary to rescue the cocaine user from his compulsion and to reassure him about the symptoms he experiences during
the withdrawal.

As a Final Step, ``Hook'' the Patient into the Anonymous Programs

Inpatient treatment also can be useful in "hooking" the cocaine-
dependent person into the Anonymous programs, Narcotics Anonymous and Alcoholics Anonymous. A new member of the Anonymous
families has been created recently: Cocaine Anonymous. The increasing cocaine problem in the United States is reflected in the rapid
growth of this movement, which sponsors 35 meetings a week in Los
Angeles alone. This self-help, over the long haul (one or more meetings
a day for the first 90 days is a good rule to start with), not infrequently
spells the difference between recovery and relapse. Once the cocaine-
dependent person is drug-free and is rooted in the Anonymous programs, then productive psychotherapy can proceed. I tell recovering
drug-dependent people that they will probably not feel themselves to
be "normal" for at least a year after becoming drug-free.

While there are no firm figures yet, the common clinical impression
is that, after treatment, relapse is even more common among cocaine-
dependent people than among other drug abusers. This may be
partly because of the intensity of the cocaine high, but I think that
many times it reflects the often-ambivalent view of both the therapist
and the patient about the seriousness of the cocaine habit. Relapse is
less likely to occur if the full, life-threatening gravity of the disorder is
faced squarely and relentlessly.

SUMMING UP

- Cocaine, more than any other drug, merits this admonition: Don't Try It; You Might Like It!
- If you have not used cocaine, don't start it. If you use cocaine, stop. If you cannot stop, get help.
- If someone you know is using cocaine, help him or her to stop. Don't take no for an answer if you care for that person.
- The glitzy image of cocaine, combined with its undeserved reputation for safety, makes cocaine the drug most likely to show an epidemic rise in the 1980s.
- As with any drug, the initial use of cocaine may be inconsequential or even negative. One use does not an addict make. But, socializing with other drug takers, the novice cocaine user is commonly taught how to get high. From there, the novice moves into the supposedly safe, easily controlled honeymoon stage of regular cocaine use. Later, if use continues, comes the crash: compulsive cocaine dependence with multiple physical and psychological problems and an inability to stop cocaine use.
- For many of America's 22 million cocaine users, about one of five who have tried the drug so far, it was a passing fancy. They appear to have stopped cocaine use. For those other 80 percent—a total of more than 17 million Americans—cocaine use is continuing. Nearly 2 million new cocaine users are added each year in the United States and about a quarter of these are 17 years of age or younger. These people are the ticking cocaine time bomb in the American drug scene.
- The consequences of continued cocaine use range from a runny nose to a sudden, unpredictable death.
- Financial problems brought on by cocaine use can be severe and relentless. Aside from health considerations, the most likely consequence from continued use of the drug is loss of control over money as the illicit substance assumes an ever-greater priority in the user's life. Compulsive users will often go to any lengths to get it. Formerly law-abiding men and women will steal from their employers and starve their families. Broken homes are common.
- Coke, as in cocaine, is not "The Real Thing." It is the great deceiver and the great destroyer, as Americans first painfully learned 100 years ago and then again 50 years ago, but seem to have forgotten today.

PART THREE

How Can Families Prevent and Treat Drug Problems?

CHAPTER
SIX

Parents and Kids:
Kids Can Be Kids Only If
Parents Are Parents

WORKING TOGETHER, IN FAMILIES, to help children grow to adulthood free of drug and alcohol dependence, is the subject of this chapter. Having described, in Chapter 2, the Drug Dependence Syndrome and having explored, in Chapters 3, 4, and 5, the three GATEWAY DRUGS through which virtually all Americans who become drug dependent begin their drug use, we now explore the family as the best resource for drug abuse prevention. Drug use is often first identified by the user's family because many of the first and most serious consequences of drug use occur in the family. The family is also the key to solving a drug problem once it has begun.

I define *families* as all the people usually living with and related to growing children. The people who care for the growing child and the maturing adolescent and who live under the same roof, plus those who are related to the child, I call family. The most prevalent pattern even today in America is the nuclear family of two parents and one or more children, with or without nearby aunts, uncles, cousins, and grandparents. The reality of family life has, of course, always been far more complex than that simple model suggests. Complicating this picture of American family life are such recent changes as increased geographic mobility, which has reduced the available family network, increased the number of women in the paid work force, increased rates of divorce and remarriage, and reduced the number of children parents have. Nevertheless, virtually all children in the United States today have adults living with them and caring for them. As I have observed them, these adults, usually parents, love their children and are highly motivated to help them grow up healthy. Similarly, most children recognize their dependence on the adults in their family and are eager to have family support and love. This chapter is written to strengthen and enhance these positive, shared family goals.

A FAMILY WORKS TOGETHER TO SOLVE
A DRUG PROBLEM: AN EXAMPLE

In developing these goal-centered principles, let me begin by describing a real-life family facing the problems this chapter is designed to solve. Charlie was 14 years old when he was brought to me by his mother and father, Susan and Bill. They had been divorced six years, and both had remarried and started new families. Charlie lived with his father except on Thursdays and alternating weekends, when he lived with his mother. Charlie had been doing well in school until this last year when, in the eighth grade, his academic performance fell noticeably. One night, dead drunk, he came home to his mother's house. She put him to bed. The next day she called his father for a family conference. They discovered that Charlie had become involved with two friends who lived near his mother's home and who were heavy users of alcohol and other drugs. They also learned that this behavior had been going on for several months. Charlie said he got bored from time to time and just went along with the other boys when they drank. He said he had only smoked marijuana a couple of times because he feared he would get caught. He was afraid of what his father would do if he found out he used pot.

Insofar as possible punishment for drinking was concerned, however, Charlie said, "I wasn't really scared of Dad. He has never hurt me or anything." Charlie had an uncle who was, at age 33, a severe alcoholic. Bill and Susan drank very little and never used other drugs. Charlie, who had recently been reading a great deal about drugs and alcohol, described how a few months earlier at band practice he had pulled out some antidrug pamphlets he had picked up at a local pharmacy. They listed a "whole lot of drugs most of us had never heard of," he explained. "We laughed about wanting to try them all. We didn't do it, but that was the first step."

Bill spoke in the initial psychotherapy session of his long-remembered experience when he was Charlie's age. His own father had been both very strict and emotionally cold. Without any discussion whatsoever he had told Bill that if he ever drank he would "kill" him. Bill had a hard childhood. From an early age he worked diligently, first in high school and then to put himself through college. He was now proud of his well-paying job. "I wanted," he said, "to make Charlie's life different from mine. I did not want him to be afraid of me. I did not want him to have to go out to work right away, because I wanted him to have a chance to do a lot of things I never did get to do, like being in sports and having fun with friends. Now I see that, by trying to make life easier for him, I have hurt him."

Charlie said he knew that drugs and alcohol were dangerous but that those possibilities were far off and seemed not to apply to him. Susan said she felt helpless. Her other children were still preschoolers, but Charlie was bigger than she was. She felt he would not obey her if she set limits on him, that "He would just walk out and say 'I'm doing it anyway!' or run back to his father's place." In reacting to this, Charlie insisted, "You never did tell me not to do anything."

I met with this family only three times in psychotherapy sessions over a six-week period. We reviewed the problems of drugs and alcohol in modern America, especially for young teenagers. I told Bill, Susan, and Charlie that many children of this age had unstable identities and unstable emotions; that not only were they volatile, but they also were easily influenced by whomever they are with. We talked about family values and the need for Charlie's parents to establish clear expectations and limitations for his behavior, including saying no to drug and alcohol use. They must enforce their rules swiftly, I told them. Charlie's totally unacceptable drinking and subsequent behavior had to be connected directly and immediately to a *consequence*, a penalty. That is, Charlie must be made to understand fully that he does not have to wreck a car or get cirrhosis of the liver to figure out that something bad will happen to him if he drinks.

Wondering if he had done his son a disservice by being so reasonable, Bill was understandably concerned about making a strong commitment to talking all these problems over with Charlie. Charlie himself provided the answer: "I like the talking, and I am glad you respect me, but I need you to be tough on me."

When I last saw this family, Charlie had not had a drop of alcohol for six weeks, his grades had improved, he had joined the baseball team, and he had stopped seeing his drinking friends. I asked him why he had stopped drinking. "I am afraid of my dad," he said, "Plus, I wanted to stop all along. Besides, baseball practice is more fun than drinking. I am still bored sometimes, and I think about doing it again."

We spoke together of the importance of values and rules in life: how important it is not to lie or cheat or steal. How important it is not to use drugs or alcohol. How important it is to work hard, including studying, doing work around the house, and working on athletics. We also spoke of the importance of Charlie's parents being strict enforcers of their rules and not just "discussion group leaders" or "good buddies." We spoke of the importance of those with whom we spend our time because we are all likely to adopt the values of our friends.

Six weeks is not a long follow-up period in situations of this kind. Nevertheless, I felt good about this family. They had worked through something together. Their commitment to sharing and to loving each other was more likely to work now that they had added a concern about drug and alcohol problems and had set up a family program to discourage the use of such drugs.

WHAT DO TEENAGERS WANT?/WHAT DO PARENTS WANT?

Recently, when I spoke to a group of parents and teenagers about problems they shared, I asked the audience what they wanted from each other. The teenagers had one major message for their parents: they wanted to be *listened to*. They wanted concern and respect. They wanted time and attention from their parents. If the kids did not feel listened to at home, they said, they felt listened to by their friends. The parents, too, had one predominant message: they wanted their children to *behave*. They were preoccupied with their children's behavioral problems—or threats of behavioral problems. These included poor grades, disrespect for parents, neglect of teen- agers' responsibilities around the home, use of alcohol and other drugs, early sexual activity, and delinquency. The enemy for the parents was the "peer group."

The next day, in my private practice, I saw a family in which the 31-year-old son, who had never made it as an independent adult, was hooked on a narcotic which he got by forging prescriptions. His parents had spent $50,000 during the preceding year on legal and psychiatric bills for their son, and—since he seemed no better—they wanted my advice. Two days later I saw a family concerned about a 14-year-old daughter who was using marijuana and threatening to run away from home if her parents placed what she considered unreason- able restrictions on her. Both of these situations reflected failed ad- olescence. To many Americans today, adolescence is a mess. When alcohol and drug use are added, the mess becomes deadly.

Although every family situation is unique, in the United States today there is an easily recognized pattern to the problems faced by parents and teenage children beset by drug abuse and its attendant problems. Teenagers, for example, rarely present themselves to par- ents or other adults, including psychiatrists, saying, "I have a drug problem and I need help." In fact, from the teenager's point of view, the experiences are defined not in terms of his or her drug use, but in terms of the "hassles" imposed on the teenager by "unreasonable" adults, most often by parents and teachers. Parents, on the other hand, almost invariably define the conflict between them and their teenage child as being the result of drug use, thinking that if only the drug use would stop, all problems would stop.

After years of work with hundreds of families, I am convinced that both are right and that both are wrong. The most important need is for clear guidelines which can be shared by parents and teenagers, based on easily understood principles both can respect. What follows is my attempt to provide such guiding principles. These basic, practical guidelines are designed to help families to think together about what is going wrong and what they can do to make their families function better. For some whose pain is most severe, they may seem remote; however, even these families will find the principles useful.

This is not a "cookbook" approach for solving all family problems; it is a set of simple guidelines which can be applied to specific family problems. My hope is that by reading these pages and by thinking quietly, families will be able to understand the source of their pain and will be able to find their own unique ways to set things right. In my own practice of psychiatry, I have had the privilege of working with many families facing difficulties involving drugs and other problems. Those who have succeeded in solving them have used the principles I describe here. In fact, this chapter reflects my collaboration with these families. It is dedicated to all of them with my thanks for what they have taught me.

What follows in this chapter are my suggestions for structuring relationships between parents and children, along with my strongly expressed views about the importance of establishing the goal of helping children grow to adulthood free of drug use. Many experts do not agree with me. Many families function well by using different organizations and sharing different goals. I am not so narrow-minded as to think my suggestions are the only right way. I do believe the guiding principles I have suggested make sense, and I have seen them work. I have worked with many families in trouble who have adopted these guidelines and found them useful. However, even if you disagree with my suggestions, and even if you adopt different guidelines for your family, I ask you to do two things. First, consider my suggestions. Second, think through your own values, relationships, and goals, making a conscious and shared *family* decision about how you plan to help your children grow up. If your approach works, fine. If it does not work for you, consider making a change to better achieve your family's goals.

CHILDHOOD—LATE ADOLESCENCE—ADULTHOOD: SOME ESSENTIAL DISTINCTIONS

In seeking a simple, understandable structure for the crucial life stage called adolescence, we need first to define two basic terms, childhood and adulthood, and draw some careful distinctions. Childhood is defined as the age, usually all of those years leading up to and including the 18th year, when the young person lives under the parental roof and is supported and "raised" by the parents. In the United States, for most families, that means childhood extends through the high school years. In terms of what happens during childhood—before age 19—it is important to recognize that *the period of adolescence is a part of childhood and not part of adulthood.* This means that parents have not only the right but also the responsibility to set limits on the child's behaviors, behaviors ranging from allocation of studying time, to conforming to curfews, to the use of alcohol and other drugs. During this period, when and if a child finds parental rules and expectations onerous or unbearable, the solution—ultimately—is for the child to assume, prematurely, adult status. This means that the child leaves home prior to age 19.

Here I am not describing the all but universal outbursts of frustration and rebellion which characterize adolescent-parent interactions from time to time. These are usually managed by letting time pass so that tempers cool by reasonable discussion and—in many cases—by compromise based on mutual respect for the purposes of the rules sometimes considered by the teenagers to be intolerable. Rather, I am raising at this early stage the ultimate and too often paralyzing threat feared by parents: sustained teenage rebellion against parental rules *after* time has passed and *after* all efforts at discussion and compromise have failed. For a variety of reasons, I strongly discourage the radical course of action of children leaving home. Leaving home prior to age 19 puts the adolescent at a considerable disadvantage in competing with his or her peers for jobs and for marital success. This is a serious drawback, not only for the short time period until the "home leaver" reaches 19, but for many years beyond. Among its many other disadvantages, such premature adulthood usually puts an immediate end to formal education and, often, leads to unfortunate involvements in premature sexual behaviors, as well as raising the risk of long-term drug and alcohol dependence.

Identifying and resolving conflicts between parents and teenagers will be dealt with extensively in later sections of this chapter. As I have just said, I strongly discourage forcing teenagers to leave home;

I strongly encourage resolution of conflicts between parents and children. But it must be clear that the final decisions remain the responsibility of the parents, and if these cannot be accepted by the teenager or if compromise cannot be worked out, *then* the parental authority is preeminent. Here, at the outset, let me clearly state what I do *not* recommend: an approach to conflict between parents and teenagers which concludes that, no matter what the problems the child has and no matter how rebellious he or she may be against the parents' requirements, the child must be permitted to remain at home because the alternatives in the community are so negative. This, in my view, is accepting blackmail, and sooner or later it will undermine *all* effective family solutions to drug and alcohol problems.

Adulthood, as I define it, is reached when the maturing child assumes financial responsibility to support himself or herself. This definition is central to my approach, so I will repeat it. Adulthood arrives when the young person is no longer financially dependent upon parents for food, shelter, clothing, health care, education, transportation, or any other benefits normally provided by parents during childhood. Again I stress this point: late adolescence is *not* a part of adulthood; rather, late adolescence is a transition interval between the two life stages of childhood and adulthood, and it is a part of childhood.

I strongly recommend that families plan for the age of 19 to be the time at which the child becomes an adult. The specific date for this transfer, the 19th birthday of the child, should be talked about, understood, and agreed upon by all concerned members of the family *early* in the child's growth to maturity—no later, certainly, than his or her entry into teenhood. It should come as no surprise or sudden jolt to anyone. *Planning* is the key word. This means, of course, that both the parents and the child fully understand that at age 19 the child leaves the parental home and assumes the responsibilities of *self-support*. Of course, the lifting of the parental yoke does not mean that, after adolescence, parents cannot help their children or that children can no longer depend on parents. It does mean, however, that when adolescence ends, the relationship between parents and child changes profoundly, and the primary responsibility for the child's behavior shifts from the parent to the now young adult.

Admittedly, some young people are not ready to support themselves financially at age 19 because they want to pursue their education at college, in specialized job- or career-training programs, in apprenticeships of one kind or another, or in some other line of educational endeavor. For many youths this is desirable because additional education or training will assist the young person in his or her functioning as an adult. Therefore, for many American families today—perhaps as many as half of them—the timetable based on age 19 needs to be modified. In cases of this kind, I suggest that an extension of adolescence beyond age 19 is reasonable and, often, even desirable for both parents and offspring. However, if such an extension of childhood is agreed to by parents and child, then it carries with it the explicit understanding that parental guidance and responsibility are likewise extended, voluntarily and by mutual agreement, beyond age 19.

More specifically, if such an extension is worked out, it must be clearly understood by all concerned that the young person agrees to accept continuing parental supervision over such typical behaviors as acceptable scholastic achievement as measured by grades, the nonuse of alcohol and other drugs, and the avoidance of other potentially harmful behaviors. If all or part of the necessary financial support is to be provided for the child beyond the age of 18, parents can and should set the conditions for this. Such an extension is, moreover, to be granted only if both the youth and the parents consider it in their best interests. If a mutually satisfying agreement cannot be worked out along these lines, then the extension should be denied and the child should become an adult at age 19. This extension principle has important practical implications for the roles of both parents and children which will be dealt with later; here, only the principle needs to be understood.

Before proceeding, however, some clarification is in order. Some readers may conclude that I am suggesting the college student should relate to his parents just as the junior high school or high school student relates to his parents. Far from it. As the child matures, the relationship changes and the child becomes progressively more independent. However, if the parents continue to support the child financially, then this growing independence should be exercised *within* the values of the parents. Successful parents and children generally do this almost instinctively. However, it is also, sadly, common for college youths to accept parental support and then to violate the parental rules and values. Parents may choose to accept this. I have found that such acceptance generally reduces the child's chances of actually completing college and successfully establishing himself or herself as an independent adult.

The parents should think this issue through carefully and make a conscious choice. The choice, at least, belongs to the parents. Too often in recent years parents have simply failed to consider the issue, acting as if their child were entitled to such financial support despite the child's behavior. The criterion for deciding what to do should be the parents' judgment of the child's own long-term interests. When that criterion is applied, I believe, many parents will decide to make college financial support for their children far more conditional than they have in recent years.

Adolescence and Its Purposes

After years of working with young people and their families, I am convinced that among both parents and children the major problem is a failure to understand what adolescence *is* and what it is *for*. Let us return, therefore, to some basics. Chronologically, *adolescence* extends roughly from the ages of 12 through 18 years (see Figure 2). Conveniently, but not entirely accurately, I have referred to it as a

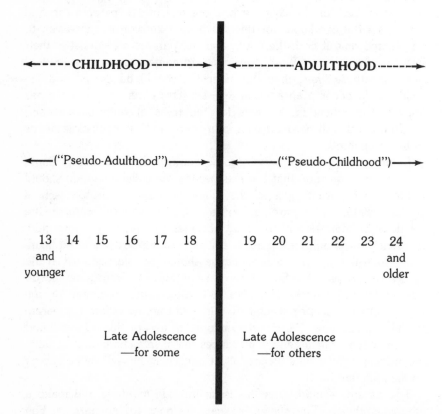

FIGURE 2.   Childhood and Adulthood: Some Chronological Distinctions

transitional period or phase. But, though it passes in a short span of years, it is neither temporary nor transitory in its effects. More accurately, perhaps, adolescence can be described as a living, swiftly alternating mosaic of chronological, academic, biological, emotional, social, and intellectual elements which young people struggle bravely and often desperately to piece together. As one teenager explained it: "Adolescence is something parents like to forget they ever went through. I feel like I'm too old to be a child and too young to be an adult. And that's hard to live with."

This "too old to be a child and too young to be an adult" segment of late adolescence is the principal focus of this chapter. This period usually extends from about ages 15 to 18. Considering that the human life expectancy of the average American is now more than 70 years, the most remarkable characteristic of the period between the time the maturing child feels stirrings of wanting to throw off parental control and the time the young person can become independent as an adult is surprisingly short. In fact, of all the phases of the human life cycle, the late-adolescence phase is one of the shortest. For an individual child, the period of late adolescence usually lasts no more than three or four years.

Late adolescence is the time of development to "make it on your own—away from parents." During late adolescence, most intense are the tensions between freedom and responsibility, between new and often personal or peer-centered values, and the values of the family and its traditions. Late adolescence is the period of forming a personal and, frequently, life-long identity. The most basic decisions relating to life's two great purposes—love and work—are made by most people during their late adolescent years. In the sense I am using the term, late adolescence is the time between the youth's first wanting to leave parental control and the time when the control is removed by the parents. The most significant and momentous part of this process is the end, for the end, in a very special sense, of this fateful phase is the beginning of adulthood. It is that moment when parents say to their child who in years past has been their responsibility: "We've given you our best. From here on, it's up to you." That moment is the end of childhood and the beginning of adulthood.

Thus the late-adolescence period, if successfully completed, always ends the same way: the child becomes an adult. It is at that point— the end point—that I want to begin our understanding. The goal of this stage of development is the same for both parents and children: *to do all that can reasonably be done to help the growing child acquire the skills, including educational skills and interpersonal skills and self-*

control skills, which will maximize the young person's ability to function as an adult. That is to say, the single, overriding purpose in this roughly four-year span of life which I have called late adolescence is the highly important preparation which the young person—assisted by parents, teachers, and others—must make in order to be able to leave home and make his or her way in the world as a responsible and contributing grown-up.

The Time-Limited Nature of the "Growing Up" Process

Much of the alienation between parents and children during the last two decades has come about because this basic goal has been lost sight of. Many of the recent and current problems we have had with adolescence have arisen because of the widespread failure to understand clearly the purpose of this brief episode in the overall life cycle, as well as to grasp fully the time-limited nature of the growing-up process. In contemporary America, much dismay, doubt, and even despair have crept into relationships between parents and teenagers because of the failure to distinguish between childhood and adulthood and the extremely crucial years of late adolescence.

When I see adolescents who are in deep conflict with their parents over rules and expectations, my clear articulation of the purpose of adolescence—"to do whatever is reasonable to prepare the young person to function as an adult at age 19"—has a sobering effect. For parents who feel exhausted by their struggles with their children, putting an end-date to these struggles—"your job ends when your child reaches age 19"—is often a great relief. Many parents have said to me, in effect: "Oh, I didn't realize this pain had an end. I can hang on *that* long." Frequently, their children are similarly relieved as they realize: "Well, whatever my parents say or do, it's not too long until I'm free." Not far below the surface, however, is the realization by both parents and children that—together—they have things of great importance to accomplish prior to the time when the youth is to assume adult status, and they had all better settle down to the hard work that requires.

"Pseudo-Adult" and "Pseudo-Child": To Be or Not to Be?

Too many parents have given their 12- to 18-year-olds too much responsibility for their own behavior. Too many teenagers are treated by their parents (and expect to be treated by their parents) as "Pseudo-Adults" who have the rights and independence of adulthood, but without the responsibilities that go with that status. Too many American young people in their 20s and 30s are still being treated as "Pseudo-Children" by their well-meaning but misguided parents who try to protect them from the consequences of their misbehaviors and rescue them from their self-created and often illegal messes. "Pseudo-Adulthood" and "Pseudo-Childhood" are, in reality, terrible distortions: they are crippling to the child and exceedingly painful to both parent and child. Pseudo-Adults do not learn how to discipline themselves. They turn virtually all their life problems into conflicts with their parents, as do Pseudo-Children.

Rather than establish and enforce firm rules, some parents—when confronted by the desire to treat their dependent children as adults rather than children—hide behind the rationalization that "Children need to learn to be adults by making their *own* decisions." This is a parental cop-out. Sure, kids need to learn to be adults, but not by doing anything and everything they please. That is poor preparation for adulthood. Children need to learn to become adults by understanding, accepting, and working within reasonable rules for behavior, including participation in a family life and avoidance of alcohol and other drug use. An intelligent parent does not teach a three-year-old about the dangers of crossing the street by "letting her learn for herself," any more than a parent should teach a 16-year-old about the dangers of drug use by "letting him learn for himself." Family rules and moral values in general are distillations of countless generations of learning. They are to be respected and treasured.

The wise and effective parent not only enforces necessary rules and worthwhile values; he or she helps the child see beyond them to the working principles which underpin them. It is in these principles that we find our full humanness—and our strength. Parents not so wise and effective will sometimes say they would rather have their teenage children use marijuana and alcohol at home than somewhere else. In this fashion, they rationalize allowing underage children to have alcohol at parties given in their homes. This, too, reflects a tragic misunderstanding of contemporary American law and of immutable biology. It makes about as much sense as for parents to conclude that "Since kids will have sex anyway, why not give them the master bedroom for the evening so they won't be cramped in the backseat of the family car?" Age-specific and role-specific rules for behavior are not only desirable, but also essential for both parents and teenagers. Without them, Pseudo-Children remain dependent on their parents and virtually helpless as the rewards and punishments normally built into life are mitigated by parental protection.

Put in its simplest and most direct terms, what I am saying is this: *Parents should treat kids who are 18 and under as kids, and they should treat young persons who are 19 and over as adults.* Parents holding tenaciously on to Pseudo-Children, children over the age of 18 who are unable to manage their lives and who remain dependent on their parents, are confronted by an especially difficult dilemma. How can they turn their child "out into the street"? Many times I encounter families who, because of love or guilt or misplaced compassion, try to justify treating their dependent adult-children as children rather than as adults. This does no genuine good for either the child or the parent, and there would be far less of it if children knew at a young age that they will pass from the role of child to the role of adult at age 19 and that, when they attain that age, parents will not rescue them from their own inappropriate or bad behavior.

Families seeking help with this problem can find it in the self-help movement. Both Families Anonymous and Al-Anon, the family support group for members of Alcoholics Anonymous, deal predominantly with this issue, and both are listed in the telephone book. These organizations help families put a stop to their enabling behavior, behavior which actually encourages drug use by overage Pseudo-Children by protecting them from the consequences of their use of alcohol and other drugs.

At this point I should mention also that, although this chapter deals directly with parents and teenagers coping with the use of alcohol and other drugs, the basic principles are generally applicable to many other family problems. I have seen families where distortions of the role relationships between parents and children do not involve use of alcohol or other drugs but where the same careful maintenance of sensible roles and goals can provide the resolution of chronic conflicts generated by failed relationships.

The Drug Dependence Syndrome as a
Factor in Teenager-Parent Relationships

Because this third part of the book, "How Can Families Prevent and Treat Drug Problems?" is fundamentally *a survival guide* to drug abuse prevention, the Drug Dependence Syndrome has some far-reaching implications which we need to explore at this point. It is especially significant because it is basic to the new approach to parent-teenager relationships I am advocating in this chapter. A clear and unflinching insight into the consistently detrimental and potentially destructive workings of the Drug Dependence Syndrome can guide both parents and teenagers in seeking intelligent solutions to problems arising from the use of alcohol, marijuana, and other drugs. From your reading of Chapter 2, you will recall that, aside from the four fateful steps which the drug user is almost invariably tempted to take, the Drug Dependence Syndrome has a number of unique characteristics which bear heavily upon the roles and goals of teenagers and parents.

The first of these characteristics is that virtually all initial drug use occurs between the ages of 12 and 20. Second, the Drug Dependence Syndrome is particularly seductive for teenagers because the initial stages of drug use are relatively free of painful consequences. Third, and finally, without strong, forceful intervention, few young people are able to avoid drug use or stop it if they start it.

A NEW APPROACH TO STRUCTURING RELATIONSHIPS BETWEEN PARENTS AND TEENAGERS

One teenager who heard me review the Drug Dependence Syndrome within this parent/child framework said, "It sounds like you are favoring a tyranny of parents over children." I readily agreed. But I was quick to explain that the tyranny I am advocating has a benevolent purpose—to help the adolescent become an adult—and that the tyranny is temporary, lasting only until the child reaches age 19. Parents need hardly apologize for this purposeful and temporary tyranny. It is, after all, a reflection of the basic strength of human society. The human childhood is by far the most prolonged in the entire natural world. How long does the parent of a dog or a cat or a monkey nurture and protect its young before they are adult in the sense I have described here? Most dogs get very little such parenting; for kittens, the growing up process lasts only a few weeks; for monkeys, it lasts a few years at the most. Not 19 years for those or for any other nonhuman species. Fortunately, this prolonged human childhood is adaptive: we humans have a great deal to learn about ourselves and our world before we are ready to function as adults in a complex society.

Practical Implications of This New Approach: Some Examples

To see something of the functional nature of this new approach to managing parent-teenager conflicts, turn for a moment to the exam-

ples I used in introducing this chapter: the crisscross messages of
parents and of teenagers. The teenagers, you will recall, said they
wanted to be *listened to*. And rightfully so. To satisfy this need,
parents have to face the reality that their teenagers need even more
time—and high-quality time—than they needed as preschoolers.
Among other things, this means parents taking time to help their
teenage children accurately discern, define, and solve problems. This
means parents who are willing to get involved with active problem
solving. It means parents who are honest about themselves and about
their own childhoods. But, most of all, it means parents who clearly
understand their unique role and unique function in helping their
children grow up to sensible, productive, and enjoyable adulthood.
"Listening," as those teenagers used the term, means all of these
things—and more.

For parents who want their children to *behave*, my message is
equally definite: parents must be involved directly and daily in their
children's behavior. There is no possibility of solving the problem of
adolescent misbehavior if parents believe they have met their responsibilities merely by spending 30 minutes each week lecturing the child
about what he or she is or is not to do. More is needed than that.
Much more. The process of goal-directed parenting must start early
and persist. For the parents who have turned their child loose at age
15, allowing him or her to get kicked out of school for pushing pot, it
is late, but not quite too late, in the process to get involved.

For parents of the rebellious 14-year-old girl (who threatened to run
away) and those with similar problems, the new approach I am
advocating means using the levers of power they have as parents to
define what she will and will not be allowed to do. I have never seen
parents who got tough—and stayed united—who did not succeed
with a child having behavioral problems at this age. Children are just
not ready to be on their own at age 14, and most of them know it.
Many will bluff, but if the bluff is called, they will shape up. However,
if the child persists or proves uncontrollable even after strict and
consistent limit setting by parents, then the courts or the psychiatric
hospital is the next stop for the beleaguered family. This may shock
you. But I have seen many families stabilized when seriously disobedi-
ent or unruly children have been placed on probation, with a credible
threat of imprisonment behind it. I have also worked with a few
families who could only work together successfully after the rebellious
teenager left home and floundered or drifted aimlessly for months or
even years.

For parents like those of the 31-year-old prescription drug addict, my message is equally straightforward: *stop saving your child.* Let him feel the full consequences of his own behavior. When I said this to the mother of that young man, she protested, saying, "You mean we should not get him a lawyer and try to keep him out of jail? He might be killed!" "Yes," I said calmly, "or worse." This woman and her husband should not only stop paying legal bills and apartment rent for their 31-year-old son; they should also refuse to provide food, school, or work for him. If that means he is to be jailed—or worse—that will be the result of *his* choice, not theirs. Their enabling behavior in repeatedly rescuing him only served to perpetuate his addiction to drugs and his failing behavior.

The pattern of enabling behavior observable in this family's experience with their 31-year-old child is one I see with some frequency in my day-to-day clinical practice. It is widely prevalent—almost rampant—among families who, having much wealth, seek to share it with their teenage and adult children. In doing this, unfortunately for them, they cannot grasp the implications of the time-limited nature of their children's growing-up process. They find it difficult, if not impossible, to confront squarely the problems caused for them and their children by their misdirected generosity. These problems are compounded by their failure to draw necessary distinctions between Pseudo-Children and real adults. These parents, because of their wealth, often have a special view of the value of money and the worth of work, and this has a powerful, continuing, and often devastating, impact on their children.

One mother, for example, was perplexed when I explained that she and her husband would have to stop supporting their 33-year-old, unemployed, heroin addict son if he were to have any chance of recovery. Talk turned to the matter of his car. Currently, he had the use of a Mercedes leased for him by a family company. I suggested to his parents that they take back this car. His mother protested, "But how will he get around? He'll be helpless!" She then proposed giving him an Oldsmobile as a "cheap car." Later in our conversation, her husband suggested that their son had, on occasion, worked well in one of the family businesses. He suggested buying him a company to "give him an incentive to get straight."

Another family had arranged trust funds for their five now-adult children, four of whom had serious drug problems. On becoming teenagers, each had been paid $30,000 a year, tax free. Not one of these five children had finished college, and not one had established an adult career identity. The most enduring and urgent concern of these children was finding sharp, shrewd legal help to gain access to the principal of their trust funds so they would no longer be restricted to living on its income alone.

For those of us who are not wealthy ourselves, these may seem like ludicrous situations. Let me hurriedly interject this thought, however: the fact that some people are rich should not mean that the rest of us cannot learn from their mistakes; nor should it mean that the affluent cannot suffer and bleed just as the rest of us do. I can assure you that these families, both parents and children, experienced terribly agonizing conflicts over these problems. They were people who had everything money could buy. The one thing they lacked was what they cared most about—successful families.

Think, for a moment, how much simpler, even if not easier, it is for families who lack wealth to direct their children's attention to one of the real challenges of adulthood: to be able to support oneself by one's own work. Wealthy families often face the crippling reality that nothing—absolutely nothing—the children can do to earn money is likely to come close to the financial rewards of cashing in on the family wealth. How many of us could complete our schooling and establish successful adult work identities if we did not need to earn the money?

Such families have limited options. The heads of such families—the parents usually—can deprive their children of the money they can so easily give (at least as long as they are alive). But even this can be exceedingly complicated and difficult. For one thing, if the money has been in the family for a long time, it is common practice by parents and grandparents to establish trust funds which become available to children at certain specific ages—usually at ages 21 to 25. Assuming that not all of the children have failed at an early age, if their wealthy parents do deprive their adult children of financial support, then they face the dilemma that some of their children are being treated one way, and some another. Moreover, if families blessed with appreciable wealth get tough on immature and irresponsible Pseudo-Children, as advocated in this book, they must face what, for them, is a lonely and terrible problem: having to renounce one of their greatest pleasures—giving to their children from their own abundance. On the other hand, if they do give their children money in any significant amounts, then the parents frequently must pay terribly frustrating prices by being compelled to stand helplessly by and watch their beloved children fail still again in their often half-hearted and even sometimes pathetically grandiose schemes modeled on their parents' fabulous success. As a homespun philosopher, whose name has long been forgotten, once said, "Bein' rich ain't easy—even when you're rich."

One must admit that family wealth makes heavy demands on both parents and children as the children mature through adolescence. Fortunate and rare indeed is the wealthy family who is able to work this out without losing one or more of the children to the ravages of alcohol and other drugs. One way in which I have seen this problem handled with good success is for the parents to begin, at an an early age, to raise their children with a sense of what used to be called "noblesse oblige"—an intense and generous family pride in the *responsibility* of wealth. This can help the children realize that not less but more is expected of them, not so much for their own good as for the good they can do for others. It also helps when affluent parents are able to emphasize the real threats to achievement that their children will face. In my experience I have seen that this hurdle is more often overcome by families with long-standing wealth, perhaps because they have already lost so much productive capacity to drug and alcohol dependence in previous generations.

Although it seems unlikely at first, a similar problem often arises in families of more modest means. When a child is handicapped—for example, deaf or physically deformed—there is an understandable and almost overwhelming urge to enable and protect. Here, too, the temptation is for well-meaning parents to take over and unwittingly undermine the child's own potential for independent adulthood. Here, too, since these children often do face the prospect of dependence and income potentials lower than that of their parents, there is a common assumption by both the parents and the rest of the family that the growing child will never, because of the handicap, be fully independent. This assumption all too often stifles the necessary confrontation of both parent and child with the hard truths of the world "out there." Parents are powerfully inclined to team up with handicapped children in order to buffer the blows that come when the child attempts to be independent. Thereupon, a variety of unhealthy dependencies develop, and sometimes these include impulsive and destructive behaviors such as drug taking and alcohol abuse.

There is no easy solution. There is, however, one thing which both wealthy parents and parents of the handicapped must do for their adult child or their handicapped youngster: they must sit down with the child and thoughtfully and patiently discuss the difficulties the child faces in life and the commitment and effort required to live with and, if possible, overcome them. At the same time, they must make clear, as honestly and directly as they possibly can, their parental commitment to helping the child become self-dependent, self-sufficient, and self-confident. As impersonal as it may sound, they must help the child to understand that failure to face up to problems, including the use of alcohol or other drugs, will lead to parental withdrawal of certain supports and possible infliction of parental punishments. Above all, such responses to problems must be made openly, calmly, and with genuine—not maudlin—compassion.

Three Basic Principles Underlying the New Approach

1. Firm Parental Control Leads Eventually to Teenage Self-Control. Admittedly, on first glance this approach to parent-child relationships may appear somewhat negative, especially to teenagers. That is understandable because almost all of us—even as adults— chafe at the thought that obstacles are being imposed on what we often mistakenly suppose to be our "absolute freedom" to think and behave as we please. Realistically, however, as we grow through teenhood and beyond, we come to the realization that there is no such absolute. Gradually we learn that whatever freedom we eventually exercise is largely an earned freedom which exists almost exclusively in the context of detailed rules of family and community life. Adolescence is a time of earning this much-cherished freedom of choice, but even that freedom, as adulthood so frequently and dramatically demonstrates, is hedged in by people and regulations and limitations beyond the individual's control. It is during this earning and learning and this slow realization process that true parental guidance should come naturally and powerfully into play.

Many teenagers, mistakenly seeing adulthood as the ultimate freedom, are shocked (I could say "sobered") when they realize the severity of the limitations placed on the behavior of adults by others almost every day in modern life. When you get right down to it, adults generally accept and live with far more rules and limitations than teenagers do. If teenagers think their parents are "on their case," they should know about the control typically exercised by spouses and employers, to say nothing of the controls over day-to-day behavior necessary to meet the monthly bills. One important difference, of course, is that for adults these behavioral controls reflect a more or less personal choice, whereas for teenagers the family-based controls are usually imposed upon them—not chosen by them. Successful passage through this stage of development by parents and teenagers helps soften the teenagers' pain of having the rules imposed. The successful family negotiates rules so that all members of the family feel they own the rules and that, on balance, these rules work to meet personal as well as family needs.

Parents—by reason of their wider experience, their greater maturity, and the love and concern they hold for their children—are best qualified to guide children toward the hoped-for mastery of one of the major lessons we all must learn: *self-control*. Through rules and controls parents impose early in adolescent years, we learn to manage our impulses and sort out those wants and needs which we can sensibly satisfy from those which are best left unsatisfied. This process of sorting out goals and the process of mastering self-control are two of the primary tasks of childhood and, especially, of adolescence. Parents who, with some success, have lived through these experiences themselves should be recognized as knowledgeable and helpful guides for their children. It is both sensible and practicable, therefore, that the first principle of my approach to clarifying parent-teenager relationships is control: control by the parents for the child under 19, and then self-control by the child when he or she reaches age 19 and goes beyond.

Some readers may find my emphasis on control to be heavy-handed and even objectionable. Others may find my emphasis on financial dependence and independence too simplistic. The first objection reminds me of a high school girl who heard this account and said, "In my family, my parents never exercise control; they trust and respect me. Your emphasis on control would be hurtful to me; it would make me want to rebel." I asked her a few questions: "How was she doing in school? Did she have any problems with drugs or alcohol or sexual activity? What kind of hours did she keep? What was the quality of her relationship with her parents?" She responded in a straightforward fashion: She was doing fine in school, she had no problems of the kind I mentioned, and she almost never went out at night except occasionally on the weekends. She felt close to her parents. She said this was true *because* she had no rules. I asked her if she thought she would have rules if she had a drug problem, failed at school, stayed out until 3:00 A.M. on weeknights, and frequently fought with her parents. She said, "I don't know, that's not me." Although she did not seem to recognize the fact, she obviously lived according to many rules—rules that were shared and respected if not articulated. This "nice guy" approach is fine as long as it works as effectively as it seems to have worked in this case. However, behind it—in successful families—are genuine authority and the determination to identify and overcome problems, if and when they occur.

To the second objection, that my emphasis on "economic determinism" in parent-child interactions is simplistic, I reply, "Yes, but it surely helps everyone focus on an underlying reality. And when ignored, it can lead to disastrous consequences for all concerned."

There is indeed more to family life than money, but that is not a bad place to start getting realistic—if the kids are ever to grow up.

2. The Family Is a Team—with Roles and Goals.   The functioning of all family members as a team is fundamental to successful interaction and productive problem-solving within the family. One of the principal problems of adolescence in America today is underemployment, or even outright unemployment. While inability to find paid work can be a serious problem, that is not the type of unemployment I am about to describe. Here I am concerned with the "unemployment" of a family's capabilities for defining family roles and for solving some of the problems of adolescence. A properly functioning family is a *team*—a system, to use the modern idiom—which has well-differentiated roles and well-defined goals. Although the family often creates problems for its members individually and collectively, when it works as a team, it can also be a highly effective problem-solving system. By working within the family system, playing on the team, the adolescent child in a family can feel needed, useful, and important. Such feelings take on an even greater significance when the adolescent is the direct focus of the family's efforts and teamwork to help him or her mature into sound adulthood. If this sounds a bit abstract, keep in mind that family teamwork is not limited to solving the teenager's problems. Teens can usefully help do such family work as cooking meals, cleaning and organizing the household, and doing yardwork. In many families, teenagers' incomes can help meet some of the family's urgent financial needs. To treat teenagers as "pampered guests" in the family is to do no family member—most of all the teenager—a favor. Teenagers require, perhaps more than anything else, the feeling of being needed and respected. It helps if they earn these feelings through hard work.

In assigning responsibilities, it is important that all family members see the fairness of the assignments. It is no more reasonable for parents to sit around lounging while teenagers work than it is for teenagers to lie around while adults work. The work of the family needs to be fairly apportioned in ways that everyone can understand. While it is possible that families overwork their teenagers—a kind of Cinderella pattern—I have never seen this in my psychiatric practice. What I often see is families which assign no responsibilities whatsoever to teenagers. When confronted about this, some parents, like Bill in the example at the beginning of this chapter, respond that they do not want to make life too hard for their children. Other parents justify their actions by saying, not without reason in many cases, that it is easier for them to do the household chores than it is to get their teenagers to do some of them. Whatever the reason, unemployment of teenagers in the family is likely to be destructive to the entire family—especially to the teenager.

3. Communicate with a PURPOSE to Explore and "Negotiate" Family Conflicts. Much popular psychology deals with the need for communication in the family, especially communication between parents and teenage children. This, surely, is an appropriate concern. But the frequent flaw in this well-meaning advice is that the *purpose* of such communication is often left unspecified. Although passive listening by parents is, in itself, better than entirely ignoring or leaving the child in total isolation, a principal purpose of family communication is to talk with one another, to interact in order to identify and resolve problems which arise as the child grows and moves toward adulthood. The problems to be dealt with in this way certainly include the harmful use of alcohol and other drugs and the infinite varieties of potentially negative peer-group pressures.

The starting point is, however, more basic. The great goals of human life, I think we can agree, are to love, to be loved, and to work. For both teenagers and adults, this requires development of the communication and problem-solving skills needed to establish and support a positive relationship with others in the family and with peers. It also requires that the teenager be able to communicate clearly in order to sustain successful functioning in school—the principal worksite of adolescence. If the family team is to "win," there needs to be clear and continuing communication regarding such matters as the definition of roles, the redefinition of the expectations of each family member, and pertinent information which enables each member to function intelligently in face-to-face interactions with one another.

For this process to work as it should, it is, of course, essential that efforts be made on all sides to protect and nurture the self-esteem of everyone in the family. In particular, this means that parents have to nurture the positive self-esteem of their adolescent children with the clear message that not only is success expected, but that the parent is confident that the child can achieve this success. Such success is achieved with much effort, with the support of the family, and, often, with frequent failures. Failures are best seen as the inevitable consequence of trying, as well as important learning experiences. All of us adults have abundant examples of such failures from our own lives with which we can educate teenagers and empathize with their struggles to maintain a sensible self-esteem in the face of many frustrations and disappointments.

In brief, then, these three principles are basic to all positive interactions, meaningful relationships, and productive problem solving within and by the family: (1) teenage acceptance of parental control as leading to eventual self-control; (2) all members of the family functioning together as a team; and (3) the employment of purposeful communication to achieve sound and mutually agreeable solutions to specific problems. These principles are the vital "engines" which start a necessary family interaction and move it toward a desirable and mutually desired destination: helping the child become an adult.

ROLES AND GOALS OF PARENTS

If we are to make understandable even a small percentage of all the interactions between parents and growing children, we need to hold steadily in mind a clear differentiation between the roles of parents and the roles of teenagers. The keystone for the basic structure of parent-teenager relationships is, of course, the distinction between the rights and the responsibilities of the child, on the one hand, and those of the adult, on the other. This distinction underpins all parent-child interactions, both those that work and those that do not. In defining family roles, goals, and responsibilities, I find it useful to focus separately on those of parents as distinguished from those of teenagers.

Let's start with parents because their roles and functions are the foundation of the family system. They were in the home before the children were born, and they will be there when the children leave it. The "family," of course, may take numerous forms. Some families are large: two parents and many children. In modern America today, many families have a single parent in the home with the child or the children. Some teenagers, because of parental divorce and remarriage, have four parents. Some families have grandparents and other relatives available; some do not. The challenges, opportunities, and frustrations for one- and two-parent families are quite similar, and the differences are fewer than you might expect.

Goals of Husband and Wife as Persons—And as Parents

Parents need a clear vision of their many husband-and-wife goals, goals which include maintenance of good working relationships with each other—relationships which have purposes beyond the needs of their children. The parents also have the primary and often exclusive responsibility for earning the income to support each other and the rest of the family. Outside their immediate household, parents have goals affecting a wider community: relatives, friends, neighbors, and work associates. They have, in addition, responsibilities for setting reasonable role models for their children. If all of this sounds like a heavy burden, that's because it *is*. It is a large and demanding task which no parent—and, of course, no couple—ever performs with complete success.

Parents have personal objectives as well as family goals. Parents are also a team, on their own, without consideration of the children in the home. Parents have conflicts and imperfections. How all this is sorted out, managed, and communicated has a great deal to do with what children, including teenagers, learn about what "family" means. Some who read this will rebel, thinking that I have set too high a standard for parents. Precisely the opposite is more nearly the case. As a psychiatrist and as a parent of teenage children, I fully respect the imperfections of all parents and all parent teams. All of us enter this process of living in families with limitations and handicaps. The issue is not our "perfection"; it is how well we cope or fail to cope with our imperfections, including the inevitable imperfections in the relationship between the parents themselves. My approach is, in fact, based on an assumption of imperfections and problems.

Families with two parents do have an advantage because when one parent gets into a blind alley with a teenager, the other parent can often help find a way out of the dilemma and reach a more productive resolution of the conflict. Also, with two parents, there is potentially more parenting power and often more parental time available to guide the teenager. With a one-parent family, especially if that parent works outside the home, parenting time is more limited. On the other hand, many single parents I have worked with are more disciplined and effective in their parenting, partly because they know they have to be in order to make the family work. Knowing there is no one to "backstop" them, they do it right the first time, if possible. Two parents can sometimes generate conflict and disagreement which can make parenting more difficult because rebellious teenagers are quick to exploit parental disagreements, playing one parent off the other. When there is only one parent, there can be no parental conflict, at least not in the home.

Similarly, divorce can be a problem, especially if the parents harbor continuing resentments. By contrast, if the parents can focus constructively on the needs of their child or children, they can often be highly effective as a team, even though they live under separate roofs. The modern, merged families living together with multiple marriages and mixed parents (with children who are "his, hers, and theirs") can also be either a liability or an asset, depending on how parents and children use them. In other words, do not let the advantages or the disadvantages of being married or divorced or remarried, of being a "single" parent or a "double" parent, or whether you live together or live apart blind you to the fact that your child needs strong, steady parenting if he or she is to grow up with reasonable success.

Coping with the Midlife Crisis.   Sometimes I think adolescence is a contagious disease. It shows up in adults as what is now called the midlife crisis. This crisis is no pop psychology myth, and it has hit America hard. Millions of husbands and wives between the ages of 35 and 50—the parents of today's teenagers—are facing a major crisis in their own lives which, in many ways, parallels the crisis being felt by teenagers. The question most asked by adults in their midlife crisis is "When Do I Get *Mine*?" The problem many adults face in midlife is a crisis of self-confidence and career direction. Having made their basic life decisions about work and love some years ago, these adults find that both love and work, as realistically experienced in their own lives, have many frustrations and have been disappointing. If you, as a parent, are facing a midlife crisis, learn to cope with it with the comforting recognition that you have a lot of company among other adults your age.

Many parents respond to this midlife crisis by making large and small changes in their lives. Job and even career changes are common. Many women who are between the ages of 35 to 50 and who have stayed at home to take care of the children respond by developing new careers and working outside the home. Women who have worked at jobs outside their homes throughout their 20s and 30s often wonder about their earlier decisions to do so, and some of them change careers or drop out of the paid work force. Moreover, men and women facing midlife doubts raise difficult questions about their marriages, and many seek divorce. The issues of identity, relationships, and responsibilities which so inflame the adolescent years are also in the forefront of the adult midlife crisis. In my view, in both of these life stages, the resolution to many of the important problems lies in renewed commitment and deeper personal investment in the areas of love and work, including recommitment to many of the

traditional roles and values. It is often more helpful—and more difficult—to think about what one wants to move toward than what one
wants to move away from. Easy, or apparently easy, pleasure and
freedom from responsibilities are dangerous seductions at both of
these stages of the life cycle. The later consequences of pleasure-
seeking in mid- or late life are often more unpleasant than are antici-
pated. They can be disastrous if pleasure is sought in drugs or
alcohol. In both the late-adolescent life stage and in the midlife crisis,
change is often needed, of course, but at the same time, it is reassuring to remember that much strength can be derived from the most
fundamental of all human support systems: the family. Talking over
these shared problems with each other and communicating across the
generational gap can help both parents and teenagers make better
adjustments to these difficult and closely related challenges.

Child-Rearing Goals of Parents

Having thus set the stage, let me turn now to some specifics of
parental goals in child rearing. As a friend of mine said recently, "For
most of us it is easy to *have* children; the challenge is *raising* them."
As almost every parent will admit, raising children is a long-range goal
which is seldom fully or satisfactorily realized, but the effort to
achieve it is one which most parents eventually consider to be the
most important activity of their lives.

In retrospect, most parents have some regrets, often fairly substantial regrets, about their own performance as parents. But if, as parents, we can comprehend the importance of the task of child rearing
and have the humility necessary to approach it constructively, we can
take encouragement from the fact that raising a family is a goal-
oriented, time-limited function, beginning with conception and ending
when the child leaves home as a self-sufficient, self-supporting adult.
In most families, as we have seen, the fulfillment of that function
takes from 18 to 22 years, from beginning to end. Throughout this
interval in their lives, parents need to keep their eyes and their minds
open to the problems their children encounter in growing up. It helps
to be aware that some of these problems are physical in nature and
that others are psychological. And, above all, if parents can fulfill
their parental destiny by helping their children identify their goals,
recognize the nature of their problems, and seek sensible solutions,
the rewards can be vast and enduring.

Some may say this is a simplistic, short-sighted view of parent-child
relationships, that these relationships do not end when the child

leaves the home. In many families, the most positive and sometimes the most important family interactions take place after the child becomes an adult and leaves home. Surely, this is true. My purpose here, however, is to focus on the period of *primary* parental responsibility. Once the child becomes an adult, then the parental role changes dramatically from one of teaching responsibility to one of offering advice and support. When parents fail to recognize the limits of their responsibility for their adult children, they do almost as much harm to themselves and their children as they do when they fail to recognize the virtually unlimited nature of their responsibility for their preadult children.

Your Child's Problem-Solving Intelligence. Sometimes parents worry that their child may lack the fleetness of mind—the "intelligence"—to run life's obstacle course safely and successfully. My suggestion is this: never underestimate your child's mental agility and capacity because there are many different "intelligences." I ask you, as a parent, to consider for a moment how your misunderstanding or misevaluation of this notion of intelligence or I.Q. might seriously impede the functioning and adversely affect the life of your child. I often hear parents talk about their child's "intelligence" as if it were an inborn, biological attribute that nothing much can be done about. A more realistic assessment of intelligence is to see it as a *measure of real-life problem-solving capability*. This capability, or even its potential, involves not only biological functioning, but also the capacity to seek, get, and use appropriately help from others; the capacity to define and complete a task; the capacity to focus one's attention on a problem and work to its solution. This is a "workaday" intelligence. Common sense, maybe.

Two contrasting examples may serve to illustrate that parents should not be too quick to over- or underassess the intelligence of their children. When I was a psychiatric resident, one of my first patients was a 25-year-old woman with an I.Q. of 140 (the genius level) who had been unable to graduate from high school because her life was in disarray. She was unable to focus her mental and physical abilities. She had never held a job for more than a few months, and she had moved randomly from one dependent relationship to another. She was not psychotic; she was not schizophrenic or anything of that sort. Although a "genius," she was handicapped—apparently for life—by what psychiatrists call a "character disorder."

Later in my life, I knew a mentally retarded girl with an I.Q. of 80 (seriously below average). This girl's retardation was the result of a poorly treated case of meningitis when she was two years old. Her retardation was not, therefore, genetic and would not be passed to her children, if any. Even so, as this girl grew to adulthood, her parents worried about whether to have her sterilized because they felt she could not take care of herself in social situations. Later, when she was 21 years of age, she managed to get a job, working in a special office situation which had been set aside by the government for the purpose of helping the handicapped. She was a pleasant and responsible worker who not only did a good job, but was also well liked by her co-workers. When her family fell on severely hard times economically, this girl literally supported her parents with her salary. Still later, she married a loving man of normal intelligence and enjoyed a happy adult life, including having two healthy children.

In comparing these two young women, which one—would you say—was truly handicapped in terms of intelligence, in the sense that intelligence reflects problem-solving ability?

Guiding the Child by Setting Limits and Providing Direction. How can parents help their children develop good problem-solving abilities? By guiding them toward self-discipline and self-control. These are ideal tools for aiding and encouraging young people to make the best possible use of their own talents as they progress from one life stage to another. To guide their children toward self-discipline, parents should skill themselves in setting limits and giving directions while, at the same time, doing those things in ways most likely to increase the child's self-respect, not to undermine it. This can be done by explaining and, if possible, showing that parental limits are designed to help the child function eventually as an independent adult. In this business of setting limits, providing directions, and giving instruction, be careful always to try to build up the youngster's self-image and self-esteem and not tear them down—advice that bears repeated emphasis.

When deciding to set particular limitations on their children's behaviors and activities, parents should think twice about the possible outcomes. They need to ask themselves if the limits they are about to impose will really help the child grow and mature. Equally important, they should be able to explain the connection between the limits, on the one hand, and the desired growth and maturation, on the other.

I enunciate these goals, roles, and functions not to encourage feelings of parental guilt, but to underscore the challenge in the overall role of parenthood. It is true, as I have emphasized, that most people view their efforts in raising their children as the most important and rewarding of all the work they do. When we imagine lying on our deathbed and looking back at our life, I suspect that most of us would consider, as the first criterion for judging our achievements, our degree of success or failure in raising our children.

SOME RIGHTS AND RESPONSIBILITIES OF TEENAGERS AND PARENTS

Thus far in this chapter I have defined the roles and functions of both parents and teenagers within a broad and general framework. In the following pages, these roles and functional goals will be examined within a somewhat more specific frame of certain rights and responsibilities pertaining to each. This time, let's start with the teenagers.

The Rights of Teenagers

A young person has a right to expect that parents will recognize and respect the teenager's natural and healthy desire to rebel and test limits: the right, as one teenager said to me recently, "to learn for myself." The teenager, as I have been emphasizing, also has the right to be heard, the right to expect that parents will be willing to listen to and respect his or her uniquely personal views, values, and desires. Teenagers also deserve respect for the fact that they are not "perfect." Many children today feel they must live out their parents' fantasies for the "perfect" teenage life the parents never had. The kids feel themselves pressured to get great grades, to be great at sports, to be leaders of their schools, to have great friends, to be in a great mood all the time. When they are confronted, as they all are routinely, with evidence of their failure to achieve such greatness, they feel disappointed in themselves and angry with their parents.

The Rights of Parents

Yes, even though they are often reluctant to admit it, parents have rights, too. Parents, even parents of adolescent children, have the right to have needs and feelings and a life which does not always center on the demands of their children. Parents have a right to some peace and some time for their own needs. They also have the right to be respected for what they are. After all, they are imperfect, too, in their own eyes and in the critical eyes of their teenage children.

The Responsibilities of the Teenager
to Accept and Abide by Family Rules

The questions of What, When, and Why of teenagers' responsibilities often produce battles between teenagers and their parents. There are certain expectations which have to be fulfilled if families are to work effectively for the benefit of both parents and teenagers. Teenagers have a definite responsibility for civil and helpful behavior around the home. They should be willing to assume a fair share of the burden of making the household function properly. This involves such responsible tasks as cleaning up their rooms and the common living space, keeping responsible hours for coming and going, and—in general—abiding by reasonable rules set by parents.

A single parent from Richmond, Virginia, recently explained to me how she had raised her two sons, boys who towered over her before they were 15 years old. "I set rules," she said, "and I expected them to be obeyed. If they weren't, I had my YMCA solution: I told the boys they could leave any time they wanted to and move into the YMCA to see if they liked the rules there any better." Years later, when her sons had successfully established themselves as adults, they frequently came home to visit their mother. As mothers will on such occasions, she sometimes rebuked them for something they did or said. Jokingly, they would respond, "Now, Mom, we know what's coming next. You are going to tell us about the YMCA!" She told this story with an embarrassed, but proud, laugh at herself. The important point here is that this woman had enforced rules in her family and she was willing—and her sons knew she was willing—to have them leave home rather than have the rules broken. Both parent and children benefitted from these rules and lived to laugh together about them.

The Responsibilities of Parents to Set and Enforce Guidelines,
Including Nonuse of Alcohol and Other Drugs

Today in America, I am convinced that alcohol and other drugs constitute the single greatest threat to effective family functioning. Alcohol and marijuana also constitute the greatest threat to growing children's ability to function outside of their families as adults. Most of the 20- and 30-year-olds I see who are still Pseudo-Children, unable to support themselves and still dependent on their parents, are handicapped by their use of drugs of various kinds. Parents, therefore, have the responsibility to set clear and enforceable guidelines for the nonuse of alcohol and other drugs as long as the child remains at home, or as long as the child accepts the financial support of the parents. The best rule, in my view, is "No alcohol and no other drugs—period." No underage drinking and no use of illegal drugs at all is the best policy.

This is a jarring restriction to many modern teenagers who consider the use of alcohol, especially beer, and marijuana to be normal at any age. The peer group encourages this attitude, and—as we know all too well—many economic interests also reinforce this prodrug posture. Nevertheless, if the teenager has problems with drug use, as have many of the youths I see, then this strict prohibition is even more vital. Unfortunately, parents cannot expect their drug-using children to see that their problems are related to drug use. Teenagers deny this connection. One boy said to me recently, "Sure, I started using marijuana almost every day about a year ago and, sure, my grades fell from A's and B's to C's and even F's. Sure, my parents are on my case. But pot has nothing to do with grades. I don't get good grades anymore because I don't want to. There's no point; I don't want to compete. As for my parents, they just don't understand me. They haven't been through what I have."

In recent years the public debate about drug use has taken a surprising turn, a turn which directly affects families' abilities to cope with drug problems. The pro-drug forces have abandoned their earlier claims that drugs are harmless and have refocused their arguments on the premise that drug use is a "civil right." They now argue that drug abuse prevention efforts, in the family and in the community at large, are violations of rights to privacy. Families, especially, need to weigh the civil rights argument carefully because it is increasingly appearing as a barrier to clear thinking about drug abuse prevention.

We all need discipline and rules, we need help and direction, and the family is the basic source of all these controls and the values they reflect. Fake civil rights arguments should not distract families from dealing firmly and decisively with threats of alcohol and other drug use. Such arguments should not be allowed to detract from the genuine right which allows and encourages all citizens, young and old, to participate positively and fully in the life of the family and of the community. Nor should specious arguments be allowed to weaken and betray the full range of family and community responsibilities that underpin these rights. Among these is the responsibility to obey the law as it bears upon drinking and drug use. If one disagrees with a law, one should attempt to change it but obey it until and unless it is changed.

The Responsibilities of Parents to
Resolve Conflicts As They Occur

Conflicts do occur. Between parents, with other adults including relatives and neighbors, and between parents and teenagers. Parents should, in my view, have the last word, but they are not, in fact, always necessarily wise or right. To be wise, parents will be slow to invoke their ultimate right. When conflicts arise, families are well served by keeping an open attitude toward conflict resolution. By that I mean a willingness of the parents to talk problems over, rather than for one parent, or both, to react hastily or arbitrarily. Take time to listen to your teenager's point of view. Talk the problem over with your friends. Get in contact with other parents facing similar problems. Counseling, either from a religiously oriented counselor or from a professional mental health worker, such as a psychiatrist, can often be useful. Keep the goals and problems clearly in view, and demonstrate to your child your willingness to work the problem through to a mutually acceptable solution. This will not only demonstrate your toughness and your love, but it will also be a useful model for your child to follow later when he or she is an adult faced with conflicts. The danger, in my view, lies in parents who either deny and ignore problems or who feel so guilty and ashamed of their problems with their children that they fail to look outside their family for help. Far better to open up the family to the support that is out there all around us.

In this regard, many parents find working with the parents of other teenagers especially helpful. It takes courage to speak up. When it comes to drug and alcohol problems, in particular, remember that they affect *all families* and that such problems are an unavoidable part of modern life in America. They do not reflect badly on your parenting, or even on your child.

The key to success for the family is to have a clear sense of the roles of parents and children and the goals of these family relationships. When threats to these goals emerge, they should be directly and consistently confronted and resolved. Having considered in some detail the basic structure of the relationships between parents and teenagers, let us now turn to some suggestions specifically addressed to teenagers and, separately, to parents. I hope both will read both sets of suggestions because self-understanding is easier when we have a clearer comprehension not only of our own problems but also of the problems of those with whom we live and interact.

FOR TEENAGERS: SOME SUGGESTIONS

Weigh the Present Against the Future

The teenage years are tough for many people. It probably was a tough time for your parents, too. You feel a desire to be adult and independent, to be free, but you also know you have a lot to lose by leaving home and starting your adulthood too soon. You feel strong at some times, and weak at others. It is hard to think beyond your intense feelings and your thoughts about the present, to think about your future needs and interests. In fact, the emphasis everyone puts on thinking about the future—hard work and discipline, for example—can be a real hassle. At the same time, you are probably discovering the excitement of more independent living and the pleasures (and frustrations) of relationships with your peers, both boys and girls. You are probably doubting many of the things you took for granted when you were younger. You want to find your own place in your own world. You probably have moods that are not easy to cope with—for you to live with and for those around you to live with. Probably, you are also discovering strengths—intellectual, physical, and personal strengths—you never thought you would have.

Set Goals and Explore Possibilities

Try to find some quiet time to think for yourself. Also, find time to talk with your parents and your trusted friends about what is happening to you. Talk about your strengths and weaknesses and about your goals and your fears. Dare to dream for yourself. Think, quietly, about what you want for yourself in the next 10 years. What kind of work do you want and what kinds of relationships with family and friends? What will it take to get you where you want to go? What are the steps between where you are and where you want to be? Do you know any people who have some of the abilities and opportunities you want? Talk to those people and see how they got them. What advice can they give you? What can you do now to make it more likely for you to realize your dreams?

If you are like most teenagers, the gap between what you have and what you want is just too big. You cannot see how you can bridge that gap. You may have had a lot of painful failures recently, failures in relationships, in athletics, and in schoolwork. If you are like most teenagers I know, you have probably had plenty of successes, too, but those are quickly forgotten, while the pain of failure seems to persist. This may sound unrealistic, but you can build on the success and learn from the failures. The biggest danger for you now is to give up on your dreams and to fail to build, bit by bit, the necessary bridge to span that gap between where you are and where you want to be. Do not underestimate what you can achieve by persistence and hard work!

Sure, your parents are imperfect. You probably are only now fully realizing that they are "just people," and that they, too, have strengths and weaknesses. You may also be aware that certain things have happened in your family—and to you—that were not ideal and that caused you pain and even handicaps. Without trying to take away from these painful realities, past and present, how can you best face them and overcome them—to make them work for you, or at least to do what you can to keep them from getting between you and what you want? Surely, no matter how difficult your parents are (and I've seen some tough customers), they have some good—something useful—to offer you. How can you help them to be good parents to you in ways that will enable both you and them to win in this game of growing up?

Meet Your Responsibilities and Think About Long-Term Strategies

You have some specific expectations—for work and play and for life in the family. What can you do to meet these expectations and expand your sense of being in charge of your own life? If you have to clean up your room or study for an exam, how can you do it as painlessly and positively as possible? If you have a conflict with your parents, how can you talk with them about it? If you cannot get the answer you want, can you see behind their position in the argument? Can you see their real concern in a way that enables you to make a reasonable and responsible counterproposal so that you can now, or later, get what you want?

I spoke recently with a 17-year-old named Don, who wanted to travel to a nearby city to attend a concert by the Grateful Dead rock group on a Monday night. His parents said no, giving as their reasons the fact that the concert was scheduled on a school night, Don's grades were mostly F's (he'd been getting mostly B's until this year), and he'd come home one hour after curfew the previous weekend. Don felt terribly frustrated, saying to his parents: "But you just don't understand how important this concert is to me!" He was determined to go, even though his parents told him that if he did, he could not return home.

Stepping back from this difficult situation and carefully weighing a long-term strategy, Don might have effected a compromise by reasoning somewhat along these lines: "Obviously, my parents want me to do well in life and in school. They are worried about me. It is my responsibility to do reasonably well and to reassure them. If I tell them I'll work harder in school, getting at least B's and C's, and abide by their curfew, then maybe after two months or so of such proof, they'll let me go to the next Dead concert." This, alas, was not to be a success story. Don did not see things that way. He could not see that it was in his best interests to change; he could not delay his gratification for even two months. All he could think about was next Monday's concert. He was prepared to lose the support of his family to have exactly what he wanted when he wanted it. I don't know for sure, but I would bet that if Don had been able to think more clearly and had proposed to his parents the kind of compromise I've outlined, he would have been able to attend—in the long run—all the Grateful Dead concerts he ever wanted to hear!

Decide What You Will Do Personally About the Use of Alcohol and Other Drugs

You must take the time to decide your own personal strategy for responding to evidence of drug abuse around you. I asked a 16-year-old boy recently if he was using alcohol or other drugs. He resented the question but, finally, said grudgingly, "I had about six beers last weekend, and I think I did pretty well not to drink more." I asked if he knew that drinking beer at 16 was illegal. He said, "Yes, but that doesn't matter to me." He then went on to explain that he felt he could pick and choose which laws he wanted to obey and that he deeply resented any suggestion that the police, school officials, his parents, or I might try to enforce the laws against underage drinking or against use of drugs like marijuana. From this boy's point of view, all he could see was that he wanted to do what he wanted now. When I asked how his life would be harmed if he waited to begin drinking until he was of legal age, he replied that that was his business.

Jim, a 17-year-old student, was brought to me by his parents because of conflicts over his use of marijuana. He was failing in school and increasingly isolated from friends and family. Jim changed over the course of a year of hard work, in treatment and out. He stopped using marijuana and all but stopped using alcohol. When he came back to see me a year or so later, he looked like a different person. He was brighter and happier. He had finished high school and was waiting to enter college in the fall. Meanwhile, he was working full-time to earn money to help pay his college expenses. He said he was too busy for drugs and his drug-using former friends. He said some other things, too—things well worth pausing to think about: "My drug use," Jim said, "made me a liar, and it made my parents into narcotics agents right in our own house. They could never believe me, and they always searched my room and my clothes, looking for drugs. They used to listen to all my telephone conversations and give my friends the 'third degree.' The only way I could change all that was to stop using drugs." He added, "My family is now the most important part of my life. I love to spend time talking with them and being with them. I realize how lucky I am and how much I'll miss them when I go to college this fall."

Play—and Work—on the Family Team

Jim had captured the essence of a major point I made earlier: the family is a team, and the game the team plays is "Raising the Children." In this game, as we have seen, there are important roles for children and young people. No one on this or any other team is perfect. The challenge is to blend the talents of the whole team so that it will be more effective than any one person could be on his or her own. There are, of course, strengths and weaknesses in each family, just as there are in each individual. Even so, I have never seen any family, however structured and whatever the characteristics of its members, which—when united and working together—did not have enormous strengths and assets with which to build a winning team.

When the family team does not function well, however, everyone loses. I recall one particular family I worked with. Susan was 16 when I first saw her. Her mother and father were divorced when she was five. She lived reasonably happily with her mother and older brother for several years. Then her mother remarried. Susan hated her step-father. He was an alcoholic and, she said, a mean man. She began regular use of marijuana and alcohol and frequently fought with her parents about wanting to stay out late at night. At age 16, Susan left home because she "couldn't take it anymore." I did not see her again for three years. When I did, I learned that she had dropped out of high school in her sophomore year and that during the past three years she had occasionally held low-paying jobs, the longest of which had lasted four months. Soon she found the only way she could support herself was to live with men, one after another, most of whom were unstable providers who did not treat her well. She had known her current boyfriend, with whom she presently lived, for only five months.

She continued to use drugs occasionally and pondered from time to

time about what her life might have been like if she had not left home
when she did. With some sadness, she told me, "You know, sometimes I even wish I'd never used drugs, had graduated from high
school, and was still a virgin." While this is not a happy story, it is not
an uncommon one. However difficult Susan's relationship with her
stepfather was, I am confident that it would have been in her own
best interest to have stayed at home and finished her schooling. Now
handicapped and trapped, she has already paid and will continue to
pay a high price for her premature independence. Her parents, too,
are deeply saddened by how it has worked out for her—and for
them.

Susan's story illustrates one other important lesson. She left home
seeking her independence. She rebelled against the dependence she
felt in her far from perfect family. What happened to her was not
what she wanted. At the age of 19, she was not independent. She
was dependent in a far more troublesome way than she had been in
her family. She was dependent on a man she had known only five
months—a man who did not love her and who treated her poorly. If
she had not rebelled at age 16, if she had stayed at home and
finished high school, if she had learned how to hold a job and work
her way up to a better salary, she would have stood a good chance of
being truly independent at age 19. As it was, by seeking a kind of
fake independence at age 16, she sealed her dependence—probably
for life.

Establish Trust in Your Family Relationships

I strongly recommend that teenagers and their families openly
discuss *trustworthiness* and *lying* and the ways they affect family
relationships, and the responsibilities of all family members for developing trust and rejecting lying. "Trust," so eagerly sought but so
quickly abused, is the inevitable victim of lying. In thinking through
the family's role in drug abuse prevention, the problem of *dishonesty*
or *deceit* needs—above all others—careful thought. Lying is often
excused on the basis that it is "universal." It can be trivialized—and
often is—just as drug use, underage drinking, reckless driving, and
other illegal behavior can be trivialized. Who has not exaggerated
some personal achievement or hidden some failing? This normaliza-
tion of the act of lying, like the equally common trivialization of illegal
drug use, reflects a peculiar and abhorrent brand of "sophistication"
prevalent in our society, especially as it relates to the functioning of
teenagers and their families. Among adults, lying and the resulting

problems arise most frequently from sexual infidelity. Sexual affairs, outside of marriage, have a decidedly negative and almost totally destructive impact on family life.

In terms of our immediate concerns in this chapter, however, lying and cheating are among the biggest destroyers of friendly and productive relationships between teenagers and their parents. Lying about teenage behavior involving drugs, alcohol, and sex is as common as parental denial. What frequently happens is that parents simply do not *ask* their teenage children about their use of drugs, and—if they do ask and if, indeed, their youngsters are using drugs—the likely answer will be not the truth but a *lie*. Lying, like denial, serves to undermine the effective functioning of the family's problem-solving capabilities. Teenagers often tell me, "Of course I lie about drugs. If I told them the truth, I'd get punished!" What a straightforward and revealing summation of a complex and, in this instance, sadly distorted thought process. Behind the statement is the recognition of the conflict between teenage and parental values on drug use and the unmistakable assumption that the existence of potential parental punishment justifies the teenage lie. When I say, "But that is dishonest. If you want to use drugs, you ought to have the courage to do it openly in your family. Otherwise, you are cheating," my statement usually produces a cynical grin or wide-eyed disbelief.

The Big Lie, ineptly concealed, is so common among drug users as to be overlooked or ignored. It is based on the misguided assumption that "Anyone who seeks to punish me for my drug-using behavior has, by his or her commitment to the punishment, forfeited the right to the truth." This assumption has been carried so far among some prevention and treatment programs in the drug and alcohol field that they insist that parents sign a formal statement that they will not punish their children *if* they tell the truth about their use of alcohol and/or other drugs. This approach buys into the falsely distorted concept that the fault in such interactions between the parents and teenagers is with the punisher, not the liar. Nothing else, it seems to me, so eloquently expresses the moral confusion that has brought us to the sad state in which we now find ourselves with the problems produced by alcohol and other drugs.

The lie—the concealment of truth for either negative or positive reasons—plagues us all, regardless of age or occupation. Physicians and therapists dealing with drug problems, as well as other dilemmas, must confront this issue almost every day. When they are treating a drug-involved teenager, for instance, when—if at all—do they tell the parents the child's "secrets" about drug taking, alcohol drinking, and premature sex as those hidden behaviors are revealed in therapy? And, in the beginning, how does the therapist explain to teenagers and parents what will and will not be revealed? This is delicate and vital stuff.

My approach to these problems in psychotherapy is simple. I start by telling both parents and teenagers that I will not keep secrets which I believe are important for all members of the family to know. When I find out things from parents that I judge to be of vital interest to teenagers, I will tell the teenagers—having told the parents I will do this. Similarly, when I learn things from the teenagers which I believe their parents should know, I tell the parents after I have told the teenagers I will share these facts. I assume the family is a team and that the basic facts of what is going on simply need to be understood for the team to work together successfully. That *does not mean* that every embarrassing fact about the parents or the teenagers will be shared. There are many facts of life for all of us which are best kept to ourselves, and many of these are the stuff of working with a therapist in psychotherapy. But when information is revealed which has a vital impact on the functioning of the family, that information must not be kept secret. All this, if it is to work, requires a trust that parents, teenagers, and therapist share values and goals. If this is not the case, in my experience, therapy is not likely to be successful.

Trust, I think we can all agree, is unquestionably important to the successful functioning of all family relationships—especially so in the emotional, impulsive years of adolescence. How, then, do we *sustain* it and make it *grow*? If we are not trusted, how do we become worthy of trust? Above all, I think, we need to understand its foundations. The only lasting basis for trust must be an uncompromising honesty— and a willingness to pay the required price for deviations from family rules. This brutally simple rule is, of course, as applicable to adults in the family as it is to children. Dealing every day, as I do, with deviations from this rule, I can tell you that the deceitful, lying family member eventually and almost invariably pays an exorbitantly high price for the lies he tells. Lying, like drug use itself, is a way of trying to get something for nothing. It is a way of trying to get what you want *now* by sacrificing what you can hope for the *future*. The price of lying, like the interest on an unpaid loan, just keeps growing as the lie persists.

Confession of the violation of rules, whether inside or outside the family, is the only way to heal the wounds caused by lying. At the risk of seeming simplistic, I believe the old-fashioned values are the best basis for clear and constructive action: tell the truth. If you cannot tell the truth to those who have a close and personal interest in your life, then you have no business doing what you are doing. This is as true for a doctor as it is for a parent or a teenager. I am reinforced in this conviction by something I have learned from the wise workings of Alcoholics Anonymous: When it comes to recovery from addiction, the lying and the cheating and the stealing that are characteristically a part of the problems produced by dependence on alcohol and other drugs must be met head-on by the making of a fearless moral *inventory*. As an outgrowth of that inventory, the liar, the cheat, or the thief must make direct amends to those who have suffered from their dishonest actions. The only acceptable reason why he would be excused from doing so would be the very strong possibility that by making such direct reparation he would further injure the victim to whom the amends are due.

Up to this point, among the other conclusions I hope you have drawn is the fact that one of the biggest problems faced by teenagers today is the lack of trust by their parents who are deeply concerned about their children's use of drugs. As a teenager, you have only one real solution to this problem: acceptance of a foolproof method to demonstrate beyond any doubt that you are not using drugs. The only way to establish trust on this point is to agree to take urine tests. True, some teenagers resent urine testing as demeaning and as an invasion of their privacy. A few see urine testing itself as a manifestation of a lack of trust. On the basis of my experience as a psychiatrist, however, I must say that the issue of teenage drug use needs to be faced directly by both teenagers and their parents. That means agreeing on a "No Drug Use" policy for teenagers and using urine testing to *verify* that the agreement is being kept. When teenagers refuse testing, I can only conclude they have something to hide.

A much more constructive approach is that used by a 16-year-old who—when the issue of trust about his possible drug use came up—simply said to his father, "You can have all the urine you want, anytime you want it." Tossing the issue back to the parent in this way ended the problem. A series of negative urine tests, indicating nonuse, will usually end parental mistrust. If, on the other hand, you say you will stop drug use, but secretly intend to continue using drugs, then urine testing is a real threat. This position I consider dishonest on the teenager's part and not worthy of respect. If you want to continue drug use and are willing to pay the price, that position I strongly disagree with, but at least it is honest. When there is any question of drug use by a teenager I work with, I strongly urge urine testing as a way to get beyond this mistrust and to reestablish trust.

Determine Not to Let Impulses and Grievances
Block Your Long-Range Goals

It is important for you as a teenager to understand that you must—to protect your interest and your future—think clearly about your real goals and not let your impulses and your grievances get in the way of accomplishing those goals. You will, one way or another, be an independent adult soon. That is not the issue. The important issue is *how* you get to adulthood and *what you have going for you* when you do become independent. Your parents can help you if you will help them. If that means cleaning and organizing your room more often than you would like to, or missing a concert or two, or getting in earlier at night than you want to, or not using marijuana or alcohol, that hardly seems like too high a price to pay. Remember that all the skills you learn by disciplining yourself to be responsible and reliable will help you when you are an adult.

One Final Point to Remember: In Spite of
All Its Problems, Adolescence Can Be Fun

This part of your life is not all trouble and pain or even all effort. When you think about becoming an adult, you do not have to become just like your parents or any other adult. (In fact, you *could not*, even if you wanted to.) Being an adult, you will discover, demands much responsibility and a lot of work, both for yourself and for those who depend on you. Building good work habits and establishing close personal relationships are a challenge. But, surprising as this may sound, attaining and using these skills can be a fulfilling experience. Many of these tough adult responsibilities prove to be the most rewarding parts of one's life. There is also plenty of time for relaxation and fun. The challenge is fitting it all together and making it work: your way, for you, and for those you care about. For everyone of all ages, this process of fitting life's pieces together is always an unfinished but exciting and, at times, inspiring challenge.

FOR PARENTS: SOME SUGGESTIONS

Don't Forget to Listen

Remember that at the beginning of this chapter I pointed out that the most commonly expressed need of teenagers from their parents is to be listened to. Teenagers, even those who rebel and appear to reject their parents, often want to be listened to. It is tempting for adults to begin interactions with teenagers with lectures or self-related stories. Sometimes this is appropriate. Most often it is not. What is needed far more often is quality, and quantity, listening: a genuine effort to understand what the teenager is going through and a sympathetic effort to help clarify *his or her feelings* without imposing, prematurely and inappropriately, parental opinions. This can, I believe, be done without the parent turning into a wishy-washy "buddy" who lacks both values and toughness. Work at being an active, problem-solving partner in the shared family enterprise of helping your child grow up happy, healthy, and productive.

Think Back Over Your Own Teenage Years, and Recall Your Special Vulnerabilities

You know that kids can drive parents crazy. But the reverse can also be true. Think back to your own late adolescence. What did *you* want? What did you feel? What did you understand? What did *your* parents do which helped you, and what did they do which—now, with 20-20 hindsight, you can see—did not help you? What were your strengths, your weaknesses—your vulnerabilities? As you think about these questions and come up with your answers, you might continue to ask yourself: How is my son, my daughter answering these self-same questions about his or her late adolescence today? How is the image of *their* world reflected in the answers they might give?

While we might profitably zero in on any number of such questions, for purposes of illustration let us take a few moments to bring the spotlight down on just one of them: *the special vulnerability of young adolescents.* Recent scientific studies have demonstrated what parents have known for generations. Children going through puberty, roughly ages 12 to 16, are riding on a scary roller coaster of physical and emotional changes. Children, who are sensible before the age of 12 and again after the age of 16, become emotionally unstable during those intervening years of change. Impulsive, emotional behavior seems to come out of nowhere. Like a summer thunderstorm, emotions blow up with a tremendous force, only to disappear minutes or hours later. Self-image and feelings toward parents (and peers) are unusually volatile during these years. I need not remind you as a parent that these are the years when good sense and control—both self-control and family control—are often the weakest. They are the years when the young person's ability to cope with emotional storms is lowest. The highs are higher and the lows lower because the child aged 12 to 16 has so little perspective on his feelings and his experiences. When down, it feels like forever. When up, it feels like walking on water would be easy.

When you, as a parent today, look back on your own adolesence, you will be quick to realize that you did not have to face one terribly difficult question which your children find nearly inescapable: *What shall I do about using alcohol and other drugs?* And they must try to answer it at a time when they are most vulnerable—when their emotionality and impulsivity are the hallmarks of this special period in their young lives. It is no accident that these are the years for the start of most of the drug and alcohol use in this country: the years when the brain's pleasure system gets turned on—or at least turned up—in your youngster's head. That turn-on is both normal and inevitable, of course. It is also understandable and survivable. That is why it is so important that parents talk with their children about what is happening to them and their peers. And that is why, too, that it helps you, in your parental role, to go back in your mind and see your children's vulnerabilities from the perspective of your own adolescence.

During the past two decades, the traditional family and community controls over young people in the 12 to 16 age bracket have been weakened, in part, because young people have been treated as Pseudo-Adults, a treatment which makes kids seem—and want to be—older and more "adult" than they really are. This, as I have observed it, just makes children of this age more worried and more vulnerable, and it makes this period in their lives more dangerous. Whatever you, as a parent, may think about drinking at age 18 or 21, or even about marijuana use by adults, you will almost surely agree that early adolescents between ages 12 and 16 need to be protected from these dependence-producing and impulse-releasing drugs. The saddening statistics cited early in Chapter 1 show that it is precisely this age group which is now first victimized by drug and alcohol use.

Not only are these children highly susceptible to the lures of drug use, but they are also especially vulnerable to *drug dependence.* Studies show that they have less resistance to the adverse effects of drugs, as well as to other feeling-producing behaviors like sex and depression. This makes even more important the support and guidance which only you as parents can give them. Young people who experiment with drugs at a later age—say, in their early 20s—have a much better chance to find their way out of the dependence trap.

Also, as you have probably noticed, youngsters who become heavily involved in alcohol and other drugs during their early teens are more likely to wander far off the track in their lives. And, even if they do stop drug use later on, the chances of their recovering the momentum of their lives are discouragingly low. These are among the many good reasons why you need to be deeply concerned about your children during these vulnerable years. The stakes are high.

Give Your Best Efforts to Raising Your Teenager

Your job as a parent is to raise your children. As I have emphasized, this is your most important responsibility. It is a responsibility you assumed even before they were born. You owe your best efforts to them. And, like them, you too can take courage from the realization that, however painful the child-raising process, it is time limited: it will end soon. One parent unintentionally but aptly summed up this time limitation factor for me when she said she found herself screaming at her 16-year-old son one night about his coming in late: "Don't you understand? I'm doing this so you will someday be free of me, not to keep you here! My greatest fear is that 10 years from tonight we'll be standing right here arguing about your allowance and your hours and your drug use, and I can't keep it up for that long!" So . . . parents, your goal should be to give the child-raising process your best effort now, while you still have a chance of success.

Help Your Child Grow Up Happy, Positive, and Productive

Think about what your child needs to help him or her grow up as a reasonably positive, reasonably happy, and reasonably productive adult. What will help your child develop his or her skills to work and to love? For teenagers, having rules to measure their intellectual, psychological, and social growth against and having a meaningful role in family life are both important. It is important also that your child know you. Spend enough time talking and *listening* to your teenager to know, as kids say today, where he or she is "coming from." That does not mean that you will always agree with your children, or that you are to change the rules to satisfy them. But they must know you have heard them. Talk conflicts over together and also talk them over with your spouse, with older and younger children, and with others you trust: friends, relatives, parents of peers, and religious leaders. Do not be afraid to ask for advice and help. And do not get yourself stuck in a corner. Show your child that you are willing to think a problem through again. But also remember that, as the parent, the decision is yours. You can do all the listening and get all the advice you need, but in the end the decision remains yours and yours alone.

Have Fun with Your Teenager: Play—and Work—Together

Families can have fun together, once they begin to function better. Think about things you can do which will include your teenager along with others in the family. These can be work projects, as well as recreational activities. It is much better to work alongside a child than to tell her or him to "go and do it." I recall one father, a single parent, complaining to me about his 16-year-old daughter because she did not always willingly carry in the groceries, put them away, cook some of the meals, and clean up the kitchen. I asked him if he did these things with his daughter. He looked at me, shocked, and said, "No. I buy the groceries! She has to do something." I did not talk with his daughter about this, but I can imagine the feeling she had about these chores: if her father was not willing to do them with her, he was saying something about the value he placed on the work and about his values for himself and for her. In her mind, I suspect, there could well have been a thread of deep resentment that ran something like this: "This is bad duty. And if I'm smart, I'll find some way not to have to do it." I think this father—and his daughter, too—would have been better off if he had worked amiably with her, realistically showing her that many things in life have to be done, whether we like them or not, and that it is a lot better to do them cheerfully than to try to push them off on someone else. That someone else is not likely to feel good about a job unfeelingly dumped on her or him.

Criticize Fairly and As Often As Needed, But Mix in Plenty of Praise, Too

Parents give a lot of criticism to their kids. Kids deserve and need criticism. A friend of mine, a middle-school principal and father of five sons, gave me some good advice about criticizing children: give them as much criticism as you want to and as much as they need, but always balance every criticism of bad behavior with at least two "praises" for things they have done right. His two-for-one rule is a good one for parents dealing with kids. I have found that it works well in relationships with others, too. It is also not a bad rule for kids who criticize their parents.

Be Alert for Signs of Drug Use and Related Problems

Knowing whether your teenage child is or is not using drugs can be a serious difficulty for parents. Always begin by trusting your child, but do not blind yourself to possibly painful reality. There are some common signs of drug use, but they are not usually obvious until use is occurring at a frequency of three times a week or more, and usually not until it has continued at that level for six months to two years.

These signs include failing grades; increased conflicts with people in authority, especially parents and teachers; pulling away from the family and centering life on new friends who share these new values; and, for many drug-using teenagers, lying and stealing. Drug paraphernalia and drug-related T-shirts and posters are the teenager's personal advertisements of pro-drug values. If you have reason to connect your teenager with possible drug use, it makes sense to ask him or her directly about it, because many drug-using children will confess immediately when asked. However, such a direct approach does not always work. Conning and lying often become the drug user's methods for handling anyone who tries to get between him and his drugs. This is, sadly, true even for children who have previously been quite trustworthy.

Urine Testing as a Detector of Drug Use. Although I strongly recommend direct asking and answering of the question about drug use, if use is denied, there is only one foolproof way to know: urine testing. A urine sample should be taken and checked by a laboratory for as long as there is an issue between the parents and the teenager about drug use. A positive test, indicating recent use of a drug, should lead to direct, reasonable punishment. Appropriate penalties are earlier curfews, reductions in allowance, and withholding use of the family car. The teenager should fully understand the possible punishments before testing begins, and the penalties should continue only for a limited time—say, one to four weeks after a positive test. Once the tests turn negative (indicating no recent drug use), the punishments should stop, and the child should be praised. The urine testing for drug use should continue until several consecutive tests are negative, thus confirming cessation of drug use. Tests can then become occasional and may even be stopped completely if trust is reestablished.

While urine testing is not the most fundamental part of family-based drug abuse prevention, it is one of the the most controversial. It therefore merits careful review. Urine can be tested for all commonly used illegal drugs except LSD. Newer technology may permit similar tests using saliva. Blood tests for recent drug use are also available. Only alcohol can be tested at this time by a breath test, but alcohol can also be tested in urine or blood samples. These objective drug tests are positive (showing recent drug use) for periods ranging from a few hours after use until several days afterwards. Results depend on many variables, among them the specific drug used, the amount used, the concentration of the urine, and the sensitivity of the particular test employed.

As a practical matter, I suggest that families concerned about teenage drug use consider, with their physician or other advisor, having a number of urine collection bottles in the home so that, if a question of drug use arises, a urine sample can be taken promptly. The closer the sample is taken to the time of suspected drug use, the more likely it is to be valid. Thus, taking it late Saturday night or early Sunday morning is more likely to produce a positive result than is a test taken Tuesday afternoon. Insofar as the teenager in question is concerned, the timing of testing should be unpredictable; he should not know when he will be tested. Maintenance of a random and uncertain timing is an important part of the drug prevention effect of urine testing.

Remember also that tests will be done only for those drugs which you specifically ask for, and, in general, you will be expected to pay for each separate question to which you are seeking an answer. The test usually costs from $5 to $25. For practical purposes, unless there has been a problem with another specific drug, the most likely intoxicating drugs used by today's teenagers are alcohol and marijuana. It is usually necessary to have a physician order the urine test and issue you a prescription for it, although some clinical laboratories are now providing this service directly to the public. When you obtain the urine bottles to be used for the sampling, ask for advice about the proper procedure for storing the samples of the urine between the time it is collected and the time when it is delivered to the laboratory for analysis. Above all, of course, be absolutely sure that the sample of the urine to be tested actually comes from the person you intend to test. You will, in fact, need to accompany the provider into the bathroom and observe the actual taking of the sample. This new technology enables families to know whether drug taking has ceased or is continuing, and for that reason it is one of the most powerful new tools in family-based drug abuse prevention. Urine testing alone, however, is not an adequate response to the overall problem of drug use; urine testing can be no more than one of the several important steps in the total family program needed to solve a drug problem.

Two issues dealt with in this chapter are likely to provoke controversy and alienate some families. The first, coming early in the chapter, was the discussion of the possibility that a child under the age of 19 may have to be controlled by the use of the criminal justice system and/or by actually leaving the family home. These are unpleasant, and fortunately, relatively uncommon outcomes. However, parents need to think these issues through and be prepared to take whatever steps are necessary, including using the powers of the law or the prospect of withdrawal of family support. If families are not willing to consider these painful options, they are likely, in my experience, to be pushed into accepting adolescent drug use. The drug-using child, in effect, often says, "You cannot stop me. I'll do what I want!"

The second difficult problem is urine testing. Most families who have not been hit by a drug problem find even the discussion of such testing to be unpleasant if not positively repugnant. If you do not need urine testing in your family, fine. Consider yourself fortunate. But if drug use is a problem, and if you believe you need to know the facts, as a practical matter there is no alternative. It is well, therefore, to think this painful issue through thoroughly. As with the use of the law and/or the threat of family rejection, it is often wise to think about the issue of urine testing early. A clear-minded, goal-oriented approach to these issues can often prevent drug problems from developing in the first place, or, if they do develop, such an approach can often hasten the solution. Avoiding these difficult issues by wishful thinking is unlikely to be useful. Avoidance can, in fact, be dangerous given the widespread and life-or-death nature of the problem of drug dependence. I believe that the approaches I am recommending are not anti-child or even pro-parent. They are, for many families, simple matters of survival in difficult times.

To Test or Not to Test: Some Pros and Cons. Some experienced therapists disagree with the recommendation of using urine testing as part of family prevention and treatment of drug dependence. One senior colleague, for example, made the following comments to me: First, there are objective changes resulting from acute intoxication with drugs producing specific alterations in thinking and behavior, especially after chronic drug use, that a concerned parent or counselor can observe. Second, there is open communication between parent and child which can help identify drug use. Third, if a urine test is positive, what, he asked, has been gained besides resentment (since it could be ascertained anyway that the youth had used drugs)? Fourth, if the urine test is negative, does this undermine the parents' position since it may vindicate a rebellious child? Fifth, what about false positives and false negatives—in other words, laboratory errors? Sixth, he suggests youngsters can read my book and turn to LSD. All in all, he thinks urine testing is better left to industry and the military. This critique, he emphasized, was not meant to question the focus on the family or on the strictly enforced drug-free goal for children. This therapist, from his experience, simply felt that urine testing was not necessary or desirable.

My colleague makes important points. To his suggestion that there are objective behavioral changes resulting from intoxication with drugs, I respond, "Sometimes. But often not until late in the process." I am reminded of all the times I have worked with people addicted to and acutely intoxicated by drugs ranging from marijuana and cocaine to heroin and tranquilizers. I, myself, have been unsure as to whether or not they were then using drugs until I tested their urine. If I have this much trouble, after nearly 20 years of experience in this field, is it realistic to expect untrained, but concerned, parents to reliably make this determination?

To his contention that open communication often gives parents all the information they need about teenage drug use, I respond, "Often so, but not invariably. Sometimes lying by a drug-using teenager gets in the way of open communication."

To his third point, that a positive test may lead to resentment, I respond, "Indeed it can. But at least the facts are clear to everyone." When he says that a negative urine test can undermine parental concerns and vindicate a rebellious child, I reply, "A negative test can be a problem because relatively infrequent use of drugs at relatively low levels can go undetected. When the urine test comes back negative under these conditions, it can actually undermine parental concern and falsely encourage teenage drug use by suggesting to the child that he can beat the urine test." The simple solution to this problem is repeated testing, since subsequent urine tests are likely to prove positive if drug use continues.

My colleague's fifth point about the unreliability of laboratory procedures is well taken. Although the tests themselves are quite reliable, there are many human and mechanical sources of error. In my experience, however, when used as part of a family drug abuse prevention program, urine testing is sufficiently reliable so this is not a serious problem. Although I am prepared to accept the fact that errors are made, the simple assumption is that a positive test is more likely to be correct than is the denial of use by a suspected drug user. Furthermore, drug use can be validated by subsequent retesting. With an accuracy of between 80 percent and 100 percent, the tests are good enough for me and most parents I have worked with.

His sixth point, that teenagers can read the book and switch to LSD, a drug which cannot now be tested for, receives this reply: "I have never seen that happen. Moreover, I expect that tests for LSD are not too far in the future."

I labor these points, not to put my colleague-friend down, but to say that I have seen the approach I am recommending work, and I have seen a more informal and trusting approach fail. My experience has convinced me that a structured, firm urine-testing policy can be useful and necessary.

Whatever approach a family uses, it should be well thought out and systematically implemented. A casual or naive approach is unlikely to achieve good results for either parents or teenagers.

Go as Far as Necessary to Keep
Your Teenager from Using Drugs

Parents frequently ask, "How far should I go to get my child to stop using drugs?" The answer is: "As far as necessary." "Necessary" can mean simply establishing rules and enforcing consequences for their violation. It can mean outpatient treatment for the drug-using child. Or it can call for more intensive and prolonged treatment. How far up this scale the family must go is determined by the teenager's commitment to continued drug use. The teenager should be made to understand completely that he or she holds the key to this escalation: the parents will go as far as necessary to ensure that the teenager stops using drugs.

To many families, my recommendations may—at first thought—sound harsh and mistrusting. But my experience with using this approach is quite the opposite. Generally, such a direct approach, which usually includes at least the possibility of urine testing, solves the problem of distrust, ends searches of the teenager's room, makes listening in on telephone calls unnecessary, and reestablishes a more compatible working relationship between parents and child. It also gives the teenage child a strong, direct reason not to use drugs because the consequences are unmistakable and inevitable. This clearcut policy will help teenagers in dealing with their peers, too. I have talked with many teenagers months or years after their families have instituted this type of "get tough on drugs" policy, and almost all of them have agreed that the results—in the end—made life simpler, more forthright, and more satisfactory for them.

Learn When to WITHHOLD Support from Your Late-Adolescent Child and When to GIVE Support

One final point for parents: On both sides of the Great Dividing Line for your teenage children, the line between childhood and adulthood, it is important to be clear and strong. For your children, that means you must be the parent, demonstrating that you are in charge. That can be difficult because some children severely test their parents. It may come, as it did for the woman with the "YMCA solution," to the point of giving your child the choice of living by the family rules or leaving the family. In most families, however, once the parents make this point firmly and calmly, the child will settle down and abide by the family guidelines. However, the old admonition to "shape up or ship out" cannot be an idle threat. If, in your parental role, you make it, you must not hesitate to carry through on it, and the child needs to know that you will. If your child decides to leave the home, you must make it unmistakably clear that the child is *choosing* to leave because he or she chooses not to accept the family rules. When and if the child is ready to accept these rules, you should welcome the child back. In any event, it should be completely understood by all that the decision to leave is the child's, and the child's alone. Children should not, in other words, be forced out of the family prematurely.

On the other side of the bridge between childhood and adulthood, there is often an equally difficult dilemma for parents: the failing adult child who wants and seems to need rescuing. Avoid—strictly avoid—the temptation to attempt such a rescue. If your child is 19 years of age or older and is arrested for drug possession or sale of an illegal substance, I urge you not to bail him out, and I strongly recommend that you do not pay a lawyer to get him off.

Similarly, even if you can afford to do so, you should not contribute to the support of adult-age drug-using children who are not supporting themselves. I make only one possible exception: you might decide—if justification is ample—to pay for the treatment of the drug-abusing adult child, especially if that person is making a positive effort to support himself or herself by holding a full-time job. Despite any compassionate concerns you might have to the contrary, the adult child should not be allowed to live at home, making use of free room and board services provided by the parents. If the child, after reaching adulthood, wants or needs to come home for a brief visit or a short vacation, fine. But such occasions should be explicitly limited to short periods of time. If the adult child is to remain in the family's home for a longer time, he or she should pay full value for room and board and whatever other services may be provided. In such circumstances, of course, the adult child should, in addition, abide by all family rules about hours of coming and going, about drug and alcohol use, about personal health and grooming, etc. For the Pseudo-Child who is allowed to remain in the home but does not follow these rules, dependency is likely to develop, and eventual adult functioning will become all the harder. In contrast, the adult child who is functioning well can and should be encouraged and supported in a variety of ways. Families who are able to support adult children financially are fortunate, but they should do so only if the child is fulfilling his or her role as an adult.

A useful distinction needs to be drawn between parents and their children in terms of their functioning relationships. Parents often disapprove of some of the actions of their adult children, and when they do, they owe it to them to make this disapproval known. Regardless of the age of the children, parents should, in other words, be clear and vocal about what they approve and do not approve. At the same time, however, they should recognize that decisions which affect the adult child now rest with the fully functioning adult, not the parents. This distinction between adult and child means, further, that both adult children and preadult children should be able to criticize fairly and make suggestions to their parents. Insofar as the preadult child is concerned, however, the decision to act or not to act on the suggestions or criticisms continues to rest with the parent.

Extend Your Jurisdiction if Your Child Goes Away to College

A special case arises for parents and children when the child is supported by the parents in college or even in graduate school. Here the child has intentionally and purposefully extended his or her childhood, and I strongly recommend that the parents retain their role as supervisor of the child's behavior for the agreed-upon duration of that extension. This includes monitoring grades and other behaviors, especially those involving the spending of support money and the use of alcohol and other drugs. Parents can and should have standards, and when their college-student children do not meet these standards, there should be serious consequences.

An incident which I observed several years ago exemplifies this point. Sally, a 19-year-old sophomore, was away from home at college. Her older sister had married and settled in this college town after having graduated from the same college herself. Shortly before Thanksgiving, Sally's older sister telephoned her parents and told them that Sally was using marijuana and probably other drugs, and that she was doing poorly in school. The parents, after talking this over together, called Sally the following day and gave her two choices: (1) return home immediately, dropping out of school to satisfy her parents that she was drug free, or (2) expect no further support from the parents for her education. Sally came home the next day to argue with her parents, asking for another chance and explaining that she was being "misunderstood." Despite Sally's pleas and tears, the parents stuck to their position.

The following morning, Sally got up and asked to go to church with her parents. Accepting their first option, she got a job and began paying for her room and board at home. Between November and the following June, she held several different jobs and learned a great deal about the kinds of work she did not want to do. In June she returned to college, and three years later she graduated. She told her parents and her older sister that they had saved her life by their intervention. How many families could have done what Sally's family did? How many children could have done what Sally did?

SUMMING UP WITH AN EXAMPLE: A FAMILY TEAM WORKS AT SOLVING ITS PROBLEMS

As many of the vignettes I have included amply demonstrate, not all families are successful in overcoming their drug problems. In closing this chapter, I would like to describe how one family worked as a team in an effort to solve its problems with alcohol and other drugs. Bud was 17 years old, a high school senior, when I first saw him. He was the second son of a government official and his wife. Bud's mother brought him into treatment, labeling Bud's marijuana use as "the problem." But, at the first session, she also expressed her concern over her husband's drinking, which she considered "alcoholic." Bud's father denied this, but he did concede that he drank too much. Bud said he smoked marijuana "at least three times a week" and admitted that his grades had fallen over the last two years from mostly B's to mostly D's and F's. His peer relationships were limited to going around with drug-using "friends."

After several sessions, during which we discussed the problem of drug dependence generally and those in Bud's family in particular, Bud agreed to stop all drug use, including marijuana and alcohol. Bud's father did not want to stop drinking, but agreed to quit smoking—something he considered a more serious threat to his health—and to limit his drinking to "no more than two drinks an evening." Bud's mother played the "heavy" in these discussions, putting pressure on both Bud and his father. They, in turn, reinforced each other's resolve to "get off drugs."

Six months after successful treatment had been completed—including regular urine testing, which confirmed that Bud had stopped drug use—I spoke with Bud's mother. She reported that Bud had improved his grades to A's and B's, that he had made the high school soccer and frisbee teams, and that for the first time ever he had gone out on some dates. He was cheerful and had been accepted at one of the two colleges he had hoped to attend. Her husband had completed a smoking-cessation program and had stopped cigarette smoking entirely. He was proud of this, as were his wife and son. He still drank two or three drinks every evening and, according to his wife, "turned nasty" when he did. She was pleased with the changes in the family: "We're back to the way we were before Bud got into drugs." But she also realized, now that she was less concerned about her son and her husband, that she had neglected some problems of her own. As Bud was about to leave home to go to college, there was more pressure on her marriage, and she felt she needed to get a job to keep herself busy and to help pay for Bud's expenses in college. She felt scared and a bit depressed about the prospects because she had not worked at a paying job since her children were born.

That's it. Unfinished. Not the stuff of which fairy tales are made. Bud was, according to his mother, "still not out of the woods." She was worried, with good reason, about what would happen to him when he went away to college. She was not entirely happy in her marriage, and she still felt strongly that her husband should stop drinking entirely. (I agreed with her and told all three of them my views.) She was also dealing more directly with the issues of her own life, some of which had nothing to do with her son or her husband.

While this is not a tidy story, it is a moderately happy one. Bud is back on track; his father has stopped smoking and cut down on his drinking. The family, in a word, is again functioning successfully as a team, dealing with their individual and shared problems with reasonable effectiveness. Taken together, their experiences highlight one other lesson: without Bud's mother's determination, it is unlikely that any of these successful changes would have been made. She, the "nonuser," blew the whistle on family drug use. Trying to deal courageously with the teenager's drug problem brought to the surface a family problem about a parent's drug use. That, too, is common.

There is a darker side to this story. Although intervention by Bud's mother did accomplish a great deal, it did not totally solve either her son's or her husband's problems. On the other hand, it did open the door to some personal problems she needed to work on. Her intervention did get the family talking and working together. It did lead to positive changes in both her husband and her son. My greatest concern as I left this family was my doubts about Bud's father's alcoholism. In a real sense he dodged a bullet by his unwillingness to confront his more serious problem with alcohol. By cutting down on his drinking, he took the momentum out of the family system. Based on my past experience with similar situations, I must conclude that it will take a major (and potentially disastrous) crisis in the life of Bud's father for him to again face his unresolved and terribly destructive alcoholism. Drug problems, obviously, know no age limit. As I have stressed so strongly, they are—after all—family affairs. And even though such problems almost always start and are often most severe in teenage years, let us reach no falsely happy conclusion that, as we grow older, we more or less automatically "grow out" of drug danger or that it will "just naturally fade away."

This chapter has focused on tensions and conflicts, but not because they are a necessary or an inevitable part of the relationships between adult parents and their teenage children. Many families escape the worst of these conflicts. My observation, however, is that those families which appear to have escaped have adopted and lived by principles similar to those I have outlined here. It is also a product of my experience that I believe such families should count themselves lucky rather than superior. For all families, these are difficult times to go through a difficult stage of the human life cycle.

CHAPTER
SEVEN

Making Drug Abuse
Treatment Work

A N OUNCE OF PREVENTION is worth a pound of cure. Nowhere is this well-worn proverb more apt than in the soul-testing domain of drug dependence. Three conceptual notions, each developed in Chapter 2, underlie all successful efforts to resolve drug problems. The first is the "Addiction Switch." The second is summarized in the words, "Two Heads Are Better Than One." The third concept, borrowed from Alcoholics Anonymous, is "Easy Does It." By way of review, let us look briefly at how these notions work to stop drug problems.

Three Guiding Considerations
Underlying Drug Abuse Treatment

Do NOT Turn on the Addiction Switch. Dependence-producing drugs are chemicals which, when taken into the human body, produce feelings the user learns to like. We call this "pleasure," but the experience ranges from the intense "rush" from intravenous cocaine use to the dreamy relaxation following the smoking of marijuana to the reduced sense of social awkwardness following a few drinks of alcohol. As we have seen all too often, after a short or long period of escalating apparently controlled use, some users of all dependence-producing drugs become dependent daily users. They have thrown their Addiction Switch to the *on* position. Their drug use then goes from casual to compulsive. Drug-caused problems mount even as the drug blinds the user to the extent and negative consequences of that use. Once he or she is dependent, there is no realistic possibility of returning to controlled drug use. The problem of drug dependence for the user, however, is far larger than mere pharmacology. His whole life becomes drug centered while he uses drugs. All feelings and relationships—good and bad—are filtered through his drug habit.

The only practical hope for him or her is to become and remain entirely drug-free. But, unfortunately, as we know from long observation, dependent users cannot of their own free will and effort call a halt to their dependence. They need support, direction, and encouragement, which—when combined—I call *social control.* The primary and most effective source of social control, when it comes to drug-induced, pleasure-producing behaviors, is the family. This leads us to the second of our conceptual notions.

Two Heads Are Better Than One. The first mental function affected by drug intoxication is self-awareness of the negative effects of drugs. The user's mind is clouded by the drug or drugs he is taking. It is clouded to the point where he is not likely to make wise or intelligent decisions about preventing further dependence even if he wanted to. He needs help. Therefore, it is the *nonusers,* especially nonusers in the family, who must step in and take action. That two heads are better than one has still another and wider implication: Drug use by one family member can, in time, figuratively if not literally drive the whole family crazy. Thus, it seems that families, too, need support. They can seldom confront and resolve a family member's drug problem alone. This support can come from meeting with other similarly affected families or from working with treatment programs and professional therapists. In fact, working in conjunction with other families having similar problems can be one of the most effective steps that the drug-affected family can take. Al-Anon, the adjunct to Alcoholics Anonymous, is the largest and most effective of these family-support groups, and one to which I will be calling further attention from time to time.

"Easy Does It." Perhaps this third concept should be elaborated to "Easy—and *Steady*—Does It." A chaotic, confused, emotional response to a drug problem will seldom be helpful for the drug user or his family. Cool heads are needed, working together as a team over a long period of time, to share in achieving a cure for this progressive, terribly serious, potentially fatal disorder called drug dependence.

PREvention and INTERvention: Review and Preview

Drug abuse treatment begins after prevention has failed. *Prevention* means stopping a drug problem before it begins; *treatment,* as I am using the word, means stopping dependence after it has become firmly established. There is a middle ground between the first use of a drug and the point at which the drug problem has become serious and chronic. This largely uncharted zone between initial experimentation and the onset of dependence is the time between that first, usually problem-free fling with the drug high and the problem-filled nightmare of total dependence.

Although many professionals prefer to call remedial efforts in this time zone *intervention,* I call them Family Action. From long and intensive experience with drug-dependent people, I realize that there are vitally important roles which the family must play during both prevention and treatment. During the crucial period between experimentation and dependence, as we shall subsequently see, Family Action is the dynamic most likely to make the difference between success and failure.

Drug abuse prevention was the central thrust of Chapter 6. The basic concept of drug abuse prevention was described as the promotion of the family working together as a team to solve problems, to meet challenges, and to do whatever is necessary to ensure that the children in the family grow to be drug-free, effective, and reasonably happy adults. To achieve this goal, we emphasized, requires a combination of clear antidrug values and actions, plus positive progrowth efforts to make this stage of the family life cycle work for both the parents and the children. I pointed then to twin dangers to be avoided. First, do not treat children under the age of 19 as if they were adults; at that age, they are still children, not "Pseudo-Adults." And, second, do not treat family members 19 years of age or older as if they were still children; at that age, they should be adults, not "Pseudo-Children."

While some, I admitted, will see the discipline and family preeminence in value-setting which I strongly recommend for those who are 18 years of age or younger as being too adult-oriented and adult-dominated, my contention continues to be this: *By learning to function successfully and happily within this framework of family discipline, children learn the self-control which is essential during their own adulthood.*

Similarly, some will object to my "hands-off" attitude toward troubled, drug-abusing family members who are 19 years old or older, arguing that it lacks compassion and love. That is not the case. Far from it. I contend that this tough-minded approach is essential if young adult family members are to learn from the consequences of their own decisions and behaviors. How else will they be able to function effectively as interdependent but self-responsible adults? These principles are basic. They are the foundation of all successful drug abuse prevention I have ever worked with or witnessed. In this chapter on drug abuse treatment, we focus on how the family can use these same guidelines when prevention has failed to stop drug problems.

Some "Energizing" Terminology

Before proceeding further, we need to pause and think about some terminology. Consider, for instance, the common confusion about such terms as "drug use" and "drug abuse." Is the person taking drugs a "drug user" or a "drug abuser?" Or, a related question: Is the drug-dependent person "sick" or "bad"? These distinctions are more important than mere semantics. Terminology is a powerful determinant of—and, often, a deterrent to—successful endeavors in drug rehabilitation. Distinctions need to be drawn and definitions made clear, for they represent the ebb and flow of public attitudes toward drug use and, hence, the treatment of drug dependence.

Currently common words and phrases can become keys (albeit sometimes rusty ones) to approaches to treatment for those entrapped in self-destructive drug use. Calling a person a "drug user" and considering the drug user to be "sick" often creates confusion and a stumbling block to effective treatment. Considering all drug users to be, by definition, drug abusers and considering drug abusers "bad" and therefore subject to punishment creates conflicts which extend into our society's deeply held views of privacy and individual liberty.

How, then, can we understand which people—and which drug problems—should be treated? So that there will be no misunderstanding, these are the precepts which govern my practice:

> Any continuing use of an illegal drug is drug abuse. Any continuing use of alcohol which produces problems as defined by the user, his or her family, or society at large is also drug abuse. To the latter I add the strong personal conviction that alcohol intake beyond the level of two or three drinks per day likewise constitutes drug abuse. I consider all drug and alcohol abuse to be both sick and bad.

Therefore, I believe, drug abuse treatment is desirable for anyone who uses any illegal, psychoactive drug or whose drinking of alcohol is excessive, reckless, self-destructive, and in any way uncontrolled. I believe, moreover, that treatment is in order for anyone who uses alcohol or a prescription dependence-producing drug *if* that use produces any problems for the user or for those around that user.

Setting Goals for Intervention and Treatment

Before outlining the drug dependence treatment process, we should return to a clear statement of goals. The goal of all drug abuse treatment is to return the drug abuser to the drug-free state. Sounds simple? It is not. The process of achieving it is often tremendously difficult. From the beginning, at the goal-setting stage of the process, those who would help the drug-dependent person are confronted with an almost insurmountable obstacle. Most drug-dependent people are, of course, eager to be free of whatever problems their drug use is causing them, but they see the goal as being somewhat different: they want to achieve this objective without stopping their use of drugs. They seek, almost without exception, to return to the state they were in when they initially used drugs without probems. They know other users of the same drug who do not appear to have problems, and they recall when they did themselves not appear to have any as a result of their own drug use. They are, in addition, quick to see their drug-related problems either as accidents or the result of somebody else's lack of understanding of them or their drug use. Rather than acknowledging that their own drug use is the problem, most drug users prefer to believe that the problem is *someone else*—family members, their physician, the police, and/or others who intervene to stop their drug use. In short, they want to be problem-free, but not drug-free. They want their problems solved, but they are seldom willing to give up the drug use that *caused* their problems.

What many drug-dependent people fail to recognize is that setting the treatment goal of becoming and remaining completely drug-free is quite different from setting the goal of being *problem-free*. Frequently, the drug user is not the only one who is caught in this distinction. Families and others often fall victim to the same wishful thinking. They, too, want to believe that it is possible for the drug-dependent person to become again, as he once was, a controlled, apparently problem-free drug user. My experience convinces me that this is a dangerous delusion. It delays and, all too often, actually prevents the actions necessary to solve the drug problem. Too many drug users who seek to return to controlled drug use do not survive to come back to treatment a second time around. Far more frequent, and almost as tragic, is the deplorable fact that the drug-dependent person who rejects the goal of becoming completely drug-free and delays making use of effective treatment pays a terrible price in terms of health, employment, and family solidarity.

Alcoholics Anonymous has a wise way of dealing with this problem of establishing the goal of life-long, drug-free living. They never say "never" about future drinking but say only "one day at a time" for sustaining sobriety, thereby taking some of the pressure off the recovering drug abuser. On the other hand, AA is strictly uncompromising about the common wish of the recovering alcoholic to return to being a social drinker. Acting on long and painful experience, AA declares clearly and unequivocally that such a goal is impossible. When alcoholics insist on trying to return to controlled drinking, AA's attitude is "Okay, you may have to do some more personal research on that question. When you've completed your studies, come on back. We'll be waiting for you. We know what the result will be." Toughened veterans of many long and hard campaigns, the people at AA know that the odds are distressingly high that the dependent person will indeed be back. Drug dependency is a chronic disorder which, both during and after treatment, is no stranger to repeated relapse.

Returning to drug use after long and/or short periods of abstinence is so common as to be almost universal. In fact, successful recovery usually comes only after repeated failures in treatment. How can this dismal reality be squared with the goal of becoming totally drug free? *Time.* It is important to understand the importance of time and the productive, reassuring value that the passage of time can offer. Maintain a sense of time and have the patience that must go with it. Be sustained by the realization that a surprising number of good things that happen in the world happen in due time. This does not mean abandonment of the goal of drug-free living. What it does mean is that the user, the user's family, and everyone who relates to the user must be both tough-minded and patient.

IDENTIFYING THE DRUG ABUSER AND ATTENDANT PROBLEMS

Identifying the Early Adolescent Who Is Developing Drug Dependence

Treatment begins with identification of the drug problem. This is often a slow and painful process. Neither the drug user nor his family members really want to know the truth about drug dependence. This is the old cop-out, *denial*: the pretense that the drug problem does not exist. Poor school or work performance, failing family relationships, auto accidents, or even arrests are seen as unfortunate accidents or as the result of adolescence or difficult relationships—almost anything but the direct result of drug use.

It is seldom the drug user himself who identifies the drug problem, since he is usually too bellicose or too befuddled. The task of identifying the dependency falls on the shoulders of the family. The job becomes their burden and their responsibility.

The structure of the Drug Dependence Syndrome, as illustrated in Chapter 2, serves to emphasize that its early stages can be difficult to detect with certainty. Since these early stages of the syndrome ordinarily occur in adolescence, changed attitudes and relationships within the family are common. A lowered interest in family and long-standing friendships is also common. A raised interest in less conventional friends and in teenage culture, especially rock music, is typical. A reduced interest in school and long-range goals is also typical. Secretive behavior, new friends who are not introduced to the family, and changes in dress and hairstyle are also characteristic of this early stage of drug dependence. The ages of 12 to 16, when initiation of drug use is most likely, is a time of intense physical and emotional growth and of reduced reliance on the family and greater reliance on friends.

While observing all of these various manifestations of drug dependence, be sure to remember that it is also common for normal teenagers to go through a "difficult stage," most often in the age range of 12 to 15 years. During these years, children often fluctuate unpredictably, with an emotional instability and a self-concept that bounces uncontrollably between grandiosity and abject hopelessness. The key to clear differentiation of normal from pathological adolescence is to step back and study the experience more carefully. Do not lose sight of the reality that the work of children is school. If school performance fails, there is a reason. Perhaps it is a drug problem, perhaps something else, but there is a problem which should be addressed. If the ties to the family are ruptured or the relationships turn sour, then there is a problem which should be solved. Again, there may or may not be a drug problem. If the teenage child has lost his or her sense of direction for the future, there is a problem that needs to involve, and to be solved by, the family as a whole.

Sometimes, even at this early stage, a drug problem is not difficult to identify. The drug-using youngster may flaunt a T-shirt which screams out "Do Drugs!" Or he may come home drunk or stoned, have an accident in the family car, or get himself arrested. Accidentally or on purpose, the drug-using teenager may leave a trail of telltale signs such as drugs, drug paraphernalia, or a revealing diary around his room, as if asking to be found out. Or the first sign of trouble may be a phone call from a parent of one of your child's friends: "Hello, Mrs. Smith," a voice may say. "I'm Helen Toms,

Ricky's mom. We just found out that Ricky has been into drugs. Since your son, Bill, spends a lot of time with Ricky, we thought you would want to know."

Surprisingly, many families pass through this stage without coming to grips with the problems of their drug-using child. Even though the parents have known that their offspring has had problems for a decade or longer, that young person may be in his 20s or even 30s before he enters drug abuse treatment for the first time. By the time he reaches the later stages of the Drug Dependence Syndrome, the drug user will have drifted far off his expected life course. This readily translates into failed school opportunities, failure to establish a career identity, and failure to establish loving relationships inside and outside the family. Usually, it also signals failure to become self-supporting financially after leaving school.

Although some people I have worked with in this later stage of drug dependence have had earlier experiences with drug abuse treatment, they all have one thing in common: families who blindly *enable* their drug use to continue over a long period of time. Families do this for many reasons. Some permit continued drug use because they have never clearly identified the drug problem for what it is. Some enable continued drug abuse because they have not clearly identified the only goal which is compatible with recovery: complete abstinence from all intoxicating drug use by the drug-dependent person. Some families blithely go through the early warning signs of drug problems in their adolescent children because they confuse the concepts of "use" and "abuse." They know their children drink alcohol and use marijuana, for example, but they mistakenly view this as a normal part of adolescence. They shrug off failing grades and poor family relationships as "just part of being a teenager."

While it is true that teenagers do grow up as distinctly different people from their parents—an inescapable fact that shocks numerous kids and parents—it is strange that no one in these families seems to care that any use of intoxicating drugs (including alcohol and marijuana) is *illegal* for teenagers throughout the United States. It is also strikingly odd that both parents and children can close their eyes and their minds to the indisputable truth that not only does drug taking violate the law, but it is also unhealthy and unwise. Furthermore, while kids do differ from their parents in talents and goals, they need to have clearly identifiable life objectives to motivate and sustain them in self-supporting work and to help ensure stable, loving human relationships. When teenagers get off these tracks, families need to react strongly and early. Delay is dangerous and expensive. Opportunities missed in teenage years can never be fully recaptured no matter how successful the drug-dependent person's treatment may later prove to be. Time is vital. Seldom, if ever, are drug and alcohol problems simply outgrown. They mar for life.

Identifying the Pseudo-Child Who Is Drug Dependent

Family enabling behavior often takes the form of inappropriate financial support for their drug-hooked adult children. Sometimes money is simply given outright; other times, enabling takes on more subtle guises. For example, room and board are provided for years and years after the "child" should have become a self-supporting adult. At still other times, family enabling consists of hiring lawyers to defend the drug abuser after he or she has been arrested. Enabling can also mean finding jobs for the drug-dependent individual over and over again. In all cases, the enabling behavior has one pernicious result: it gets between the drug user and the consequences of his drug-using behavior—never between him and his drug. Most insidious of all, blind parental coddling blunts the potentially educational blows of reality. In short, it prevents the drug user from learning from his own mistakes.

There can be an odd and perhaps well-deserved twist of fate in all this. Family enabling prompts the drug user to turn against the overly generous parents. This is especially likely to happen when things go wrong in the drug user's life. The real culprit, of course, is the drug use. But the drug user blames his father or his mother or both, insisting that they did something wrong or failed to do something right to prevent the problem from occurring. On the day a 35-year-old heroin addict finally went into a hospital for detoxification, he told me, "My real problem is that my parents favored my brothers over me. They just never gave me support—they always put me down." This after his parents had supported him completely for the 16 years since he had dropped out of college at 19!

A drug-dependent Pseudo-Child who turns on his supportive family in this way may seem paradoxical. He isn't. Families who function in this enabling fashion may one day realize that they have created a monster. Sooner or later they may come to understand that when both the parents and the child focus, inappropriately, on their painful interactions as being "the problem," the inevitable outcome is sheer stupidity. When they worry, argue, and struggle over who did what for whom, about all the "shoulds" of their painful relationships, they generate heat, but no light. A family conflict of this kind can only be resolved when both parents and adult children, behaving as the adults they should be, are able to reorient themselves to an appropriate family goal: the goal of helping the adult child to function in the larger world, outside the family. Once that is clear, then the family becomes a *team*, functioning together to solve the drug dependence problem and all of the tasks attendant upon it. Those tasks are "out there," not "in here" in the family. The primary responsibility for facing those tasks belongs to the adult child, not to his or her parents. And tough tasks they are! If a job is lost or an arrest must be faced, the problem and its solution belong to the adult child, not to his parents. If a drug debt must be paid or the adult child faces a threat to life and limb, he must pay it without help from the family. If a cold night alone without shelter must be faced, then the adult child must face it, because his drug use has caused these problems. Only when he or she is drug-free and is able to handle personal problems well may the family again help. Any help given during continuing drug use will, in my experience, simply perpetuate the drug-induced problems and turn the family life into a horribly painful battleground. In it, not only will child be turned against parents, but parents, all too often, will be turned against each other. The one exception: families, in my view, can help support the cost of drug dependence treatment of adult children if they are financially able to do so.

Identifying the Drug-Dependent Youth with Sociopathic Tendencies

Tied directly into the step of identifying the drug abuser and his problem are the many adult children who fail to become self-supporting when they leave school. Many of these people have what professionals call a character disorder or an antisocial personality. For our purposes, we will call these people "sociopaths" because of their tendency to reject society's behavioral rules. It is commonly said that they fail to learn from experience. Such persons in the past have been called psychopaths because of their self-centered approach to life, their casual lying, and their frequent criminal behavior. Many of them showed these distinctive character traits even before they first used drugs. Frequently, as young children they were seen as hyperactive, extroverted, and hard to control. Often, from grade school years onward, they were clearly different from their siblings. Many theories, some genetic, some environmental, have been advanced to explain the origins of this troublesome behavior pattern.

After working for two decades with hundreds of such people, I have come up with three concepts which enable me to identify and sometimes help these difficult youngsters. First, whatever the deficit underlying this disorder, I am convinced that *adolescent drug and alcohol use makes it worse*. Drug-produced pleasures and the criminal drug subculture exaggerate and perpetuate this destructive syndrome. Young people with these characteristics are unusually vulnerable to drug dependence. For them, drug abuse prevention is especially vital if they are not to fall even deeper into an increasingly vicious cycle of problems.

Second, *it is not true that these people do not learn from experience*. They make excellent con artists, and they are often bright as well as engaging. They can, in most cases, learn in every way but one: they are unable to learn from ordinary punishment. While most children respond promptly and appropriately to punishment, whether it be a spanking or a critical glance, the future sociopath seems to shrug off punishment, apparently concluding that the failure of the moment is not the misbehavior for which he was punished, but the fact that he got caught. Thus, his solution is to do the same thing better next time so as to make sure he does not get caught. In contrast, the more normal child concludes that he must stop the behavior which produced punishment.

Third, *the most troublesome aspect of this syndrome is lying*: telling people what they want to hear so that the teller can get away with something that would not be permitted if the truth were known. Lying undermines family control, as well as all other forms of social control because it obscures the facts. As any con artist knows, the successful con works only to the extent that the person conned wants to believe it. Thus, sociopaths are excellent at sensing what the other person, "the mark," wants to believe. Having figured this out, they just tell that person what he wants to hear. One early casualty of this process is *trust*. Once trust is lost, something precious and essential to successful functioning in caring relationships is lost. Trust is hard to rebuild. If it is rebuilt at all, it takes years. Here, of course, I am not talking about the minor fibs or half-truths which are common in most relationships. I am talking about lying that goes to the heart of human relationships.

Many sociopaths mix these three characteristics in a remarkable fashion. Recently, in justifying why he lied to his parents when they asked him if he was continuing to use drugs, one of them blandly explained, "They would have punished me if I had told the truth." His meaning was clear: "If you want to have the truth, then let me do whatever I want to do, because if you don't, I'll have to lie." What he had trouble seeing was that, although lying did enable him to get his way in the short run, in the longer run, he had short-changed himself. When he was found out, what he had lost—his parents' trust—was far more important than anything he would have lost if he had told the truth and accepted the relatively minor punishment. But a central symptom of this syndrome is the tendency to focus only on the present tense. In the sociopathic view, if it is not now, it is never.

This is why the attraction of the drug experience is so powerful for the adolescent with sociopathic tendencies. It offers—or seems to offer—something (pleasure) for nothing (something obtainable without the work or effort usually necessary to gain the pleasure). This holds an almost irresistible lure for such an adolescent.

To make matters worse, the biological effects of puberty, with its intense activation of the brain's pleasure/reward system, come at a time when the youth's inner controls over impulses are weak. This also tends to exaggerate this syndrome. Some have observed that the normal state of the early adolescent is similar to the sociopathic state: focus on self-centered, present-tense pleasure, and heedlessly ignore future consequences and the feelings of others.

This sounds and *is* negative and discouraging. After working with dozens of families facing this problem, however, I have a few suggestions for these difficult youngsters (some of whom are no longer so young) and also for the families trying to cope with the complex and trying problems they generate. What can be done to prevent these sociopathic problems before they begin? And, once they have started, what can be done to stop them?

For the sociopathic person himself, I have advice that is simple to give but hard to follow: Face the fact that you have a problem, that you do not have the same warning system most people have for trouble. You tend to drive right through the useful stoplights in life. To overcome this, you must apply a simple test to any pleasure-producing behavior before you indulge your wishes: if you cannot tell the whole truth about what you are going to do to all the people who are involved, do not do it. If you do it anyway, then tell the truth and accept the consequences right away. If you do not, you can confidently expect that sooner or later you will pay the full price for your misbehavior. Cons and lies never work in the long run.

For parents who have children with this sociopathic tendency, I urge a firm approach to punishment for misbehavior. Make the punishment swift and certain, being sure that it is noticeable and effective. As you do this, take plenty of time to talk it all through in order to help your child understand that the pain that comes to him in the form of punishment is the result of his misbehaviors themselves and that he will never be able to solve problems of this kind merely by trying to be more clever. If the family pressure from this approach is too great, it is often helpful to involve others in the process. Relatives, church-related helpers, and professional therapists can all offer assistance.

Alcoholics Anonymous has an effective means of handling this type of problem through their group-support process and their 12-Step Program. Upon concluding successive steps in the program, the person under treatment summarizes the corrective actions taken. I cite a few examples: Step 8 is "Made a list of all persons we had harmed, and became willing to make amends to them all." Step 9 is "Made direct amends to such people whenever possible, except when to do so would injure them or others." Step 10 is "Continued to make personal inventory, and when we were wrong, promptly admitted it."

One question I have long pondered is why some people learn so quickly from punishment and why others are so slow to learn from it. In fact, in my clinical psychiatric practice I see many patients who are overly sensitive to punishment and react strongly to it, sometimes even when it is not present at all. These people, I have noticed, often suffer from phobias and depression. This causes me to wonder if there are not some significant biological factors within some people which prompt them to experience pain following punishment whereas other people are unable to experience pain when punished. The sociopath seems to have a tiny, if any, reaction to punishment: it seems not to hurt at all. The phobic or the depressive is supersensitive: his or her bad feelings following even relatively mild or subtle punishment are intense and long lasting. To help the sociopathic person find the answer is generally to help him understand what is going on: to assist him in finding help, especially from others (for example, in Alcoholics Anonymous) with similar problems; and to turn up the volume on punishment in order to get the point across.

Before concluding this discussion of those who are both sociopathic and drug dependent, I must emphasize that most drug-dependent people are not sociopathic, especially those who became dependent during the current drug abuse epidemic. However, drug dependence, once established, tends to bring out sociopathic traits in many otherwise responsible people. Although the principles I have outlined in this brief section are designed specifically for *sociopathic* drug-dependent people, they are also useful in dealing with all drug-dependent people. Additionally, sociopathic tendencies are not all or none. Most people have these traits to some extent, and few people are completely dominated by sociopathic traits. Focusing on these specific traits, and their relationship to drug dependence, is often useful for families coping with drug problems.

Identifying the Adult "Social" Drug User
Who Is Developing an Unexpected Dependence

So far, I have identified the typical early adolescent entrapped in drug use and the 19- to 40-year-old "child" who has, in a sense, never grown up because of chronic drug dependence, and I have described their separate but closely related problems. Those two types are comparatively easy for most families to identify. Not so easy to detect is the type of drug-affected individual about to be identified here: the adult "social" drug user who begins to develop a serious and unexpected dependence on his drug, often—but by no means always—alcohol.

Typically, this is an adult who has established himself in a career and a family as a seemingly normal, social drug user. For years, such people will have used dependence-producing drugs with no apparent problem, or—more realistically—with few apparent ill effects. Then, often in their 40s or even later, their previously benign pattern of drug use becomes malignant. Drug dependence develops, suddenly or gradually, with striking negative consequences. Early on, usually, there are deteriorating family relationships, a short temper, and a sharp tongue. Actual withdrawal from the family, if it comes, occurs later. In still later stages, this middle-aged drug dependent experiences work failure, accidents, and even arrests—most likely for driving while intoxicated. Still later comes physical illness resulting from the long-standing use and subsequent overuse of the drug of choice. This pattern of drug dependence is harder to recognize because it evolves from drug-using behavior which has for many years been taken for granted as normal. Again, as with any type of drug abuse, the nonusing members of the family must assume the responsibility for identifying the nature and severity of the drug problem and take on the task of determining what is to be done about it.

Identifying the Problem of Medical Drug
Dependence and Its Victim

A fifth and final type of drug dependence requiring identification and treatment can be seen in adult men and women who, usually inadvertently over time, have used or overused medically prescribed, dependence-producing drugs. This is generally referred to as *medical dependence,* and it also requires family identification and solution.

This form of dependence occurs with some frequency in adults who have done well for years and lived fairly well-ordered and well-adjusted lives. Often they have been moderate-to-heavy drinkers of alcohol. At some point, however, an illness develops, ranging from chronic pain to anxiety, and they are given a prescription for a dependence-producing drug: a painkiller, a sleeping pill, or a tranquilizer. Most people who obtain prescribed drugs in this manner use the medicines briefly and wisely. A minority, however, progress over a period of months or even years to full-blown drug dependence. This malignant evolution is more likely to occur if the person had a tendency to alcohol abuse prior to using the prescription drug, and also if the medical condition for which the drug was prescribed happens to be a chronic one which has gone on year after year. Arthritic pain is a good example of this.

Medical drug dependence is particularly hard for families to identify because the drug is prescribed as a medicine and because the drug user is taking it for a genuine illness. Nevertheless, the key to successful family identification of this drug problem is the same as it is for the other types of drug dependence: detecting the problem-producing use of the drug and, more often than you might imagine, its secretive use. And, as is the case with the other types, the family cannot assume that the drug user, when confronted with his or her drug problem, will identify it or even acknowledge its existence.

Limitations of Drug-Dependent People in Identifying Their Own Problems

Throughout our considerations of these five identifiable types of drug-dependent people, you have seen me hammer at the theme that identification of drug problems is a family responsibility. To assume the drug user will identify the drug problem on his or her own is to misunderstand the nature of the Drug Dependence Syndrome. The dependence-producing drug, by its nature, affects the user's brain and thereby diminishes his ability to identify his own drug problem. This is as true for those adults who take drugs for pain as it is for those teenagers who take drugs for pleasure. The drug interacting with the user's brain does not know or care whether its presence there is illegal or not, or whether the user's intent is to avoid pain or seek pleasure. Once the user is deep into his drug, only some other person can make the identification and recommend appropriate action.

This is not to say that drug users never see their own drug problems. They do. Reliably. But that self-recognition generally comes later in the evolution of the Drug Dependence Syndrome, after terrible prices have been paid by the user, his family, and directly and/or indirectly by society at large. In Alcoholics Anonymous, the phrase for such self-awareness is "hitting bottom." An alcoholic or other drug-dependent person is said to be ready for treatment when he has suffered enough to realize that his life is unmanageable and that he has lost control of his drinking or other drug use. The pain required to achieve this self-awareness is variable; some drug users have to sink lower than others. Unfortunately, it is not uncommon for death to occur before this awareness is sufficient to overcome the dependence.

The first generation of contemporary treatment for drug dependence relied almost exclusively on such self-motivation or "will power" for recovery. This, the second and current generation of drug abuse treatment, intervenes earlier in the identification process and makes more aggressive use of social pressures on the drug user to bring his dependency to a halt. Although such pressures are most powerful and most reliable when they come from the drug-dependent person's own family, if the job gets too big or gets out of hand, there are other sources of support and pressure: physicians, employers, school officials, and law enforcement personnel.

In a literal sense these social control processes "raise the bottom" for the drug-dependent person: they accelerate the emergence of negative consequences of drug use, hastening the drug-dependent person's awareness that his life is unmanageable and that only by living drug-free can he regain control over his life—and avoid the pain produced by his drug use. This purposeful acceleration of negative consequences can make the difference between life and death—for the drug user, and not infrequently, for his family. To passively await the full unfolding of the Drug Dependence Syndrome, without active intervention, or to "lower the bottom" by enabling behavior, is to risk death as the eventual outcome of the process of drug dependence.

Alcoholics Anonymous speaks of turning the drug or alcohol problem over to a "higher power." One AA member, years after successful rehabilitation, told me that for the first year of his recovery his higher power was his parole officer. More commonly the higher power is a spouse or a parent. This notion of a higher power or authority was illuminated for me by an incident related by a New York heroin addict who was told by his family, when he was in his 20s, that he could not remain in the home unless he became drug-free. He left home and lived a miserable life. One Sunday, being cold and hungry, he showed up at his parents' home at the time he knew they would be eating Sunday dinner. He asked to come in. His mother, he later recalled, asked, "Are you clean?" meaning, "Are you drug-free?" He replied, "No, but I'll quit tomorrow. Now I'm sick. Let me in." His mother gave him a plate of chicken with mashed potatoes and gravy but insisted that he eat it outside in a cold rain, saying that he could come inside only after he was free of all drugs. He told me that this encounter, as the rain poured off the eaves and on to his plate, was the moment when he finally stopped his drug use. A "higher power" had indeed intervened. Successfully.

There is one other aspect of identification of drug dependence which needs emphasis. One family member usually sees the drug problem first. Initially, he is likely to be hesitant. He may meet with resistance from other family members who are not sure the problems can be traced to drugs. Of course, it is possible that the family member who first voiced his concern may be wrong. Maybe the family member with problems is not using alcohol or another drug. Fortunately, there is an easy way to find out: a three to six months' drug-free trial period. If the family member with the problem can stop drug use for three to six months, it is often possible to find out whether or not drug use is at the root of the problem. If he cannot or will not stop, that is strong evidence that drug use is in fact the underlying problem and that stopping it is the first step toward recovery.

Family pressure to stop drug dependence is unlikely to be successful unless it reflects family agreement. A consensus must be built. That means discussion and investigation. And more family interaction. It also means some willingness to be assertive and to be skeptical. Begin by focusing on the problems that are seen, the evidence that is detectable: for example, the poor school performance, the shattered family relationships, or the chronic cough common among marijuana smokers. *The family goal, remember, is to solve the problem.* If that requires stopping drug use, fine. If not, then take whatever other steps are necessary to discover and resolve the difficulty. I recommend an open family discussion of the problem, with a continuing commitment to finding the truth and using it intelligently to solve the problem. Blame and shame are not likely to prove helpful. Even before confronting the drug user himself, I suggest that other members of the family explore together the perplexities and dilemmas they have been experiencing, and then work out a unified family response to the problem at hand. At some point, this may involve only the parents talking things over together. If it is one of the parents who has the drug problem, this circumstance may involve the non-drug-using spouse in a discussion with other adult members of the family, as well as friends, religious advisors, therapists, or even the family's adolescent or adult children since they are likely to be affected by the outcome.

In the task of problem identification, psychologically sophisticated families sometimes have a paradoxical handicap. Psychologically oriented as they are, they tend to see the failed school achievement, work performance, or family conflicts as symptoms of some deeper problem. They see the failures of the drug-dependent child as a reflection of hidden or deeper family problems. This soul-searching for suspected "root" problems can be painful, seemingly without end, and ultimately completely confusing. Families engrossed in this kind of attributive psychology end with too many conflicting and unverifiable explanations. What is worse, these are usually cleverly exploited by the drug user as excuses and easy cop-outs, and the family's problem-solving focus is diverted into unproductive areas or lost entirely. For example, families searching for deeper explanations explore long-standing conflicts between the parents, or philosophical analyses of the value of planning for the future versus having fun now, or polemics centered on generational conflicts in values. Avoid these traps.

The drug use and the failed grades are *the problem*. The so-called deeper problems are far more likely to be symptoms of the drug dependence than the other way around. My evidence? Once the drug problem is solved, most of these seemingly horrible and complex problems become irrelevant. Those that remain will be far easier to deal with when the stress of drug dependence is removed from the family circle. When drug dependence has been stopped, that is the time when more sophisticated psychiatric treatment can help families, not before.

INTERVENTION: GETTING BETWEEN THE DRUG-DEPENDENT PERSON AND HIS DRUG

Family Action: A Step-By-Step Approach

Once the drug abuser and his drug problem have been identified—usually the most difficult stage of the entire treatment process—it is followed by the next stage: action, or intervention. In Chapters 2 and 6, I have stressed the considerable significance of the family's role in all stages of the Drug Dependence Syndrome. Here, in the workings of intervention, there is a unique opportunity and challenge for the family to enlarge and extend that role. I call this Family Action. The opportunity for intervention to which I refer occurs after prevention has failed but before the drug or alcohol problem has reached such gravity or become so chronic that professional help is essential. Such an approach is more likely to work if the drug or alcohol problem has not become terribly severe, and it is also more likely to succeed if the family is reasonably effective in working as a team.

The principles of Family Action are simple. *First,* identify the drug or alcohol problem clearly and define the goal, unequivocally, as the dependent person's becoming and remaining completely drug free. *Second,* make clear that the project is a family project. Most of us are well aware that, as families, we can seldom get teenagers to pick up their rooms or do the dishes after dinner if the whole family is not visibly and regularly involved in such chores. It is equally unlikely that a drug-dependent family member will do the work needed to solve his or her drug problem if other members of the family are not willing to roll up their sleeves and make a solid effort to join in and help seek the solution, too. *Third,* get help; don't try to go it alone. The best help is often to be found in other families facing the same problem. Peer-parent groups are an admirable example. Since the mid-1970s, these groups have sprung up in all parts of the nation.

Information about how to find one and/or how to start one can be obtained from Parents Resource Institute for Drug Education (PRIDE) (Georgia State University, University Plaza, Physical Education Building, Room 137, Atlanta, Georgia 30303) and from the National Federation of Parents for Drug-Free Youth (NFP) (1820 Fanwall Avenue, Silver Spring, Maryland 20902). The "bible" for such groups is the U.S. Government's best-selling book, *Parents, Peers, and Pot,* published in 1978. More than one million copies are in print. An updated sequel, *Parents, Peers, and Pot II: Parents in Action,* by the same author, Marsha Manatt, is available in single copies, free of charge, from the National Clearinghouse for Drug Abuse Information (Room 10A56, Parklawn Building, 5600 Fishers Lane, Rockville, Maryland 20857).

In addition, there is the previously mentioned Al-Anon, the non-users' family group affiliated with Alcoholics Anonymous, which has chapters in virtually every neighborhood in America. Finally, several private and even some public family support groups have been formed by building on the parent peer group concept to offer specialized help. Two of the best of these are Toughlove and the Palmer

Drug Abuse Program (PDAP). The former has published an excellent book outlining the principles of their approach (which is similar to the approach I advocate in this book), and the latter meets in churches and other community facilities in many parts of the country.

Family Action requires little money. Most of the programs I have described are free. However, regardless of where it is initiated, Family Action does require real work and a willingness of the entire family to work together to solve the drug problem and, together, to grow from facing and overcoming the drug problem. A physician friend of mine, whose son was going through the experience of trying to overcome drug dependence, decided to join one of these family-based programs. So gratified and impressed with the results was this physician that he determined to enter the drug abuse field professionally. Recently he told me what had happened: "Johnny is fine now. It was nip and tuck for years. We almost lost him. Really, we almost lost our whole family. We all went nuts. But the most amazing thing about the whole experience, to me, was the way it brought our family together. We learned how to *communicate* for the first time ever in that program. The lessons we all learned, not just Johnny, have made us all stronger and happier. That's strange, given how awful the drug problem was for our family."

Confronting the Drug Abuser in the Family Context

The first action to take is to confront the possibly drug-dependent person in the family context. That generally means that family members sit down with the drug abuser, the other adults, and possibly the older children for the purpose of talking about the problem. This should be a preplanned event. It should not occur on impulse or when people are terribly angry. The intervention should be scheduled at a time when the drug-dependent family member is most likely to be sober or straight.

In the initial discussion, the focus should be twofold. First, concentrate on unusual or negative behaviors of the suspected dependent and other problems actually observed. Each family member should describe, in some detail, problems he or she has experienced with the possibly drug-dependent person. Try to stay clear, especially in the beginning, from drawing conclusions. Stick to the facts. I call this the "Joe Friday approach." Joe Friday was the name of the famous police sergeant on the old *Dragnet* television show. When confronted with the most emotional and confusing situations, his legendary tactic was to say, in a reassuring monotone, "Just the facts, ma'am." That is what is called for in the initial phases of intervention: just the facts. The second focal point in this opening discussion is to think together about possible solutions. Listen carefully to what the drug-dependent person says, and try to work out courses of action that might be taken to solve the problems as they are discussed.

During an intervention, it is almost inevitable for the user to hide behind the tactic of denial. If the drug in question is illicit and disapproved by the family, he will deny using it. If the drug is alcohol or a drug which is accepted by the family, he will deny that his use is a problem. While some of this may be straight-out lying, sometimes it is a truthful account of the way the user sees the situation. Pay close attention to it. He frequently does not want to stop using the drug because it brings him pleasure or reduces his pain. Expect him to see his drug use as a solution to his problems, not as the problem itself.

If the drug user denies use and the family is unable at this time to prove otherwise, alternative approaches will have to be devised. You might, for instance, redirect attention to other problems which have been identified and verified—bad family relationships, poor achievement in school, or unacceptable work performance, for example— and try to solve them. Perhaps an even more productive alternative (families will need extra courage for this) is to say, in effect, that the time has come to consider ways in which to establish, by whatever objective means are available, whether the problem-prone person has or has not been using drugs. Emphasize that this can be most accurately and easily done by regular urine testing for illegal drugs. Generally, this will involve contact with a physician who can prescribe such testing.

If the drug user admits drug use but denies that this use is causing the problem identified by his family, I suggest a drug-free trial period of 90 days. This gives both the drug user and the family a chance to work on their problems in other ways, and it allows time for the drugs to clear out of the user's brain. This should, in turn, permit clearer thinking and new and more constructive behaviors to develop. Periodic urine testing must be employed during the test period to establish that the drug user is truly drug free.

Summing up what I am recommending, when the drug abuser has been confronted with his problem in the family context, the family should (1) identify specific problems that have occurred; (2) know if, in fact, the suspected family member is taking intoxicating drugs of any kind; (3) know what phase the suspected drug problem is now in, i.e., its present state; (4) assess the damage done; (5) identify the possible solutions to the drug dependence; and (6) select the solution the family is determined to pursue to ensure a successful outcome.

Additionally, if after concluding the step-by-step intervention, the family decides that the case is severe and chronic, the family needs to be ready to take the drug user to a therapist or a program without further delay. Ideally for such severe cases, admission to treatment should proceed directly from the family intervention session, without permitting even an overnight period to elapse and harden resistance to getting help.

Despite my strong advocacy of Family Action in drug intervention, I must draw your attention to one *exception*. There is one noteworthy circumstance in which the step-by-step family approach is not desirable. If, prior to intervention, the family concludes that the drug abuse is unquestionably severe and if it feels certain that further delay in seeking definitive treatment is a dangerous waste of time, then the family needs to act quickly and decisively. It should proceed immediately to take the drug-dependent person to a good drug abuse treatment center in the community. Often this is an inpatient or a hospital-based program. In less severe cases, it may be a specifically skilled drug abuse therapist or outpatient program. More on program shopping later.

Clearing Up Some Common Sources of Confusion

Drug Abuse Is a "Family Disease": Two Views. One of the clichés of drug abuse treatment is that drug abuse is a family disease. Viewed in one way, this statement is true and helpful; looked at in another way, it can be dangerously misinterpreted. It has become common among some drug-dependent people, and an embarrassingly large number of professional therapists, to view the drug-dependent member as the victim of a "sick" family. In this unorthodox view, the concept can be carried to the absurd point of believing that the family needs the drug abuser's disorder to sustain the functioning of the family.

For my part, when I call drug abuse a "family disease," I emphatically do not mean that the family has victimized the drug-dependent person, and I certainly do not believe that families want to encourage drug abuse. Seeing the intense suffering of the very first family I saw as a therapist was enough to convince me that such a view is wrong. The pain, not to say despair, endured by the nonusers is so intense and the family disruption caused by the drug use is so profound that it is hard to imagine that anyone would want such problems to continue.

True or False? Before the Dependence Begins, the Problem Patterns of the Drug User and His Family Are Different from Those Found in Nonusing Families. False. There is no simple pattern to the problems that characterize or predict the future drug user or the family from which he comes. Before the person became drug dependent, he—like all the rest of us—had problems. His family—like all other families—had problems. Families of drug abusers are not unique in their imperfections: all families have failings and weaknesses. The sources of some of these problems are structural ones: families broken by divorce or separated by distance. Families can be educationally or culturally or financially handicapped. Some family problems are almost purely emotional: deep-seated conflicts between family members make it hard for the family to work as a team.

Taken together, these problems are as varied and as complex as the range of human experience itself. This fact alone should make it understandable why there is no discernible pattern by which to predict which families will have a drug-using problem and what will or will not happen before, during, and after intervention and treatment. Each individual case is a pattern unto itself. Would that there were a convenient compass to chart for us the uncertain paths over which the problems of the non-drug-using family travel to become the problems of the family with a drug abuser.

The only pattern we can be sure of in this endeavor is the somewhat parallel pattern seen in the Drug Dependence Syndrome: Drug use will begin and progress through the stages of Experimentation, Occasional Use, Regular Use, and Dependence. From this, we have learned that, as the drug use progresses over time, the consequences to the user and his family tend to mount progressively. Usually, as we can observe, it is only when drug-caused problems can no longer be ignored or denied, when the drug user's life and the lives of his family become truly unmanageable, that the drug problem is faced and intervention and treatment begin.

While no consistent family pattern has been found which predicts later emergence of drug problems, and no family pattern has been found which prevents drug problems, there is a predictable consequence of drug dependence. All families living with drug-dependent people are made miserable and function poorly. Thus, family problems do not, in my view, cause drug problems, but drug problems do cause family problems.

The Family Can Handle the Drug Abuse Problem Without Professional Help: Yes or No? The best answer is *maybe*. Although we cannot establish a clear pattern or the concise course the family's drug-related problems will take, we can make a few useful observations. In the early stages of confronting the drug problem, the family's determination to solve the problem is unsteady, wavering between whether to go ahead or turn back. Both the abuser and the family can expect to find themselves wishing, from time to time, that the problem would just go away—vanish magically. Predictably, they will grudgingly, but sensibly, realize that the problem will not go away until the drug use stops completely. Personally, I take solace in the thought that since drug abuse is, when viewed in the proper context, a family "disease," there must be somewhere or somehow a "remedy" for it. And that remedy, insofar as I am familiar with one, is intervention and treatment. I am convinced that the best energizing force and most compassionate giver of that remedy is the family.

When the family assumes this task, the responsibility is large. If lasting good is to come from drug abuse treatment, each member of the family must—as a part of the treatment—evaluate his or her own life and be willing to make the adjustments necessary to promote the whole family's recovery from the disorder. This demands *change*. The fact that change is painful and typically takes a long time helps to explain why treatment and recovery are so painful and have no appointed end. Fortunately, families do change and they do endure and sometimes—happily for all—they do "get well." That is the good, the kindly, side of change.

Change has its darker side, too. Whether we like it or not and whether we intend it or not, it does take place. This can sometimes seriously frustrate, even nullify, Family Action. Consider communication. By the time drug abuse has become unmistakable in a family member, communication usually will have deteriorated noticeably. The former joys of family talk will have disintegrated or been replaced by vituperative outbursts, shouting matches, menacing threats, and sullen silences—all destructive enough to drive the whole family half out of its mind. Lost almost entirely is that precious ability and willingness to talk together and to work together which is so essential to successful drug abuse treatment. Potential success thus falls victim to drug-shriveled communication. The far-reaching implications of this surface again and again.

Drug abusers whose families are willing, even eager, to face shared problems and try to solve them in an open and positive spirit are far more likely to succeed in treatment. Drug abusers whose families' attitudes communicate "We're all fine—*you* are the only one with a problem" are far more likely to fail in treatment. Unquestionably, refusal to change attitudes and behaviors can seriously handicap the operation of the entire family.

Some mental health workers despair of helping these drug-caused sick families. My outlook is different. Success in preventing and treating drug problems in the family requires a positive effort to focus on its strengths rather than its weaknesses. At the same time, however, I believe that family weaknesses should not be ignored. When they surface (and they commonly do) and seem impossible for the family to surmount, I urge the family to get outside help of the kind I have already described—from other families, a church affiliation, or a psychiatrist. The barriers to such a collaboration are seldom financial. The enemies of productive help-seeking by a family are far more likely to be false pride, shame, and that old bugaboo—denial. Whatever the sources of resistance to honest family coping, remember that although self-understanding and self-acceptance are valuable assets, they are useful in drug abuse prevention only if they lead to effective action.

There are, as noted, two *preconditions* essential for drug abuse treatment: making an accurate diagnosis of the drug dependence and establishing a shared, family commitment to solving the problem. These are the starting points if the family is resolved to do the rehabilitation job itself. Some families solve serious drug problems without professional help. Often these successful families use support from religious groups or from other families who are similarly affected by drug dependence. As a psychiatrist, I never see these families. For the families I have seen with drug problems, however, outside professional help is necessary. The main fact to face in either of these choices is that the family goal must be uncompromising: *drug-free living for any family member who has become drug dependent.* If that can be achieved without formal treatment, fine. If not, then by all means get expert help.

Intervention Geared to the Steps in the Drug Dependence Syndrome

In making this difficult decision about whether to proceed with Family Action or to call in a professional therapist, a good place to start is with an assessment of the seriousness of the drug or alcohol problem. The less serious the drug abuse problem is, the more likely it is to respond to Family Action. The more serious the problem, the more likely it is to require professional, structured treatment. Also assess the present state of the abuser's drug dependence. Is he or she in the stage of Experimentation? If so, the abuser may respond to a discussion of family values and expectations and careful supervision in the context of education about the dangers of drug abuse.

I saw this happen as I worked with the parents of an 18-year-old boy who was beginning to have a marijuana problem. They were reluctant to initiate treatment. The two parents and the son, a senior in high school, came to see me twice to talk over their concerns, concerns which included the son's failing school performance and declining interest in extracurricular activities. The boy admitted his marijuana use and said he would not smoke the drug again. His parents were skeptical, and we arranged a urine-testing program. If, at any time, the parents suspected the son of using marijuana or other drugs, they would collect a urine sample. If he admitted using pot *before* being tested, he would lose the right to drive the family car for 15 days. If his marijuana use was discovered by testing, then he lost the use of the car for 30 days. During the next year, he was caught once, and his parents followed through on the agreed punishment. That ended his drug problem. When I last heard from him, he was a college junior and doing well. He told me that having to face the threat of urine testing had helped him handle a problem he had previously been unable to solve: peer pressure to smoke marijuana. Once he could tell his buddies about his parents' program of urine testing, they stopped asking him to smoke pot. They obviously respected this parental toughness. As he later explained, "After all, my friends didn't want me to get into trouble."

Is the drug abuser in the stage of Occasional or Regular Use? If this is the case, will he—can he—stop use? How much damage has been done already to his life, his relationships in and out of the family, and to his physical health? Again, if the dependent person is willing and able to stop all drug use completely, formal treatment may not be necessary.

Or is the family member in the final, Dependent Stage of the syndrome? If so, the family must not delude itself. The abuser may say and, at the moment, believe that he himself can handle the problem, that he will be able to stop drug use without professional help. Again, assess the extent of the damage done by drug use. If it has been slight, perhaps minimal intervention is all that is really needed; if it has been extensive and prolonged, then prompt treatment is imperative.

Earlier I focused on lying as a central threat to family-based drug abuse treatment. Lying destroys trust and undermines family problem solving. There is another common, related problem which must be confronted: the tendency of the drug user when caught to say, "I'm sorry. I've learned my lesson and I'll never do it again." Many drug users think that if they just say they are sorry, then everything is forgiven and forgotten. In fact, they are often terribly resentful if they are punished once they have said they are sorry. All too often families, desperate to solve the drug-caused problems without doing the hard work necessary, will accept the apology only to see the same behavior occur again and again. It is amazing to me how often families can go through this same process over the course of many years without learning from their experiences. When families confront drug-caused problems, they must also confront their own tendency to hide behind wishful thinking—their own tendency, not to say eagerness, to accept the con job. Someone simply saying, "I'm sorry," is not entitled to avoid punishment, and families are ill-advised to accept the simple reassurance that it won't happen again. Rather, families should impose appropriate punishments for misbehavior. They should expect a verifiable plan of work to overcome the drug-caused problem, not just an assertion that it is over. Regular family monitoring of behavior, usually with treatment, is required to achieve actual recovery.

Let's assume you have carried your analysis of the drug-caused problem through the appropriate steps and have made your decision. If Family Action without formal treatment is to be tried as a first step of intervention, make it clear to everyone that there will be no compromise on the goal of total, permanent drug-free living and that the family motto must be "We Will Do Whatever Is Necessary." If you find the drug problem is persisting, strengthen your efforts to stop it. Start small and build up, but do not give in. One caveat: Do not *underreact* to the scope of the danger or misjudge the import of a crisis. I have seen many families who underestimated the seriousness of the drug abuser's problem and downplayed the seriousness of the consequences of his drug use. By underreacting, they delayed their responses, thereby—in many instances—building new layers of resistance to treatment. *Overreacting* may be equally detrimental to successful treatment, but after more than a decade of working with drug-dependent people and their families, I cannot recall a single case in which a knowledgeable family seriously overreacted to a drug problem. Prudence should tell you: don't underrate the danger. Be skeptical of your own judgment.

TYPES OF DRUG ABUSE TREATMENT

Broadly speaking, drug abuse treatment can be divided into two types: (1) *Self-Help Groups* such as Alcoholics Anonymous, Narcotics Anonymous, and Families Anonymous and (2) *Professional Treatment.* I hesitate to use the term "professional" in this context because it implies that people holding degrees have expertise in drug abuse treatment and that people without professional degrees—for example, those who may be working in the Anonymous groups—do not. That, certainly, is not the conclusion I wish you to draw. Rather, in making this differentiation between the two kinds of assistance, I am using only the two factors: the formality of treatment setting and the cost of treatment. The help and services provided by the Anonymous groups are free of financial costs. The help and services available in almost all professional treatment have a cost to the drug user, to his family, to his health insurance company, or to the taxpayer. The traditional Anonymous groups will not accept public funding.

Within the category of professional treatment, there are two broad divisions. The first is the general mental health or counseling approach. This type of drug abuse treatment may occur in the office of a psychiatrist, psychologist, social worker, nurse practitioner, or other health care professional. It may also occur in a clinic, church, or community care program. For our purposes, notice that this individual professional care is not part of an organized drug abuse treatment *program.* It is, rather, part of a more generalized mental health effort.

The second broad division of professional drug abuse treatment is the formal, usually structured, program—what most of us mean when we talk of drug abuse treatment. Programs of this kind have multiplied almost beyond classification in recent years. As recently as 1965, there were almost no drug abuse treatment programs anywhere in the nation. Except in New York City and in California, such programs were rare until the early 1970s. Today it is an unusual American community which does not have access to numerous drug abuse treatment programs. These programs can be classified in a variety of ways: by the age or other characteristics of the patients served, for instance. Increasingly common are programs for youth, for women, or for prisoners and programs for people using specific drugs such as heroin, marijuana, or cocaine. The modern drug abuse treatment program can also be classified according to the type of facility. For example, it can be an outpatient program, a residential program, or an inpatient, often hospital-based, program. Residential drug abuse treatment programs can be relatively intensive, as they are in the modern therapeutic community, or they may be relatively unstructured, as, for example, frequently is the case in a halfway house. Drug abuse treatment programs can also be classified according to the type of treatment they provide. They can, for instance, be drug free; they can offer medical detoxification or withdrawal services; or they can be methadone maintenance programs restricted to chronic heroin addicts. As if this were not complicated enough, drug abuse treatment programs differ in the extent to which they use personnel with degrees and licensed health professionals and the extent to which they rely on former drug abusers and others who frequently lack professional credentials. And finally, drug abuse treatment programs can also be classified on the basis of their source of funding: private, public, or mixed.

Confused? You are not alone. Fortunately, from the viewpoint of the consumer of drug abuse treatment services, these distinctions are by no means as complicated as they may at first appear. All successful drug abuse treatment programs have the same goal: to help the drug-dependent person become and remain drug free, and they all work in close conjunction with family-based efforts to overcome problems of drug dependence.

FINDING THE RIGHT PROGRAM FOR YOUR FAMILY

Locating the Possibilities

With these types of drug abuse treatment facilities in mind, I suggest you work the support network in your community. A good place to begin is with the yellow pages of your telephone directory. There you will find a listing of the available drug abuse and alcohol abuse programs, usually under such headings as "Drug Abuse and Addiction—Information and Treatment" and "Alcoholism Information and Treatment Centers." Another excellent place to start is with your local government. The people there are likely to have a drug abuse and/or an alcohol abuse office which can supply you with a list of reliable treatment resources available locally. They may give you some tips, too, on which drug abuse programs to consider and which ones to steer clear of. Consider also the possibility of seeking help from the psychiatric society in your area. Social workers and psychologists are among the other possible resources you can call upon for assistance, and your local public school or church may also be able to provide you with help. Still another possibility, of course, is to seek advice and help from your family physician, and if there is a medical school in your vicinity, it may be of assistance to you.

Without hesitation, I urge that you call Alcoholics Anonymous (they are listed in the telephone directory) and ask for help. If you are a non-drug-dependent family member, ask AA for the location of Al-Anon meetings in your neighborhood. Their meetings are usually held at 8:30 in the evening in local churches or community centers, and attendance varies from roughly eight to 50 people. Al-Anon members, most of whom are veterans of many drug and alcohol treatment programs, can often give firsthand evaluations of local programs.

Investigating the Possibilities

Having a list of drug abuse treatment programs, you will find that you probably do not have time to investigate all of them. So how do you pick one? If you have analyzed the drug problem of the person for whom you are seeking treatment and have assessed the seriousness of it (procedures for which I have already described), you already have a clear idea of what you want. Go with your instincts, your gut feelings. On the basis of well-weighed reasons, some families prefer the self-help approach, while others favor a more private, professional approach. Call and get the facts, costs, and program descriptions. Arrange, if you can, to visit the office or facility of the treatment program you are considering, and try to talk with others in the program and with members of their families. Remember that you are not obligated to use any drug abuse treatment program merely because you visit it or because you go for an evaluation. Be an educated consumer. Choose a drug abuse treatment program which fits your family needs and your budget and which also reflects your values and attitudes. Finally, no matter what else you do, stick to programs which have no-drug/drug-free objectives. This I underscore. If you find the therapist talking about "responsible" drug use or about "social" drug use, or if you find him or her referring to certain intoxicating drugs as problems but implying that others are okay (alcohol and marijuana are the most likely candidates for this list), I suggest finding a different therapist.

When I use the term "drug-free," I am referring to treatment program values which reject, categorically, *self-administered* drugs which have the capacity to produce dependence. This means active discouragement of any use of alcohol and marijuana, as well as cocaine and heroin. However, I make an exception for medically prescribed drugs. As I see it, once a drug is prescribed by a physician, it is in a different category. Some may think I make this distinction because I am a physician and I seek to excuse physicians, and their drugs, from blame. Far from it. For me, the central question is not the name of the drug involved or even its pharmacology, but the circumstances of whether the drug is "self-prescribed" and self-administered. When a physician controls the administration of a drug, it is— or should be—less difficult to avoid a drug problem and prevent dependency. In other words, medically prescribed drugs are different *only* if the physician is actively and continuously supervising their use, while carefully controlling the dose and duration of that use. If the physician abdicates this close supervision, then medically prescribed, dependence-producing drugs can produce the same problems as street drugs.

The medical drug *methadone* illustrates the point. This drug has been used in the treatment of heroin addicts for the past two decades and has been the most controversial of all drug abuse treatments. If the patient refuses the option of total freedom from heroin, then it is my considered judgment that even though methadone is an addicting opiate, its use is far preferable to continued heroin use. However, I would suggest that treatment only as long as the treatment personnel are fully in charge of the patient's methadone and other drug use as that control is determined by careful urine testing. However, if methadone is used recklessly, it can add to the drug problems of the heroin addict and his community.

Certain drugs prescribed by physicians as part of general medical practice also produce dependence. Among these are the tranquilizers, sleeping pills, and many of the painkillers. Use of these drugs by recovering drug-dependent people is hazardous and, as a general rule, should be avoided except for brief, in-hospital use as part of a medically supervised withdrawal procedure. If kept under strict control, however, there are a few other circumstances in which such drugs are useful in drug abuse treatment. To work safely, their use requires that the patient be educated about the drug in question and the potential problems its use may cause. And, even more to the point, it requires the active supervision of the use of the drug not only by the physician but also by a member of the patient's family. This is not easy to ensure. Many physicians themselves are still not well-informed as to the specific dangers of dependence-producing drugs for recovering drug-dependent people. Moreover, too few family members are educated and brought into the picture. But *if* all those involved understand the potential problems and *if* all understand their roles in the treatment, then, in some cases, these drugs can be made to work safely, and their use will not, in my opinion, constitute a barrier to effective drug abuse treatment.

Fortunately, most medically prescribable drugs are not dependence hazards. These drugs are sometimes used by physicians and psychiatrists to treat people who have drug or alcohol problems. Many people confuse psychoactive drugs which *do* produce dependence with those which *do not* produce dependence. For example, the antidepressant drugs, as a class, are not dependence producing. Often, these drugs—including imipramine and amitriptyline—prove useful in treating the depression which may both complicate and contribute to drug dependence. Such antipsychotic drugs as Thorazine and Stelazine do not produce dependence, and so for some drug-dependent people they are helpful.

The narcotic antagonist, Naltrexone, does not produce dependence, nor does Antabuse, the anti-alcohol drug. A full discussion of the possible drugs useful in the treatment of drug-dependent people is, of course, beyond the scope of this book.

There are three safeguards which should always be taken into consideration whenever these medically prescribed drugs are used: (1) use dependence-producing drugs rarely, if at all, for recovering drug-dependent people; (2) require the physician to take extra precautions and exert extra supervision when such drugs are used by drug-dependent people; and (3) enlist the patient's family in daily supervision of such drug use to ensure that it is not excessive and that it does not cause problems.

Regardless of the form of drug abuse therapy you elect to pursue, do not forget that the family remains in charge, not the therapist and not the program. It is undesirable and, as a practical matter, impossible for the family to abdicate its primary responsibility. Families must have the facts, and they must insist on the cessation of nonmedical drug use—period.

GETTING INSIDE A TREATMENT PROGRAM AND USING IT

Look again to the type of drug abuse program exclusively designed to deal with a drug or alcohol dependence problem—the kind of program briefly described in the preceding section. It is quite unlike the previously described Family Action approach of the Anony-mous/Self-Help concept. Nor is it similar to the mental health therapy or outpatient psychotherapy I referred to earlier. The context or setting for this type of treatment may be a part of a larger institu-tion—a hospital or a community health center, for example—or it may be a stand-alone facility housed in its own building.

Some drug abuse treatment programs are planned to last for a relatively short time, usually 10 to 30 days; others last for a year or longer. Because of the cost and the necessarily disruptive impact on the patient's community life, inpatient treatment programs are usually shorter, whereas the less disruptive outpatient programs are longer. Therapeutic community programs which last from six to 18 months are an exception to this observation. In general, the more restrictive the drug abuse treatment program, the more likely patients in it are to be assigned to treatment by a court of law. The less restrictive the treatment program, the more likely patients are to be voluntary or quasi-voluntary. As we have seen, few drug-dependent people come to treatment without some form of external social pressure from courts, employers, or family members.

Although sometimes shorter, but not uncommonly longer, most drug abuse treatment of this specific, structured kind lasts about one year, with a prolonged stage of aftercare lasting for many years or even for a lifetime. This long duration of treatment reflects the serious nature of the drug dependence problem and the great difficulty the drug-dependent person has in becoming and staying drug free. While the purely pharmacological problem of dependence can usually be overcome in a few weeks or at most a few months, the problem of changing lifestyles and reinforcement of the commitment to avoidance of intoxicating drugs is almost never short or easy.

The Four Stages of Treatment

Regardless of the setting, duration, and patient characteristics of this type of drug abuse treatment, the experience can be divided into four stages: *Intake, Structured Treatment, Termination, and Aftercare.*

Intake: What Happens During Orientation. After selecting a treatment program, the family goes with the drug-dependent family member to the program's treatment facility for admission to treat-ment. In this, the orientation stage of the program, the patient and rest of the family are informed and educated about the nature of the program and the expectations for patients and family members. The professional staff members explain the nature of the dependent user's drug problem as they see it, and they describe the program's approach to overcoming it.

My advice at this stage is to learn as much as possible. The family stands to learn as much or more than the patient. While family skepticism and even hostility to some aspect of the drug abuse treatment program is common in this stage, you are well advised to open your mind to what is being said about the program and "soak up" the wisdom that is offered. This intake stage can last a few days or a few weeks. It is often helpful for both the drug-dependent patient and his family members to reach out and involve themselves with the old-timers in the program. These veterans have much to teach, and the support they offer can make the difference between success and failure during the stages that follow.

Structured Treatment: Getting Down to Business. Once the orientation process is complete, the really hard work of treatment begins. This structured treatment stage lasts from a few weeks to a year or more. During this time, each family member involved in the process is expected to participate, bringing concerns and problems to the program staff and working through the solutions. In this stage, many of the behaviors which have caused family problems in the past will reemerge, and the family will have the opportunity to confront and solve them in the supportive environment of the program with the professional assistance of the staff.

That, from the outset, the drug abuser is faced with a gigantic job there can be no question. If he is to benefit from drug abuse treatment, he must begin by accepting certain hard facts. He must recognize that, having lost control of his drug use—and of his life—he now must work to regain that control. He must admit, or learn to admit, that his drug use is a reckless and destructive behavior and that his life has become unmanageable. He must understand that this disorder, if not overcome, will destroy his future and will sooner or later be fatal. No longer can he pretend to see the forces and the people who brought him to treatment as the problem. The family, school officials, employers, or the agents of the criminal justice system are not—and never have been—the problem. His drug use is the problem, the enemy. And, often most difficult of all, he must accept that he can never again use dependence-producing drugs with safety.

These are shocking ideas. Small wonder that they are initially rejected. The drug abuser has *other* ideas. Typically, on entering the structured stage of treatment, his first priority is to get out—to attempt to return to self-controlled, social drug use. Since this goal is not realistic, staff and family members alike reject it. Or they should. Not infrequently at this point, the abuser begins a conning campaign. Calling on the cunning and manipulative skills that were well honed from his earlier drug days, he may employ them now to deceive the people in the treatment program. Somehow, by hook or crook, he is determined to get back to his drug.

This, of course, is central to his biggest problem: the drug dependence itself. The family and program staff should lose no time in confronting it. Close supervision, together with urine testing, is continued throughout this period. Staff and family steadily, painstakingly, and patiently pursue the goal as they work to overcome the dependent person's resistance to treatment. Even he may come to recognize eventually that an honest effort must be made to come clean. But the effort—and the pressure—may prove too great.

In this, the most trying phase of treatment, numerous drug-dependent people—frequently abetted, surprisingly enough, by their families—leave or "split" from treatment and return to their former drug-taking patterns. Sometimes this happens because of what may appear, superficially at least, logical or defensible reasons: conflicts with the program staff over issues too difficult for the patient and/or the family to handle, belated realization that the sheer magnitude and cost of treatment are terribly burdensome for all family members, or (as most often happens) the family's premature conviction that the drug problem has been solved. Collectively, the family may say that the abuser's drug problems are "not as serious as the problems of the other people in this program," or they may conclude that "this is the wrong program for us—we can handle the problem ourselves."

At this point, the potential splitter will probably be doing all he can to add to the destructive momentum. Delighted with the prospect of fleeing the program, he will promise anything. If the family accepts the con and takes the drug-dependent person home, there may be a brief "honeymoon" in the family. Once outside the treatment, however, the drug taking usually begins all over again, and all the old problems which led originally to admission to drug abuse treatment usually reemerge, often in a more malignant form, complicated by the family demoralization with the failure of their treatment efforts.

In due time, let us hope—as tensions and new crises build—the family and its drug abuser decide, however painfully and reluctantly, to go back to the treatment program and give it another go. This time, the family will try harder—especially the drug abuser himself. The stakes—and the hurdle—are higher. Even if and when he manages to clear it, he must confront the long and discouraging process of reestablishing a new, nondrug existence and learn how to deal with such feelings as anger and depression. In the past, he has been able to avoid these and similar confrontations and feelings by floating over them on the high of his drug. Now, with the support of the staff and other patients in the treatment program, these feelings must be dealt with honestly and realistically. Relationships previously distorted by deception and exploitation must be faced, including a full recognition of the depths to which he has previously gone to pursue his drug habit. In the later stages of successful treatment, he knows he must build a new life, one based on a capacity to cope with feelings of pain and frustration without running away, to work at solving problems rather than ducking them, and to recognize those obligations which a former drug-dependent person owes to school, job, family, and the community. That is a tall order and is seldom accomplished easily, quickly, or fully. It is, nevertheless, a goal to be worked toward.

The family of the recovering drug-dependent individual finds itself facing a series of tasks almost as difficult. Not only must it face up to the tormenting extent of the damage already done by the offender's use of drugs, a painful task in any community, but it must also critically evaluate the flaws and sources of the tribulations inherent in the family functioning before the drug problem began. Then, having gained these insights, they must devise a workable plan for mending these cracks in the family structure. Simultaneously, they must put realistic limits on what they can do to stop the drug use and help the drug user solve his own problems. They must do what they have to do to achieve completely drug-free living for him, but at the same time, they must let him know that the job is squarely in his hands now. If they have been enabling him to get away with things he should not have gotten away with, they must have the guts to stop it. If the drug-dependent person and the family do not look these problems straight in the eye and solve them head on, they will not have a worthwhile family life. If someone else in the family—a sibling, spouse, or parent—is addicted to a drug, the family must put its foot down and insist that the offender get straight or get out. A recovering drug-dependent person leaving treatment and returning home to the unsolved drug problem of another family member is almost certainly doomed to relapse.

This account of drug abuse treatment may seem negative and painful, because treatment is often negative and painful. But if it is to work, it is far more than that. Treatment means building new values and new skills. It means having fun and growing in positive, constructive ways. For example, many recovering drug-dependent people discover, as part of their treatment, the positive pleasures of regular physical exercise, a healthy diet, and the joys of warm, loving human relationships. As they learn to think less of themselves, they learn more about the pleasures of healthy living and of caring for others. Paradoxically, this often means not pushing and demanding quick success or gratification, but a more relaxed and patient approach to life, feelings, and relationships. This is one reason AA focuses on the phrase, "Easy Does It."

The core of professional drug abuse treatment is "structured." Unlike most mental health treatment programs, but similar to the tradition of Alcoholics Anonymous, most successful drug abuse treatment programs have specific structures, or stages, of treatment. These grow out of an understanding of the Drug Dependence Syndrome and the needs of drug-dependent people. Many drug abuse programs have written handbooks for patients and families. These steps, this structure, may be fairly general or highly detailed. The focus is on rebuilding values—usually that means traditional values of love and work—and on rebuilding family life—usually that means reestablishing communication and teamwork.

Overcoming the problems of deceit and lying and rebuilding trust are central objectives. When all this works, as it often does, the result is little short of miraculous. The drug-dependent person who entered treatment as a physical and moral wreck emerges as a healthy, productive, and responsible member of his family and his community. The family which entered in a shambles of hostility and isolation emerges as a unit—a team—which is truly more than the sum of its individual members. It is a common conclusion of families to feel that not only have they returned to the level of functioning before the drug problem ruined them, but that they have gained greatly from the treatment and become more than they had even dared hope for before treatment. As a physician and a psychiatrist, among the most remarkable and gratifying of all my treatment experiences has been working with drug-dependent people and their families. When it works, it is wonderful. When, as too often happens, it fails, drug-abuse treatment is a downer which I have come to think of as a "failure this time," leaving open the hope that in the future, success will be achieved.

Termination: The End of the Beginning. By this time, after a span of a few months or possibly a year, let us assume that the family has successfully completed treatment. There have been, almost certainly, many small failures but, perhaps, one major success. The goal has seemingly been achieved, and a triumph—of at least modest dimensions—is at hand: the dependent person has become independent of his drug. Along the way, we can be fairly certain, the family and the formerly drug-dependent patient have become "plugged into" the treatment program. And from it, they have learned, among many other things, a small truth: The successful treatment program, like many another successful life experience, however hard it may have been to start, is also hard to leave. The world without the support of the program can suddenly seem cold and lonely. As a part of the termination stage, it is often helpful in overcoming these feelings to develop a family Aftercare Plan which includes setting aside some time to help others who have similar problems. Alcoholics Anonymous, basing the term on its twelve steps to rehabilitation, calls this "Twelfth Step Work."

Aftercare: The Long Road Back. This fourth and final stage of treatment takes place after the family, having completed the program, has left formal treatment. But when drug abuse treatment ends, then what? Treatment can end in only one of two ways: success or failure. If the drug abuser achieves a relatively stable drug-free state, the treatment is a success. However, a realistic understanding of the drug-dependence process supports the relevant view taken by Alcoholics Anonymous: "Once an alcoholic, always an alcoholic." Even if a formerly drug-dependent person goes 10 years without using a drug, he remains vulnerable to relapse, and he and his family are far better off recognizing this sad fact. Once that "Addiction Switch" gets thrown on, it never returns to the off position.

For the period immediately following drug abuse treatment, I strongly urge regular attendance at either Alcoholics Anonymous or Narcotics Anonymous for the recovering drug-dependent person (a position I will reinforce in a moment). As time passes, attendance may or may not diminish; this is best determined by the drug-dependent person himself or herself. Al-Anon offers meaningful, long-term support for families. As important as shaking off the shackles of dependence most certainly is, it is also important to recognize that real recovery means more than stopping drug use by the drug-dependent person. It means a whole new family lifestyle based on love and work rather than on escape into self-indulgent, chemically induced pleasure. Recovery means new friends and a new structure to life. And new values.

What if drug abuse treatment *fails?* Here I am not referring to failure of a particular treatment experience in a particular treatment program. What I am pointing to is the failure of the drug-dependent person in one treatment after another, or refusal to attend a treatment program, or refusal to even try to become drug free. This dismal outcome is all too common. In matters of failure, of course, I draw distinctions between adults and children. Adult failures are easier. Adult drug-dependent people need to be confronted directly with this proposition: you can have the family or the drug, but not both. That puts it on the line—that is "for real." For most spouses to take such a position, indeed for most parents to take such a position, requires specific support from a treatment program, a therapist, or a self-help group like Al-Anon, the world's experts at this particular problem.

When children, progeny under 19, fail, the parents simply cannot give up even if they want to. They have little choice but to do whatever it takes to help their child wrench free of drugs. In extreme cases, this may involve sending the child out of the home to a special school (one with sufficient discipline to enforce the no-drug values) or to invoke intervention by the criminal justice system. I have seen many families powerless to confront teenage drug abuse until the long, strong arm of the law intervened, and in many of those cases, the parents themselves sought the intervention. In other cases, parents may have to work out a plan of family therapy or even a short- or long-term placement of the drug-using child in a formal or informal foster home. This can mean living with a family friend, a grandparent, or another relative.

Some children, especially those in the age range of 16 to 19, are so rebellious and so persistent that they declare themselves, by their behavior, emancipated from their families and therefore legal adults. This is rare, however, because it requires self-support financially. It is an unusual teenager in America today who is willing, much less able, to support himself or herself. But if they are, and if the family has exhausted their alternatives in drug abuse treatment, then this course is all that is left. Even so, my suggestion is that the family, faced with this gloomy situation, keep the door open for the return of the child—drug-free—if that should ever happen.

Taking the more optimistic view, let us assume that our typical former drug-dependent person, together with his family, has emerged from drug abuse treatment into the bright sunshine of success. They are "out there in the Big World" again. But not quite alone. As an essential part of Aftercare, two options deserve careful consideration.

The first option is to join one of the Anonymous groups—Narcotics Anonymous or Alcoholics Anonymous—for the former drug-dependent person, and the family support groups—Families Anonymous or Al-Anon—for family members. The second option, one I earlier cautioned against for the first stages of treatment, is mental health therapy or, more technically, psychotherapy.

The Anonymous self-help groups, the first option for Aftercare, are ideally suited to fit into drug abuse treatment. This, in fact, is what they were "born" to do. Alcoholics Anonymous was founded about 50 years ago by two recovering alcoholics, one a physician. The program has now spread throughout the world and has over one million active members. It is difficult to find a neighborhood, let alone a community, in the United States that does not have an active AA group. After years of exclusive focus on the problems of alcohol, in the last 10 years AA has increasingly opened itself to members who are dependent on other drugs such as marijuana and cocaine. Only by opening its doors to admit members dependent on other intoxicating drugs could AA attract young people since this group is almost universally characterized by a polydrug syndrome. In recent years, an offshoot of AA known as Narcotics Anonymous (NA) was created. This program began in prison settings to deal with the problem of chronic heroin addiction. As Alcoholics Anonymous has reached out to include people dependent on other drugs, so has Narcotics Anonymous. The basic tenets of both organizations are similar, based on the Twelve Steps of the original Alcoholics Anonymous groups.

The companion organization for family members of alcoholic and drug-dependent people is called Al-Anon. Like AA, Al-Anon has chapters in every community in the country and, increasingly, throughout the world. The related group for teenagers is Alateen.

In the early years of Alcoholics Anonymous, it was somewhat hostile to more traditional, professional treatment programs. In recent years this has changed. The professional treatment programs reached out to incorporate AA and NA into their ongoing treatment, and AA and NA have, in turn, reached out to the professionals. In my experience in treating alcohol- and drug-dependent people, I have seen people get better without using these self-help groups. But such an outcome is unusual. The more typical pattern associated with real, lasting recovery is for the drug- and alcohol-dependent person to join AA or NA and attend meetings regularly. A typical commitment of a person leaving a drug abuse treatment program is to attend "90 meetings in 90 days." Another useful way of assessing how often a person should attend meetings is to say, "As often as you used to use drugs or alcohol."

The Anonymous groups not only offer a positive, healthy peer group for the recovering drug-dependent person, but they also offer a highly specific, well thought out, and well-implemented program of rehabilitation. Some people can overcome drug and alcohol problems by using the AA program without recourse to professional treatment. Other people—in my experience a smaller number—can overcome drug and alcohol problems through professional treatment without AA or NA. I am convinced, however, that a combination of the two, tailored to the individual and family needs, is the most likely to succeed.

Psychotherapy is the second option for Aftercare. I am aware that I have previously warned that traditional mental health or "talking" psychotherapy is not likely to be an effective treatment for drug dependence *prior to recovery.* However, in Aftercare, for many former drug-dependent people and their families, psychotherapy can definitely be useful. Psychotherapy usually does not help the drug-dependent person to *stop using drugs.* But once recovery or secure sobriety has been established, psychotherapy has much to offer. Reasonable objectives for psychotherapy in the Aftercare period include a careful investigation of feelings, behaviors, and relationships and a thoughtful, collaborative approach to making a better, more loving and productive life.

PRESCRIPTION-DRUG DEPENDENCE:
GETTING HOOKED—AND UNHOOKED

To this point we have focused on the core drug problem in America today, which is the dependent use of intoxicating drugs primarily by youth aged 16 to 35—the drug epidemic generation. Some of these drug-dependent people are still teenagers—still children in the sense I have used the word—while others are failed young adults I have called Pseudo-Children. In this section we shift our focus dramatically to consider the treatment of adults who have become dependent on prescription medicines which are also dependence-producing drugs. Most of these drug-dependent people are female and over 35, and few have had experience with nonmedical use of intoxicating drugs other than alcohol.

The person trapped in prescription drug dependence is not there for fun and not as a result of a peer-centered social activity. She is there to relieve pain, anxiety, or insomnia—a process which started out as legitimate medical treatment. One might say she is a victim of good intentions—a doctor's good, but uninformed, intention in prescribing a painkiller or sedative, or a family, with the best of intentions, trying to help the suffering woman recover, but perhaps careless about supervision and negligent about following the instructions on the pillbox or bottle. Although some people dependent on prescription drugs are middle-aged and a few are young, many are older. In fact, a goodly number of them are "the elderly ill."

Before proceeding, some readers may appreciate an explanation of the language used in this section. Since more women than men suffer from this particular drug dependence problem, I often use the female pronoun in describing sufferers. This may strike some readers as sexist. I hope not. My intention is simply to make reading easier and to point out that in the same way that males predominate in nonmedical drug use (the descriptions of which often include male pronouns) so do females predominate in medical-drug use and dependence. I intend no more criticism of women by my use of the female pronoun here than I mean to criticize men in the use of the male pronoun in describing the more common, nonmedical pattern of drug dependence. It should also be clearly understood that many women suffer from nonmedical drug dependence and many men suffer from dependence on medically prescribed drugs.

Prescribed Dependence-Producing Drugs

Many potentially abused drugs have legitimate medical usage, and most medical patients who use these drugs as medicines, no matter how intense their pharmacologic dependence-producing properties, do not become dependent on them in the sense that we have used the word "dependent" in this book. For example, the antianxiety drugs which include Valium—the most widely prescribed drug in America until it was displaced from that profitable position by a successful antiulcer drug, Tagamet, in 1980—are usually taken for short periods of time. Most people for whom these drugs are prescribed do not use all the pills they get from the pharmacist, and many do not take full advantage of the refills authorized by their physicians. On the other hand, once high-dose, frequent use persists for many months, this class of antianxiety drugs can produce—as we shall see—a full-blown dependence syndrome with a difficult withdrawal and common relapse. Before attempting to explain this apparent paradox—that most users of prescription dependence-producing drugs have no depen-

dence problems, while some users have serious dependence problems—let us review the typical pattern of prescription drug dependence.

Patterns and Dimensions of Prescription Drug Dependence

In recent years, much has been made in the media of the excess of
women among the people who are dependent upon prescription
drugs. There is a simple explanation for this, one having little to do
with exploitation of women patients by male physicians or by pharma-
ceutical companies. The increased rate of prescription dependence
among women is explained as being due primarily to the increased
rate at which women seek medical attention for problems likely to
lead to prescription of dependence-producing drugs.

The typical person who is dependent upon prescription drugs is a
woman who has a chronic, painful illness such as arthritis or headaches. She frequently has a history of either borderline or excessive
use of alcohol and often has an unusual sensitivity to uncomfortable
bodily feelings, including pain and anxiety. She may also have a
personal history of depression. Family histories of both alcoholism and
depression are common among people who become dependent on
prescription drugs. Such a person typically seeks medical attention;
her physician, responding to her distress over chronic pain or anxiety,
prescribes a dependence-producing drug. Usually this is an antianxiety drug such as Valium or Xanax, an antipain drug (called an
analgesic) such as Darvon or Percodan, or an anti-insomnia drug
(called a hypnotic) such as Seconal or Dalmane. Not uncommonly, the
physician may prescribe more than one such drug for a single patient.
Generally, after initial use, there is a prompt but modest reduction in
the patient's symptoms.

Not only does the drug partially relieve the distressing symptoms
experienced by the patient, but it also produces a moderate euphoria,
a high or a "buzz," although this is seldom noticed by the person
taking these drugs for medical purposes. As is the case with other
drug dependence, prescription drug dependence shows a progression
from experimentation to dependence that occurs over weeks or
years, the actual time lapse being determined principally by the
frequency and the size of the dose taken by the patient. In addition,
the characteristics of the drug and of the patient affect the probability
of eventual dependence.

At some point in this process, it can often be seen that the patient
not only took the analgesic or other dependence-producing drug to
cure the headaches, for example, but that—with increasing fre-

quency—the person experienced headaches or other symptoms to justify the drug use. This is a difficult concept to understand. Many drug-dependent people I have talked to are able, in retrospect, to identify a period in their drug use when they noticed that the withdrawal symptoms resulting from not using the drug prompted them to have the symptoms for which they were taking the drug.

Two distinctly different patterns emerge at this point. The more common pattern is a stabilization of the use of the dependence-producing prescription drug at about the level prescribed by the physician—perhaps a bit above, or more often, a bit below the amount prescribed by the doctor. For this group of drug-dependent people, there is no escalation in the drug use over time. This pattern of prolonged use, often despite repeated attempts to stop, can be distressing for the patient, the physician, and the patient's family. It can produce a life-long, chronic drug dependence. When the patient attempts to stop using the dependence-producing drug, the problem for which the drug was initially taken reemerges, and a new problem is added: acute and protracted withdrawal symptoms. Such patients are indeed "hooked."

On the other hand, most long-term, low-dose drug dependence of this type seems to be free of behavioral or physical consequences, as long as there is no escalation of dose and no concurrent alcohol-caused problems. When such dependent patients and their families seek help, they usually do so because they are distressed by the *idea* of drug dependence, not because of any identifiable problem they can associate with the drug's use. Because the symptoms for which the patient sought help in the first place are usually only partially relieved by such treatment, there is frequently a continuing problem with the underlying disorder: pain, anxiety, or insomnia.

The second pattern of prescription drug dependence is less common but more malignant: a progressively increasing dose of the medicine substantially beyond the levels initially prescribed by the physician. In the worst cases, those occurring among people who have shown earlier evidence of unstable or unreliable behavior, there is a movement to escalate dependence. This may cause the patient to try to acquire, in surreptitious fashion, additional prescriptions for her drug. Typically, she will obtain them from several physicians without honestly revealing the alternate sources. Sometimes this tactic requires that she involve multiple pharmacies to conceal the extent of her drug use or to hide entirely her completely illegal acquisition of the drug by using forged prescriptions or by purchasing the drug illegally.

With this second, high-dose, unstable pattern (or with either pattern if the drug use is combined with an excessive intake of alcohol), there is a characteristic deterioration of the patient's behavior. Most often this deterioration begins with irritability and poor performance of family tasks in the home. Accidents around the house and in the car are also common early symptoms of prescription drug dependence. Later, as the syndrome develops and if drug dependence persists, there are more extreme problems, including disturbed family relationships. If the person works outside the home, failed work performance is almost certain to occur.

Preventing and/or Coping with
Prescription Drug Dependence

As with other drug dependence problems, the best solution to prescription drug dependence is prevention: stopping the problem before it begins. There are constructive roles for patients, family, and physicians. The patient needs to be fully aware of the purposes of the dependence-producing medications and to know, before the first pill is taken or the first spoonful swallowed, the outside limits of use. This means knowing how much medication or how many pills are to be used per day, how frequently the pills are to be taken, and for how long the drug is to be used. Taken together, this means establishing a clear understanding by all concerned—the patient, the family, and the physician—of exactly what results are to be expected from the drug use, what the "target symptoms" are, and what the goal of the drug use is. Moreover, before beginning the use of the medication, all concerned in its administration and supervision should be aware of the likelihood of withdrawal symptoms when usage of the drug is eventually stopped.

Two warnings are important here. First, with the newly heightened family and patient concern about prescription drug dependence, there is a growing tendency to *underutilize* effective medical treatments. Many drugs about which patients and families worry are not dependence producing at all. Additionally, dependence-producing drugs are often entirely appropriate in specific situations. For example, it is usually desirable to use a narcotic painkiller for short-term treatment of pain associated with terminal illness. Such a drug may be safely and appropriately used for a painful illness that is likely to be quickly overcome. Some of these useful drugs are now underused because of the unrealistic concerns of both patients and doctors. The second warning is this: if you are afraid that a family member or you yourself are "hooked" on a dependence-producing drug, do not stop using the drug without *first* talking it over with the prescribing physician. If you continue to have doubts, get a second opinion from another physician.

Withdrawal from Prescription Drug Dependence: A Serious, But Not Necessarily Frightening, Process

When stopping the use of a dependence-producing drug, do so *gradually*. Abrupt withdrawal is generally unwise, and it can be dangerous. Abrupt withdrawal produces symptoms that are generally more severe if withdrawal is from a higher dose or from longer use of the drug. Pharmacologists often describe the severity of abrupt withdrawal as being related to both dose and duration. For example, abrupt withdrawal from relatively high doses of many tranquilizers and sleeping pills can produce severe disorders, including epileptic seizures. Problems of this nature can be avoided altogether by more gradual withdrawal, which can be accomplished by diminishing the doses over the course of one to four weeks.

Remember, contrary to what you may have concluded from watching television or reading horror stories in the newspapers, symptoms of withdrawal from medically prescribed, dependence-producing drugs are customarily mild; they are virtually never life-threatening (except for abrupt withdrawal), and they are usually temporary. Do not let withdrawal symptoms, or the idea of withdrawal symptoms, from prescription drug dependence scare you. Know what these symptoms are, face them directly, and go through them with a positive attitude. The self-reassurances I suggest that people repeat to themselves as they experience such symptoms are these: "My symptoms are distressing but not dangerous," and "I'm uncomfortable now, but it will pass."

Actually, what are withdrawal symptoms? They can be mild or severe, and they include irritability and insomnia; various gastrointestinal problems, such as loss of appetite, nausea, and diarrhea; and sweating and blurred vision. Headaches and strange feelings in the head, hands, and feet can occur. Psychotic symptoms—paranoia, delusions, and hallucinations—may develop. Epileptic seizures can occur following abrupt withdrawal. These symptoms may begin even before the last dose is taken; that is, they may start when the dose level is severely reduced, but before the drug use is stopped. They can begin within a few hours, or they can start as long as a week after the last dose is taken.

Withdrawal symptoms are hard to predict: I cannot tell which patients will have them and which will not. Many patients have no withdrawal symptoms at all while many others have very mild symptoms; only a few have severe symptoms. When symptoms do appear, they are distressing. However, they are of brief duration, generally lasting—in their intense form—for a few days or, at most, for a few weeks. They are not generally dangerous, except when there are seizures from abrupt withdrawal from high doses of depressant drugs, including sleeping pills and some tranquilizers. It is important to respect withdrawal symptoms but not to fear them. Medical care can often help reduce and manage these symptoms if they do occur.

Such withdrawal symptoms are often difficult to separate from the symptoms of the condition for which the drug was taken in the first place. In general, withdrawal symptoms are short-lived and get progressively less severe once the drug use has stopped. In contrast, reemergence of the problem for which the drug was taken tends to be persistent or even to increase in the weeks after the drug use has stopped. This distinction can help the patient and the physician separate withdrawal from the symptoms of the underlying disorder. Often patients know the difference. They commonly experience withdrawal symptoms as a new problem.

There is one major complication: Although withdrawal symptoms are real and are the direct result of the drug use itself, the characteristics, intensity, duration, and consequences of these symptoms are strongly influenced by the thoughts and the expectations of the patient and the physician. For example, if there is terror and confusion, withdrawal symptoms will be more disturbing. If there is sober, realistic recognition that they are distressing but not dangerous and especially that they are temporary, then they will be relatively easy to manage.

In my experience in dealing with thousands of people dependent on all sorts of drugs, I have found that withdrawal symptoms are usually not the major problem in becoming drug-free. The big problem for most drug-dependent people is what happens once withdrawal is complete. The use of the drug, medical or nonmedical, often becomes a way to solve problems and deal with unpleasant feelings. It can serve as a substitute for relationships and activities. It can become, in effect, a way of life. Real recovery is a long-term process of relearning to live drug-free. Recovery means finding new ways to cope with life, including life's real problems, some of which may have contributed to the initial drug use and many of which will remain as difficult obstacles after withdrawal from drug use.

I have emphasized the importance of medically supervised, gradual withdrawal from medically prescribed, dependence-producing drugs.

This can usually be done on an outpatient basis by simply reducing the dose of the drug over the course of from several weeks to as long as several months. In particularly difficult cases, withdrawal in a hospital may be required. If it is, hospitalization seldom lasts more than 10 to 30 days.

The tougher phase of recovery comes after the acute withdrawal period is ended. It has two parts. The first is the management of the underlying problem for which the prescribed drugs were taken in the first place. The recovering patient may have to develop techniques, which do not include drugs, to cope with insomnia, pain, or anxiety. This is no small task, but it can be done. When done successfully, it usually produces a substantial boost in self-esteem.

The second part of recovery is the problem of craving for the drug, which is often called the "protracted withdrawal syndrome." This occurs among all recovered drug-dependent people, whether their drug was medically prescribed or not. It can last for many months or even for years. In dealing with this problem, it is often useful to work with other people who have the same problem.

The most likely source of help is an Anonymous program such as Alcoholics Anonymous or the more recently developed program, Pills Anonymous, which is specifically designed to help people who have been medically dependent. Both self-help and professional alcohol abuse treatment programs are well equipped to help the person with a medical dependence. Sometimes such people do well in drug abuse treatment programs, but because the typical alcohol program in the United States today includes many middle-aged and older patients, and because many of these prescription drug dependents were never part of the illegal drug subculture associated with dependence on such drugs as cocaine and heroin, the typical person who is dependent on medical drugs feels more comfortable in alcohol abuse rather than drug abuse treatment programs.

FAMILY PROBLEMS COMPLICATING DRUG ABUSE TREATMENT

Returning from our exploration of prescription drug dependence to the universal issues of psychoactive drug abuse treatment, we note that problems in family life can complicate, impede, and even destroy the effectiveness of treatment. This is especially the case when so-called "healthy" family members have drug and alcohol problems of their own. In fact, one of the most common family problems encountered in drug abuse treatment is the drug or alcohol dependence of family members other than the identified patient. When this is the case, a fearlessly prepared and shared "family inventory" must be a high priority as an essential part of the treatment of drug problems within the family. How can the family be sure that a fellow member— a nonpatient—does or does not have a drug or alcohol problem? Follow the simple rule laid out earlier: any continuing use of illegal drugs, any use of prescription drugs in excess of a doctor's orders, or any use of alcohol beyond the specific limits stated in Chapter 4 are probable drug abuse problems.

In making the inventory of family drug problems, add answers to this question: Do any family members consider a drug or alcohol user's use to be a problem to him or to them? If the answer is yes, then the identified member or members probably will have to become drug free—with or without the help of treatment. If family members are to contribute positively, as they certainly should, toward successful drug abuse treatment, they must acknowledge their own drug involvement, change whatever attitudes are necessary, and decide to stop using intoxicating substances. In all adjustments of this kind, the family as a whole must be continuously open to communication and change.

When the family already has one member in drug abuse treatment, it should be sure to inventory the family's nondrug problems which may complicate his or her recovery. Parental conflicts are common, and they are frequently complicated by circumstances arising when one or more members of the family are hooked on drugs. Possibly, some of these conflicts and complications will abate when the drug problem or problems are resolved. Others will not. To reduce drug problems and resultant complications, parents—in particular—need to function effectively and judiciously in their parental roles and also in their roles as husband and wife. If that means making a real effort to solve a long-standing problem in their marital relationship, then they must make it. That, too, is a valuable and constructive benefit which can result when some other member of the family is in drug abuse treatment.

In making the family inventory of drug-complicated factors, do not overlook another significant and contributing problem: In these crucial times, when treatment is going on for the drug-dependent family member, fathers and—nowadays often—mothers tend to work too hard in jobs and careers inside or outside the home and to spend too little time with their families. This can aggravate the other family problems which require solution.

Further, family members (parents, most often) fall into a pattern of constant, negative, and usually overt antagonism toward the drug-dependent person. It is both essential and fair to ask, once a person has succeeded in completely halting his or her drug use, that a more supportive and less critical relationship be developed and maintained.

There is still another problem unique in its effect upon drug treatment of a family member: a drug-dependent "adult child," more often than not a single or divorced woman in her 20s or 30s, with one or more preschool children of her own. Such persons are usually Pseudo-Children in that they are over the age of 19, but have never successfully established themselves as effective, independent adults. They have remained dependent on their parents, usually having passed first through the rebellious stage of being Pseudo-Adults during their stormy teenage years. Typically, they have failed to complete the education required to work beyond the limits of either a minimum wage income or they have been set up in a family business. I have worked with some drug-dependent people in this category who have done quite well in school, but who have nevertheless failed to separate emotionally or financially from their parents.

Of special importance here is the fact that the presence of a young, helpless, and needy infant or child poses terrible problems for both the immature young adult and *her* harried parents. My advice, in such cases, is direct and simple: make self-support and responsible, drug-free living a precondition for family support of this Pseudo-Child. If it is not forthcoming, then withdraw family support because it will, in this case, merely enable continued drug abuse. As an added admonition, if there is evidence of gross neglect of the infant or child, seek legal intervention to remove the child from his or her drug-using, Pseudo-Child parent. Unfortunately, the most common response to this problem is a blurring of roles of the parents and would-be adult children, and this blurring produces terrible pain and seriously complicates the lives of all concerned, especially the life of the family member currently trying to recover from drug dependence.

All families, with and without drug-dependent members, have deficiencies. These deficiencies can often have a malignant impact on the drug use of one or more family members. When confronting these deficiencies, whatever their form or severity, it is important to build on the positive aspects of the family rather than to let negativism and pessimism thwart successful action. There are two ways to build this support. The first is to understand and apply the fundamental principles of family organization as developed in Chapter 6. This involves a clear recognition of the roles of various family members and the specific goals of family life, especially the goal of helping the children grow up to function as independent, reasonably happy, productive adults.

The second way is to support the family by becoming involved with other families confronting similar problems and/or to seek professional assistance, including the support of a drug abuse treatment program, which can be literally lifesaving. Of these two support systems, the guidance of similarly struggling families is usually the most useful. This is true because advice and support from families not confronting drug and alcohol problems, as well as advice from experts—however wise and well meaning—often reinforce the family's feelings of shame and failure, feelings which undermine successful coping. By contrast, guidance from families facing similar problems often builds family self-esteem. To see that other families have wrestled with and successfully overcome this difficult situation and to see that they are basically good families made up of basically good people can be vital to building the family morale necessary to solve the drug problem. For this to happen, however, the drug-involved family must come out of its isolation and become part of a specific helping community. It must share with others many of the most intimate and painful aspects of family life in order to benefit from this support. This takes real courage. It seldom happens until the pain caused by the drug problems has become literally intolerable.

THE HANDICAPPED AND DRUGS: IF LIFE GIVES YOU LEMONS, MAKE LEMONADE

By this time, you should be convinced that we are all direct or indirect victims of drug dependence. The people we have reason to be deeply concerned about in this section are a special breed of victim: *the handicapped.* The truly handicapped—whether beset by a disadvantage or by physical, mental, economic, or cultural happenstances—are the victims who suffer more and pay an even higher price in personal pain and frustrating lives than the rest of us do. It may not be immediately obvious why the handicapped should be highlighted in this book about family drug dependence prevention. This short section is necessary, I believe, for many families to overcome one of the more common and difficult obstacles to drug abuse prevention. When young people are handicapped, for whatever reason, there are two problems which must be solved before a family-based prevention program can work. First, many handicapped people are especially vulnerable to drug dependence for reasons which will be explored shortly. Second, those who live and work with the handicapped are often reluctant to confront drug problems because they think antidrug efforts may demoralize the handicapped or because they think that the handicap excuses the drug use. While severe physical handicaps are relatively rare in our society, significant, if less visible, handicaps are common. Confronting these problems with understanding is a vital part of any drug dependence prevention effort. This issue of handicaps thwarting drug abuse prevention is not limited to the severely handicapped or to any widespread and serious problem for thousands upon thousands of families. Thirty-five million Americans have significant disabilities.

As you meet the handicapped in these pages, keep in mind the more inclusive view of the term. Look beyond what the word most readily calls to mind: the deaf-mute, the blind man with his white cane, the legless person in a wheelchair—those most visibly handicapped by an unthinking twist of fate or the drop of a wild card from a genetic deck. When I use the word handicapped here, I mean all of those people put at a significant disadvantage in life's race by any physical, mental, emotional, economic, or cultural handicap whatsoever.

Hard Decisions: Quick and Easy Pleasures— Or Slow and Tough Ones?

Drug use and drug dependence affect the handicapped in many ways, but one of the most significant is simply that the handicapped people's opportunities for nondrug pleasures and success are more limited than those of nonhandicapped people of comparable age. There is almost certain to be also a lowered self-esteem growing out of the handicap, and this, in turn, reduces resistance to drug use and drug dependence. Those who have less to lose are less likely to resist drug experimentation and, later, escalation of initial use to a state of dependency. It is for these reasons that the handicapped are more vulnerable to drug dependence. Drug use, remember, appears to the new drug user to be an easily managed way to feel good. The natural ways to feel good require more work and are harder to achieve. If a student should try to make good grades as a means of feeling good, success will come only as a result of diligent study and hard work. Of course, there is always a chance that the student will fail to attain the goal, thus reducing or even eliminating the good feelings that would result from the achievement. There is no such effort and no such risk involved in getting high on pot. Compare the pleasure of getting a good grade on a final exam with the pleasure of puffing on a marijuana cigarette. Think of how much work each takes: the grade takes lots of work continued over many days or even weeks, while the drug high costs perhaps $1.00 and takes only a few minutes to achieve.

Now contrast that same calculation (seldom made with conscious awareness, but often made by young people without much thought) as it is made by a handicapped person. Compare the decision to go for a good grade versus the decision to use marijuana as that decision is likely to be made by an impoverished rural or urban minority teenager, or by a deaf youth, or by a youngster handicapped by a learning disability. For all of these handicapped people, the healthy pleasure is almost certain to be harder to choose and, if chosen, much more difficult to achieve. It would be surprising indeed if many handicapped people did not opt for the quick and easy pleasure on the drug route. That negative choice is, for some, facilitated by the strong probability that the drug pleasure is more readily available because drug usage in their peer groups is often greater than among the peer groups of the nonhandicapped.

Many handicaps also are combined with lower levels of family and community control, a combination further aggravating the problems of drug abuse. On top of this, the handicapped are burdened by the unfortunate fact that sometimes people who *could* stop the handicapped person's use of drugs fail to do so. They refrain from interfering because they mistakenly conclude that saying no will be a blow to the handicapped person's self-esteem or autonomy, both of which are often fragile.

Before we explore approaches to handling handicaps as they may be affected by drug use, a special point should be noted: the fundamental effects and outcomes of drug use and drug abuse are the same for *all*—whether handicapped or nonhandicapped. With respect to drug deterioration and ultimate dependency, it makes little difference whether the person is a mentally handicapped teenager or a brilliantly successful college professor, a wheelchair-bound paraplegic or the swaggering leader of a street gang, the poorest kid on the block or the richest oilman in the world. Drugs are no respecters of persons. The butcher, the baker, the high-tech maker—whatever the race, the color, or the creed—the basic drug dependence process is the same for all. Granted, as between one individual and another, the damage drugs do may be greater or smaller, the pain may be more or less agonizing. But the major point remains: Drugs will exact their price and take their toll whether the user is handicapped or not.

Approaches to Handling Handicaps—Without Drugs

In recent years, some observers of the drug scene have focused on the relationship of economic deprivation to drug use and have concluded that drug use (often heroin use) is a social disease which can only be cured by eliminating social inequities. There are some faulty assumptions in this position. To approach the connection between a handicap and drug use in this way is doubly handicapping for the individuals actually involved. Since the person *is* poor (an economic handicap) or deaf (a physical handicap) or culturally disadvantaged, and since this type of "disease" is not likely to change during a particular person's vulnerable teenage years, to blame the drug use on the handicap is (from the point of view of the person thus handicapped) to excuse and perpetuate the drug problem and to further reduce the ability of the handicapped person to succeed in life. It mistakenly assumes that the "diseased" drug user has no responsibility for or opportunity to overcome his handicap *on his own*. After all, if his handicap is indeed the result of a social or an economic or a cultural disease, what can the individual exposed to drugs do about it? It is not *his* responsibility that he has fallen into the drug trap. Society—"somebody out there"—is to blame. Worst of all, this outlook discourages (even takes out of the individual's hands) *self*-direction and *self*-improvement. It leaves him without hope for the captaincy of his life. It contradicts the time-tested reality that the deprived or disadvantaged person can retain meaningful mastery of his fate. This approach of excusing the handicapped and blaming the society creates a sad and sizeable additional handicap to the already handicapped.

Making Sweet Lemonade from Sour Lemons. A far more positive approach to helping the handicapped, it seems to me, is to take the view that handicaps of whatever kind should be looked at as potential opportunities. "Too unreal! Too optimistic," you scoff? Not true. To take any other view is to conclude that the handicapped person is a born loser who never has had and never will have a chance in life. That I cannot agree to. The handicapped person—boy or girl, man or woman—can win out, can have real say-so about his or her personal destiny. But the only way a deprived, disadvantaged, or incapacitated person can compete successfully with the nonhandicapped in life is *to work harder*. There is no simple, easy way. But who ever said that overcoming a handicap was a piece of cake? One inescapable truth which the person who, for whatever reason, is handicapped must accept from the outset is this: *Drug use* is almost certain to reduce the user's will and ability to work, thereby reducing the prospects for success, whether that person is handicapped or not.

If, on the other hand, the handicapped person sees his handicap as a difficulty to be overcome by hard work, then his disadvantage can be turned into an advantage. The obstacle can then be surmounted, and by surmounting it the handicapped person will grow stronger. The poor, for example, who face the fact that they are disadvantaged and then proceed to work harder to overcome this handicap, are better equipped to compete in the larger community. Because they have thus toughened themselves and learned to endure, they are often better able to compete than those who are economically better-off, who may lack the incentive and the powerful motivation provided by the handicap of poverty. How often have you heard from people who have become successful about the role that early poverty or some other handicap played in their motivation and achievement? It is a common story—one with endlessly inspiring variations.

Nor should the handicapped overlook the other side of this coin: Many who are presently poor were once well off. They have fallen from economic grace for many reasons—drug dependence being one of them. Recent studies of poverty in America have shown that most families who start out poor do not remain poor generation after generation. There is a great and continuing movement upward from poverty into the middle and upper classes. The handicapped should take a long, hard look at this upward trend and analyze why it happens and why it will continue to happen. While looking, they may find it reassuring to realize that there is an approximately equal movement of people downward from the upper and middle classes into poverty. Whether they see it or not, one of the key determinants of movement down the success-to-failure ladder is drug and alcohol dependence.

The Victims Become the Victors: Some Triumphant Models.
Do not discount what I am saying as mere Pollyanna rhetoric. I have seen this approach work over and over again. I have seen this approach work with all kinds of handicaps. One large group of related handicaps is now labeled "Attention Deficit Disorder." This disorder affects children, many of them preteens and teenagers, who have a variety of behavioral and learning problems including hyperactivity as well as reading and math problems. The kids I have worked with who have done well despite their learning disabilities and hyperactivity are kids who know they have a problem and know that the only way to solve this problem is to work harder than the "next

person." Families can help the child thus handicapped by seeing and emphasizing the unique opportunities which the handicap presents. They can assist and encourage the child to learn well the simple lesson that success in life primarily reflects not good fortune but the capacity to work hard purposefully over a long period of time.

Perhaps because of my personal history of childhood asthma, I was moved when I read in a recently published biography of Theodore Roosevelt about his sickly childhood. At the age of about 12, his father, who had previously anxiously indulged young Teddy, set him down and flatly told him that he had a weak body which might prevent him from doing all he would like to do. Clearly and in painfully direct terms, he told the boy that it was strictly up to him to do whatever he could to cope with this handicap. Despite the reality of his suffering, he was told, his family would no longer pamper him. Tough medicine? No question about it. But do not assume that compassion was lacking. Teddy responded. He became a committed physical fitness enthusiast, beginning a lifelong commitment to an active and often outdoor life. This life, in the end, benefited not only himself, but our nation as a whole. Among the host of the many remarkable successes he achieved, he promoted and extended the National Park system which so many of us enjoy today.

Recently I worked with a woman who, late in her teens, had experienced severe agoraphobia. Her mother, having suffered a similar experience in her own young adulthood, told her child, "I know this handicap is hard for you. But you just have to face your fears and get on with your life." This daughter, now middle-aged herself, reflected that if her mother had been more sympathetic and had let her avoid confrontation of her fears, she probably would have become and remained housebound by her phobia. She was grateful to her mother, as Teddy Roosevelt became grateful to his father, for an invaluable gift: the toughening-up process without which she would never have been able to work hard enough to conquer her phobia handicap.

Start SELF-Tough and Stay SELF-Tough. This is the message these victories over obstacles beam to all the physically, mentally, economically, and culturally handicapped of this world: Start *self*-tough and stay *self*-tough. No other way can you make it in our highly competitive world. Throw self-pity out the window. The only real and lasting help is the help *inside* you, coming from *within*. And, above all else—I should add—*forget drugs*. Your handicap, God knows, is already big enough.

This is certainly not to say that others cannot and will not help.

They will often do their best—or close to it. In modern America, those who are struggling to overcome their handicaps are finding another source of strength, another opportunity: the community of others having the same or similar problems offer real support. There is a potential for pride and growth in these associations. Such groups provide an opportunity to assess more realistically the true potential for functioning triumphantly with their handicap. The success stories of those who have "made it" become personal incentives for the others. For adults working with handicapped children, the upbeat and tough-minded advice we have noted must of course be tempered with a realistic assessment of what is possible. Although errors are sometimes made in overestimating possibilities for the handicapped, my observation has been that the more common error lies in the opposite direction. Our society cannot afford to underestimate the potential that the handicapped have for the effective, satisfying functioning that leads to personal, positive pleasure, and that makes a real contribution to the welfare of the family, the community, and the country. Of course, we must not delude ourselves in this regard. Handicaps can often actually block outlets for creativity and hard work. But the demonstrably optimistic news is that handicaps can, at the same time, open other promising outlets and channels. A blind person, no matter how hard he tries, will never make it as an airline pilot. He can, however, become an outstanding musician or radio personality by using well and selectively his other sensory and expressive capabilities: his hands, his voice, and his ears.

For all of us, handicapped and nonhandicapped, growing up offers us chances to fit and refit our abilities, our interests, and our opportunities into a meaningful unity. Often the closed doors in our lives present us with more important growth opportunities than the easy successes. Look at your own life. How often have you noticed that a failure or a disappointment has led you to rethink your situation, forcing you to come up with a far better solution than you had before you failed? If one can learn anything at all, one is more likely to learn from failure than from success. When you fail, you have to think and change. When you succeed, you probably will keep doing the same old thing, often missing new opportunities. For a happy outcome to occur, however, failure must be understood for what it is: an inevitable and recurring consequence of *trying*. To live with this and go on trying, the handicapped person must have—at the core—a solid yet flexible toughness, a toughness buttressed from time to time by the real and reassuring support available in the family and in the community so that the individual confronting failure can pick herself or himself up, learn, and go on.

Whatever the handicap—whether economic, cultural, physical, or emotional—it must be confronted and, whenever possible, used creatively to fashion a successful life. While it is often true that the handicap itself can be turned to an advantage, it is equally true that this will happen only if the handicapped individual has a clear understanding of the handicap itself and of the requirements to overcome it. A positive attitude and a commitment to hard work are absolutely necessary.

People who overcome handicaps not only offer hope to others with similar handicaps, but they also offer inspiration to all, including the nonhandicapped. In this shared process, the family stands at the center and holds the key to potential success. Conversely, drug and alcohol dependence stands as one of the greatest threats to success in overcoming a handicap.

Without taking anything away from the unique problems of the severely handicapped it is true that in different ways all of us are handicapped. No one is dealt a full hand of aces in life. We all hold losing cards. The challenge, for all of us, is to play our own unique cards with skill and courage. Working with the handicapped can teach useful lessons to us all—lessons focused precisely on that courage and skill, lessons about the real strength and beauty of the human spirit. Drug and alcohol dependence is the great enemy of this spirit. Family and community are its best friends.

INVOKING THE "HIGHER POWER" IN TREATMENT

As this chapter draws to a close, it is pertinent to call our thoughts back to a concept we have talked about before: the "higher power." To the extent that it can help to motivate and support drug-dependent people and their families, it can help to energize the total end-to-end rehabilitation enterprise. For those who care to think about it, it can become a strength-renewing factor, a goal-sustaining force guiding the recovery effort. Some see the "higher power" as a practical, down-to-earth idea. Others see it as more metaphorical or metaphysical. Many who are struggling to overcome drug dependency welcome it as religion.

At the psychological level, one way to think about the effect of religion is to see religion as a system of related, shared values that *transcend* both the individual person and his or her moment in time. That is as good a way as any to define the "higher power"—or, if you prefer, the "Higher Power"—that we are talking about here. It is precisely this connection with values that transcend one's personal experiences, to say nothing of one's personal pleasure, which constitutes both an important element in drug abuse prevention and an important element in drug abuse intervention and treatment.

In our modern secular society, talk of religion in relation to a drug problem or drug abuse treatment can sound old-fashioned or even narrow-minded. I take that chance. As a physician who has spent over a decade treating drug-dependent people and their families, I am convinced that this kind of religious experience is an enormously useful part of dealing with a drug problem. This is why the Anonymous groups—Alcoholics Anonymous and Narcotics Anonymous— make so much of what they call "turning the problem over to one's higher power." This kind of giving up of control is often the first step in making one's life, and one's family life, manageable, productive, and reasonably happy. In my personal experience, I have found that the precise content of the religion is far less important than that the religious values be respected.

From a public health point of view, virtually all religions, other than the bizarre cult credos of an individualistic and often seemingly mad leader, are effective in helping to stop drug problems. Thus, it matters little whether one speaks of Christian or Jewish religions or of Buddhism or Islam. The point is simply that a renunciation of personal, present-tense pleasure as the ultimate goal of living, seeing that one's life is part of a larger and more meaningful shared process, is often essential to solving a drug problem. This should hardly be surprising, given the dark and unrelenting tenacity of the Drug Dependence Syndrome. As I pointed out in Chapter 2, when it comes to preventing or curing a drug problem, the drug-burdened traveler needs a bridge over troubled waters. Religion, surely, is one of the most sturdy of bridges.

SUMMING UP

The description of making drug abuse treatment work, as examined in this chapter, does not do justice to the experience of families actually going through the process. There are as many unique experiences as there are families working their way through drug abuse treatment: now more than 400,000 each year in the United States. Even so, what has been written here should serve to identify and illuminate certain key principles which can be applied to the work of overcoming drug dependence. Admittedly, the steps I have sketched to be taken in surmounting obstacles to successful recovery may not be as complete and as practical as one might wish, but they at least point out the direction to be taken. They single out the signposts that tell us something of the scope and nature of the journey to be traveled, pitfalls to be skirted, and hazardous roadblocks to be removed before the hoped-for destination—the drug-free state—can be reached. And, having explored it, we should perhaps look back and recapture a few of the highlights:

- The first line of defense, after drug abuse prevention has failed, is Family Action, a structured family intervention to stop drug use by the family member who is abusing drugs. Support groups are often essential for this approach to work.
- The Anonymous groups, Alcoholics Anonymous and Narcotics Anonymous, and the related family support groups, Al-Anon and Alateen, are the best hope for many drug- and alcohol-dependent people and their families.
- Professional drug abuse treatment has many forms and takes place in many settings. It is often required for drug- and alcohol-dependent people in the final stage of the Drug Dependence Syndrome. It must have the goal of drug-free living, and it must involve the family.
- Psychotherapy for the individual drug- or alcohol-dependent person and his family is unlikely to lead to stopping of drug use, but psychotherapy can be highly effective as part of Aftercare in supporting positive personal and family growth.

CHAPTER
EIGHT

The Community and Drugs

I N THIS CHAPTER, we are going to look *outside*—beyond the family and into the community—for help to combat drug dependence. In this effort, we will pinpoint those community groups that are uniquely situated or constituted to prevent drug problems the school, the workplace, the highway safety system, the criminal justice administration, and the medical profession. These particular settings and populations are explored to broaden the focus of this book beyond the core drug dependence patterns of teenagers and their families. In addition, these community settings offer opportunities to reinforce and extend the role of the family in drug abuse prevention and treatment. Families are more likely, for example, to stop drug problems in their teenage children to the extent that their schools are helping students grow up free of drug use. Similarly, families are more likely to identify and treat drug problems among adult family members if drug-free values are reinforced by the parents' employers and by their family physicians.

THE COMMUNITY AND DRUGS: LIKE IT OR NOT, WE ARE ALL IN THIS BOAT TOGETHER

It is essential to project the "get tough" fight against drugs beyond the family and outward into the community. We must concentrate our attention on those resources, organizations, systems, situations, and settings that are uniquely qualified to apply and extend the special *societal toughness* needed to prevent drug use and drug dependence. Certain of these organizations and systems are, moreover, expressly designed to curb, penalize, or punish those who, by reason of drug and alcohol use, are endangering their own lives and destroying the lives of others.

Just as individuals function in families, so families function in communities. Our communities can be thought of as a series of interdependent, interlocking elements: the school, the church, the workplace, the criminal justice system, the medical practice center, and the highway traffic safety system. Some of these resources and systems are primarily instructive, guidance oriented, and even inspirational; others have been designed as basic deterrent forces within the society. As our society has enlarged and become increasingly complex, these instructive/deterrent functions have been developed in ways that can enhance their effectiveness. Because these systems come in direct, person-to-person contact with actual and potential drug-dependent people, all are vital for successful community-based drug abuse prevention. The nature of these contacts has a great deal to do with whether people become and remain drug dependent. When assessing the usefulness of these contacts, we must keep in mind certain implications—some real, some contrived. Broadening the base of drug dependence prevention beyond the confines of the family creates two fundamental problems: the conflicting and controversial interpretation of (1) privacy and (2) civil rights. Those problems become all the more pertinent here where the standards of social control are different—for example, in the schools or on the highways—than they are in the family.

Before exploring the possibilities of specific community institutions in drug abuse prevention, let us return to the most fundamental concept developed in this book: the biological basis for drug dependence. When we do, we will see more clearly why community responses are so important and what these responses must be for a successful outcome.

Recall that the brain organizes behavior around the pursuit of pleasure and the avoidance of pain. We go toward what makes us feel good and away from what makes us feel bad. The biology of this process pushes us toward such naturally pleasure-producing experiences as sex and eating, as well as toward far more complex pleasures such as caring human relationships and achievement. The problem is that these natural, or at least nondrug, pleasures cannot always be wisely managed by the individual, because the pleasure they produce tends to distort judgment. The unbridled pursuit of pleasures, even natural pleasures, is dangerous for the individual and for his community.

Take eating, for example. If an individual were to seek to maximize the pleasure of eating, without thought of consequences, not only would the individual become obese, but his diet would not likely be sensibly balanced. In fact, the increasingly individualized nature of eating in modern America has led to an epidemic rise in such eating disorders as obesity, anorexia nervosa, and bulimia. The eating pleasure is everywhere hedged in by social or cultural forces. These forces extend from an understanding of the concept of a balanced diet, to the controls involved in eating a meal, to table manners. All of these pleasure-controlling forces reflect the learning that comes from the larger community, learning that has taken place over many years—often over countless generations. Thus, the eating behavior we see about us every day is a complex, and usually reasonably effective, interplay of biology and culture. This eating behavior begins with the vitally important, biologically based experience of pleasure which is then shaped by forces outside the individual. In other words, eating behavior begins with a feeling called "appetite"—a good feeling that comes from even the thought of eating—which is then shaped and reshaped by a wise network of relationships and beliefs which I call *social control*. This same process occurs in all pleasure-producing behaviors. This process starts out as fairly simple biology and is given expression only after cultural controls have been applied.

Sexual pleasure is another good example: while the capacity for sexual pleasure is innate and generally unfocused, before it is expressed in human behavior it is shaped by many cultural controls, notably through law and religion. This must be so if the needs of the community—and at a larger level, the society—are to be met. Even more bluntly, this social control process must be maintained if individualistic pleasures are not to upset and undermine the community itself. For example, unbridled sexual activity wrecks the capacity to form families and raise children. No society can endure without explicit and strict controls over sexual and other pleasure-producing behaviors.

Notice especially that although social control over pleasure-producing behavior is expressed and reinforced in many ways by many organizations and institutions, the most powerful and effective expression of the social control process is the family. This is as true of the social control over eating and sex as it is over the use of drugs and alcohol. These social controls are often internalized in the individual as values and the conscience.

Notice also that pleasure itself is not defined as bad or wrong. The forces of social control, rather than rejecting biologically driven pleasures, act to channel the expression of these pleasures into socially constructive paths, or at least away from socially destructive paths. While the paths being rejected are labeled, depending on the process at work, as "bad" or "illegal" or "unacceptable," the underlying purpose of the process of social control is not difficult to understand. It represents the same process we have labeled "two heads are better than one"; that is, decisions about pleasure-producing behaviors are partially controlled by people whose brains are not directly influenced by the pleasure process. As is commonly observed, when it comes to pleasure-producing behaviors, good advice is easy to give but, unfortunately, hard to accept.

Where, you may ask, do drugs fit into this social control process? And how do community institutions fit into this concept? Drugs are chemicals which make people feel good. They preempt the natural pleasure-producing centers in the brain. They subvert the incentives to growth and productivity. They evade many of the social control processes affecting most natural pleasure-producing behaviors. But, of course, drugs are widely desired by many people because they work—at least in the short run—in the sense that they do produce good feelings.

When human life was lived in small villages, and when people were exposed to few, if any, pleasure-producing drugs, social control over pleasure-producing behaviors was simple, direct, and universal. Punishments for deviations tended to be quick and severe. As people lived in ever-larger, more complex communities, the direct exercise of social control was replaced by an ever-expanding network of social institutions, all having the purpose of shaping behavior. Many of these behaviors were pleasure-producing. The two most far-reaching social control systems in modern life are law and religion. As our society has beome more secular, the law has carried a heavier burden of this social control.

The principles underlying this process are simpler than the details might lead one to believe. Community institutions, ranging from the school to the workplace to the criminal justice system, all have an impact on drug-taking behavior to protect the needs of the larger community against the dangers of reckless individual activities. These community institutions are not, of course, unconcerned about the needs or feelings of individuals. In fact, they generally reflect the long-term interests of individuals. They tend to correct the distortions of judgment so characteristic of the drug experience: they raise the importance of community needs, and they raise the value of the needs of both the individual and the community for the future. In this regard, community-based social control tends to diminish the importance of individual feeling states in the present tense—at least insofar as they are contrary to the long-term best interest of the individual and of the larger community.

When social control is exercised in the family, it is not particularly controversial, although we have already seen that it is precisely the reduction of this family-based social control which has led to the drug epidemic in the last 15 years. However, when social control is exercised by formal community institutions, it is often controversial and there are legitimate concerns for the protection of both individual privacy and self-determination. It is this balancing of needs that provides the dynamic tension in the contemporary drug scene.

In recalling the far-distant past for most human communities, the time when most people lived in villages of a few dozen people, it is easy to see that behavior of all kinds was fairly easily managed. This was true for all pleasure-producing behavior, including drug taking. Everyone not only knew everyone else, but they knew virtually everything that everyone was doing. Privacy was almost nonexistent. When lying, theft, and other types of deviant behavior emerged, they were promptly recognized and punished. When communities grew, so did privacy and anonymity. And diversity of human behavior. And richness of individual opportunity.

Certainly not all of this is bad—far from it. Many people in the modern world find the social control in small communities to be stifling and actively seek larger, more complex, more tolerant communities. But, as with so many improvements, there are prices to be paid. One of the most severe is drug addiction. Youth in America today have unprecedented exposure to pleasure-producing chemicals in an environment that is far more permissive of drug taking than any existing in the past, or any existing elsewhere in the world today. Sorting this out, and solving the problems it creates, is a tremendous challenge. The way will be easier to find, I believe, if we have a clear understanding of the drug dependence process. When we do, it seems to me, we need to recognize that illegal drug use is *not a protected individual right* and that the *community has a vital stake in preventing drug dependence*. Finally, it will help to recognize that *the family is the most effective site of social control*.

When it comes to the promotion of individual freedoms and the pursuit of pleasure, it is important to be clear about the role of drug use. If drug use is seen as merely another area of personal choice, somewhat like hairstyle or, even worse, somewhat like free speech, then we have failed to comprehend the reality of the drug experience for the family and the community. We also have failed to grasp the threat to the individual. This is a threat to long-term self-interest and even, paradoxically, to the prospects for individual pleasure. While drug use begins as the search for pleasure, it typically ends in the flight from pain, the pain of withdrawal, and the pain of facing the devastating consequences of the drug use itself. This entire reality, unpleasant as it unquestionably is, must be faced before it is possible to think through the seeming conflicts of values involved in social controls which reject drug use. I believe that when drug dependence is seen clearly, it is then understandable why the goal of drug-free living is not only reasonable but a matter of life and death for individuals, families, and communities.

The community response to drug use is expressed in specific institutions. In this chapter, we will focus on those institutions which are the most comprehensive and the most relevant to drug abuse prevention, exploring how they can work better to prevent drug dependence while still respecting the value of individual rights and the preeminent role of the family. Let us begin with the largest institution most directly concerned with children: the school.

Combatting Drug Problems in the School

Sixty million Americans go to school. A higher percentage of Americans are in school than of any other nationality in the world. Today about 45 million Americans are in public schools through the 12th grade, about five million are in private elementary and secondary schools, and about 10 million are enrolled in colleges and universities.

Most use of illegal and intoxicating drugs begins between the ages of 12 and 20, with the peak age of first use being about 15. During this most vulnerable span of adolescence, most Americans are in school. School administrators and forward-looking teachers, in cooperation with concerned parents, are now recognizing the vast opportunities schools have to prevent drug dependence. Promising steps have been taken, and the outlines of a number of well thought out and productive approaches to handling drug problems have emerged. Based on my observation of these approaches, I have singled out four fundamental guidelines which, I believe, provide a foundation upon which to build a successful, school-based program to combat drug problems:

1. Promote drug-free and alcohol-free lifestyles for the students. Do not be taken in by the easy cop-out that "Everyone does it," or that "Drug use is okay, but drug abuse is a problem." All use of alcohol and other drugs by students attending high school is both unhealthy and illegal in all parts of the United States. Any compromise with this objective is self-defeating for the school and dangerous for the students. Kids are looking to adults to set the standards.

Adults have in the past two decades too often abandoned the kids, especially when it comes to marijuana and alcohol, seeming to accept the notion that "Everyone has to try it for himself" and that "Drugs are there for the kids. They cannot run away from them." These trends need to be reversed with clear statements that intoxicating drugs are poisons and pollutants to the brain and the entire human body. They are to be rejected—not played with.

2. Involve the students' families early and often in the solution of any drug problem that may arise and in education and prevention efforts.   See the family as the linchpin of prevention and treatment. When families fail, do not blame them. Help them. Families need to be informed and educated about the dangers of drugs generally, and about the dangers of the GATEWAY DRUGS in particular. Families need to understand the workings of the Drug Dependence Syndrome, and they need to comprehend their role in drug abuse prevention. Families can benefit greatly by getting together with other families to prevent and solve drug problems. Parents, by organizing Parent Peer Groups centered around their own teenage children and the peer groups of their friends, can contribute more strongly to successful prevention efforts. When serious drug problems do arise, families need to work with other similarly affected families in overcoming these problems, cooperating both inside and outside treatment programs. In all of these family-centered activities, the school should play a facilitating role. To achieve worthwhile and lasting results, families must look upon these drug abuse prevention efforts as an important, continuing part of the activities of the entire school year, not a "once-a-year" exercise.

3. Base all school drug abuse prevention and treatment programs on clearly written, widely discussed school policies and procedures.   Do not make it personal or impulsive, but carefully build drug abuse prevention into all facets of school policy. Schools need to articulate drug dependence prevention goals, express their reasons for establishing these goals, and develop comprehensive policies and procedures to ensure reaching them. To have genuine and lasting merit, an antidrug program cannot be an isolated project of some principal or teacher; it must be built into the ongoing commitment of the institution to promote the health and the education of its students. Particularly important, after the goal of drug-free lifestyles has been established, is clear formulation, dissemination, and enforcement of rules against drug and alcohol use. This is an adult responsibility—for teachers, counselors, administrators, and parents.

4. Base prevention, treatment, and all school policies on a clear understanding of verifiable facts and established truths. These include recognition that drug use is the *number one* health threat for young people of school age and that the use of alcohol and other dependence-producing drugs constitutes the single biggest threat to young people who are endeavoring to gain full benefit from their education. In other words, take the drug and alcohol menace seriously. At the same time and to the extent that is reasonable, try to "accentuate the positive." Since health and well-being are generally incontestable values, firmly root prevention of drug use in a fundamental commitment to healthy living. Relate it to performance in athletics, academics, and in human relationships as well as to exercise and diet. Stress the advantages of good mental health practices, such as coping courageously with discouragement, dealing constructively with stress and pressure, and maintaining a realistic self-confidence. And, throughout, continue to emphasize the view that drug abuse prevention is less "anti-drug" than it is "pro-youth."

An in-depth exploration of these guidelines and their practical application are beyond the intent of this book. However, for those readers who wish to pursue further the dynamics of drug abuse prevention in our schools, I recommend, without reservation, a recent publication which deals directly and knowledgeably with this subject: *A School Answers Back: Responding to Student Drug Use,* by Dr. Richard A. Hawley. Dr. Hawley, a leader in the drug abuse prevention field, a published poet, and an excellent writer, is the Director of the University School, Hunting Valley Campus, an independent high school near Cleveland, Ohio. His book not only describes practical drug prevention programs for schools, but it also elevates the drug abuse problem to the appropriate intellectual level, making it easier for educators to take action. It is sold by The American Council for Drug Education, 6193 Executive Boulevard, Rockville, Maryland 20852.

Combatting Drug Problems in the Workplace

Even larger than the schools, in terms of the number of Americans involved, is the world of work. More than 100 million Americans have paying jobs. Drug abuse not only constitutes a serious threat to the health of American workers themselves, but it also poses a threat to their productivity and safety on the job. From the employer's point of view, drug and alcohol abuse also constitute a security threat—a constantly escalating threat to the financial well-being of business and corporate enterprise. Petty theft from the cash register and stolen merchandise are commonplace, while the stealing of corporate secrets and financial data that are marketable to competitors occurs with alarming frequency. It is now estimated that drugs cost the American economy $60 billion a year because of lost productivity, increased absenteeism and medical claims, increased accident rates, and employee theft. For example, about two-thirds of all absenteeism is the result of drug and alcohol use. Drug abusers take advantage of three to four times as many company-paid medical benefits as do nonusers. And let us not forget that you and I—as consumers of services and products—must foot this bill.

Health care costs, in general, are now rising about 15 percent a year—one of the most rapidly spiraling costs of doing business. To cite just one disturbing instance, the cost of health care for workers now accounts for a bigger share of the cost of a new car than does the steel which goes into making it. Businesses must also pay the substantial hidden costs attributable to drug and alcohol problems. Included in these buried costs—to name but a few—are increased turnover of personnel, lowered morale among nonusers because of problems and inequities caused by drug users, loss of product quality, and deteriorating relations between employers and employees.

It is time that American business, both employers and employees, got tough on drugs, and a few of them—still far too few—are starting to do so. As yet, however, few companies in the United States have clear, comprehensive, and ongoing drug abuse prevention programs. Why? Because both employers and employees have failed to recognize their shared interest in solving the drug problem. That solution can have only one basis: no worker, at any level of the company, can be at work with intoxicating drugs or alcohol in his or her body. Any equivocating on that battle line and the war against drug and alcohol problems is lost. For example, once the company says that alcohol on the job is okay as long as the employee is not "drunk," the floodgates to on-the-job drinking are open. Once a company says marijuana or cocaine use is okay, the illicit-drug problem mushrooms out of control. Once a company says executives can drink alcohol at lunch, but workers below that level cannot drink during the work day, the fairness and effectiveness of the policy is compromised. Once a company says it will only investigate drug or alcohol problems after there is measurable employee failure, the barn door is being closed only after the horse is gone.

How, you may ask, can a company establish and enforce a fair and workable no-drug and no-alcohol standard? How can the company deal with alcohol use during the work day at top levels of the corporate or business structure? How can the company deal with employees' dependence on medically prescribed drugs? These questions are not easily answered. But the reason why answers are not easily found is not that appropriate technology and the scientific knowledge are unavailable, but because these are tough questions to face after decades of what has been tolerated by American industry.

The failure to deal toughly and fairly with drug and alcohol problems in the workplace stems directly from the unwillingness of the appropriate people to establish the goal of working while free of drug use. Often this goal has not been established because the true costs of drug and alcohol dependence at the worksite have not been recognized. Or the necessary implementation of a program may have been sidetracked because of a mistaken concern for poorly understood civil or privacy rights which blunted effective action. There is no civil or constitutional right to use illegal drugs, and it is well within the rights of a corporation to establish the principle that the work force, from the corporate president to the night watchman, must work drug-free. In fact, it is the company's responsibility to provide a safe work environment.

One employer has recently taken effective action against drug abuse: the United States military services. After years of inaction, the military—led by the Navy—got moving in 1981. Their slogan was: "Not on my watch, not on my ship, not in my Navy!" The principal enforcement technique was a program of regular, random urine testing for drug use, with strict, clearly defined punishment for those caught having illicit drugs in their bodies. This program was coupled with a powerful and broadly based education campaign. The results have been predictable: A prompt drop in drug use among the military and a *rise* in morale, with appreciable increases in enlistment and reenlistment rates and broad support for the new drug abuse prevention project from all segments of the service.

In 1982, at the annual Navy Dinner at the New York Waldorf Astoria Hotel, it was my pleasure to present an award to the Chairman of the United States Joint Chiefs of Staff, General John W. Vessey, Jr., honoring this achievement in taking action against drug abuse and commending it as a model for other employers. Thus, the U.S. military, as the nation's largest employer of young people, is leading the way. I anticipate, however, that another decade will pass before all American workplaces implement a comprehensive and effective policy for preventing drug abuse, but the direction in which we need to move is clear. Companies, like schools, need a clear, easily understood drug abuse prevention policy. They need to communicate it effectively, and they need to enforce it vigorously and fairly.

One of the most visible struggles against drug dependence is taking

place today in the area of professional sports. Like military command-
ers, owners of professional sports teams are employers of young
people who are particularly vulnerable to drug and alcohol problems.
There are unmistakable signs that a movement is underway in professional sports to implement regular, routine urinalysis as a test for drug
use, as is now the practice in Olympic competitions. If professional
sports organizations adopt the same or a similar approach, not only
will it protect the image of the sports and their stars, but it will also
literally save the lives and careers of many of the athletes themselves.

Urine testing for drug use in the workplace shares with urine testing
on the highways two difficult problems. First, there is no generally
agreed-upon standard by which to measure impairment or intoxication
for drugs other than alcohol. As I will explain when we consider
highway safety programs, the standard for measuring intoxication or
impairment from alcohol use is itself faulty, but at least there is a
standard. Second, whereas alcohol is quickly eliminated from the
body after the drug is consumed, this is not true for many illegal
drugs. This is especially not true for marijuana use, which can be
detected in the urine for days and even for weeks after initial drug
use. A positive test for drugs is more difficult to interpret than is a
positive test for alcohol.

Questions are raised about the best way to devise a test, but they
are not answerable with the techniques and knowledge currently
available. "Is the person impaired by his drug use or just 'using'?"
"Did the actual use of the drug itself take place on the job or off the
job?" While not everyone will agree with it, I have a simple answer to
these complex questions. It is the one used by the military in their
drug abuse prevention program, and it states: *The presence of any
amount of any intoxicating drug, or the breakdown product of any
drug, which can produce impairment, and which is not prescribed by a
physician for a specific illness, is by definition unacceptable in the
workplace.* Thus, when an employee, at whatever level in the company, comes to work, he must be drug-free. If he is not, he is to be
sent home, referred for treatment, or made subject to disciplinary
action, depending on company policies. On-the-job presence of a drug
in the body is contrary to safe work habits and presents a risk that
need not be taken by the company, by the involved employee himself, by his co-workers, or by the public.

There are other, less controversial steps which employers and
unions can take to reduce drug and alcohol problems. One of the
easiest places to start is to develop drug education programs aimed
at bringing to employees the facts about the Drug Dependence Syn-

drome and about the specific job-related health threats posed by the GATEWAY DRUGS which are widely and mistakenly thought of as harmless: alcohol, marijuana, and cocaine. Another step is the establishment of Employee Assistance Programs (EAPs) to identify and assist employees with possible drug and alcohol problems.

The most important drug abuse prevention action which can be taken in the workplace is to educate and empower the nonusers— who comprise the large majority of workers of all ages and at all levels in the company—to act to stop drug and alcohol problems. Nonusers need to know how much the drug and alcohol use of their fellow workers is costing them, and they need to be encouraged to act to end drug-caused problems.

One of my patients recently recovered from a five-year dependence on cocaine. Working as an assistant chef at a large and prestigious restaurant, he makes it clear to his co-workers that he will not tolerate any drug or alcohol use on the job. He told me, "I know what drugs do to people, and I don't want anyone who is high on any drug working near me with hot liquids and knives!"

The response to recent concern about "secondhand" tobacco smoke is a model which can usefully be followed in drug and alcohol prevention in the workplace. Workers who do not smoke are now making the assertion, based on scientific facts of the dangers to their own health, of their right to a smoke-free worksite. This is not a violation of the civil rights of smokers, any more than a program aimed to ensure a drug-free worksite is a violation of the civil rights of drug users. No one, in fact, has a civil right to violate the law. It is a simple matter of economics, health, safety, and self-interest. Such drug and alcohol abuse prevention efforts in the workplace are also the best hope many dependent people have of preventing or overcoming their drug and alcohol problems.

Use of prescription drugs among workers can be a serious and confusing problem, if not thought through. Once use of prescribed, dependence-producing drugs is identified, it is a relatively simple matter to verify that the use is within the levels prescribed by the employee's physician in the treatment of a diagnosed illness. If such use of a prescribed dependence-producing drug is within the established boundaries and if it is not causing a work-related problem, then no intervention is necessary. If there are possible work-related problems produced by this prescription drug use—or if the employee works in a job involving significant safety risks to himself, his co-workers, or the public—then the company's medical personnel can work with the employee and his or her physician to solve the problem in an appropriate way, in accordance with procedures I have previously described.

Before leaving the potential of drug abuse prevention in the workplace, a word of caution is in order: Almost as bad as no action is precipitous and ill-conceived action by employers and unions. Any program to prevent drug and alcohol problems must be based on scientific facts; it must operate within the laws of the community in which the company does business; and it must be backed by a thorough educational program and comprehensive, written company policies. If urine testing is to be used, then the program planners should seek professional medical and legal advice concerning implementation of this often misunderstood technique. Because our nation as a whole is only now—with much confusion and ambivalence—waking up to our drug and alcohol dilemmas, the application and sound utilization of the principles we have recommended here will, admittedly, be difficult to achieve in the workplace. However, the benefits can be substantial. The costs of inaction are large. That is one of the many persuasive reasons why the development of a steady, well-conceived drug abuse prevention program will prove, in the long run, to be sensible and economical.

Combatting Drug Problems on the Highways

The most politically visible part of the entire drug and alcohol problem in America today is the question of what to do about the drunk driver. While this attention is long overdue and thoroughly justified by the extent and seriousness of the problem, it can also be misleading. The impression is widely held that the problem is the *alcoholic* who drives when he or she is drunk. As a result of this impression, many concerned citizens conclude that the best solution to the problem—the way to end the mayhem and manslaughter—is to "get the drunk off the road." There are, however, some barriers to this seemingly simple approach. One major obstacle is that there is no scientifically valid standard for "drunkenness." Various communities adopt different standards for measuring the blood alcohol concentration as the basis for defining *legal* drunkenness. These may range from about 0.08 to 0.15 percent. In a practical sense, the legally adopted standards are ridiculously high. In many areas of the country, in order to be ruled legally drunk, a person of average weight would have to consume as many as five or six drinks in a two-hour period, and then begin driving immediately.

More misleading, however, is the assumption that anyone with a lower blood alcohol concentration is not drunk and is therefore not a hazard on the highway. This mistaken assumption has prompted the owners of some taverns and bars to install breath meters for the purpose of measuring their patrons' blood alcohol concentrations when they are about ready to depart the premises. The scientific fact is that any blood alcohol concentration at all makes the imbiber less safe for driving. There is a measurable impairment of driving which begins with the lowest level of alcohol use and which increases with each addition to the blood alcohol concentration. Campaigns that emphasize the sensible-sounding slogan "Friends don't let friends drive drunk" imply that friends *know* when friends are drunk. They do not. They cannot.

The plain and honest solution to this problem is to establish the principle that *any* measurable blood alcohol concentration resulting from drinking is incompatible with safe driving. This, in essence, is the approach now widely used in Europe. If a number must be put to this, then I suggest a blood alcohol concentration of 0.02 percent. This level is achieved by taking one or two drinks within the last hour or two before starting to drive. The local county-run liquor stores in my neighborhood have it right on the brown bags in which they send their liquor out with their customers: "If You Drink, Don't Drive." And "If You Drive, Don't Drink." Any other basis for laws and social norms about drinking and driving is scientifically indefensible and creates a confusing, and thus a counterproductive, public message.

I recently spoke with an American woman who had just returned from a prolonged official visit to Hungary. She recalled the attitudes about drinking and driving that were expressed by the Hungarians, including the senior officials, the social leaders, and the university professors (all of these, she felt, are types that in most societies are cynical about legal rules for individual behavior). Before going out each night, someone in the party was identified as the driver. That person would not touch one drop of alcohol all evening. When the American first heard about this, she was amazed. She assumed that drivers would approach the problem merely by limiting their alcohol use to perhaps one or two drinks plus wine at dinner. When she expressed this idea, expecting it to produce a sophisticated wink, she was greeted with a simple statement that it was really in everyone's interest to follow this arrangement strictly and to obey the laws about drinking and driving. She never saw it violated. No drinking—period—for anyone who was responsible for driving. This is now the pattern throughout Europe.

Surely the terrible confusion in the United States today about drinking and driving must one day have a similar solution. There is no other basis for a sensible social policy. Drinking and drug use are incompatible with driving, working, or going to school. Is that such a shocking idea?

Recent history of the problems of drinking and driving carries an important lesson to teach us: conflicting and contradictory interpretations of "civil rights" can seriously affect the possibilities for achieving a successful program for preventing drug and alcohol abuse. It used to be that only people who exhibited probable evidence of driving while drunk could expect to have their blood alcohol concentration tested by the police. It used to be, too, that anyone could refuse to have his or her blood alcohol concentration checked without having that refusal reflected in any court proceedings against the possibly intoxicated driver. No more. Those "civil rights" misinterpretations have been clarified by laws which make it a privilege rather than a right to drive a car. You can still refuse to have your blood alcohol concentration checked by a highway patrolman in most areas, but such refusal will be reported to the court if your case comes to trial, and refusal will also mean the automatic forfeiture of your driver's license. The same solution is available for schools and in the workplace, once we understand better both the drug problem and the concept of genuine civil rights. Who, after all, is in favor of having intoxicated people driving on the highways, whether they are traveling to work, going to school, or coming home from a party?

Probably the most extreme and controversial opinion advanced in this book is my suggestion that children should not drink alcohol until they reach the legal drinking age. Almost as shocking to many readers, I suppose, is my conclusion that when it comes to schools, the workplace, and the highways, the only workable standard is a *Zero Tolerance* for nonprescribed drugs and alcohol. Some will argue that this is unrealistic or that it lacks scientific authority. "Surely," it will be asked, "Is there not some level of marijuana in the urine or alcohol on the breath which is not incompatible with driving a car safely?" I am convinced that once we open the door to allow any level of these intoxicating drugs inside the body of an individual who is driving, working, or going to school, the possibility of again closing the door is gone. Equally important, if some "safe" level were to be legally established, is that we thereby give a bewildering and ultimately self-defeating public message. We need to have clear, easily understood, and widely supported public policies. The best place to draw the line, in my opinion, is here: *No use of alcohol or intoxicating illegal drugs for anyone on the job, at school, or behind the wheel of a vehicle on our highways.*

This conflict will be familiar from earlier discussions of the contrast between drug use and drug abuse. Once a social sanction, or disapproval, is limited to the concept of abuse, the usefulness of the disapproval is almost totally lost because few drug users consider themselves to be drug abusers. No universally acceptable standard for distinguishing between use and abuse for any intoxicating drug is possible. Attempting to adopt a policy of disapproval limited to abuse leads to the problem I witnessed recently when a teenage speaker was addressing a high school audience about the dangers of driving drunk. The entire discussion centered around how many drinks a person of various body weights could drink in what period of time and still not be considered legally drunk. Many in the teenage audience left that talk reassured that alcohol use up to approximately six to eight drinks in a two-hour period was legal and safe. That is precisely what I mean by a confusing public message.

One of the arguments often heard against such a view is that drug use is a private matter affecting only the drug user. Many nonusers, as well as many drug users, wish this were true. Unfortunately, it never was true and it never will be true. When it comes to drug and alcohol use in schools, at work, and on the highways, it is beyond question that the incalculable costs of such use are borne not only by the drug user but by all who are exposed to his or her actions and by all who depend on the drug user for security, sustenance, or support. This larger community has a vital stake in decisions as to whether the person shall use or not use drugs and alcohol. Just as decisions to use drugs and alcohol in these settings affect nonusers adversely, so do antidrug efforts of nonusers in these same settings affect the users positively. Let me put that another way. When a clear standard of no drug use and no alcohol use—a *Zero Tolerance*—is established in schools, at work, and on the highways, and when this standard is routinely enforced, both the drug user and the potential drug user have a powerful reinforcment for becoming and remaining drug free. And if, in the face of this, the ambivalent person decides to use drugs or alcohol, such standards push drug use toward moderation and away from dependence.

Combatting Drug Abuse in the Criminal Justice System

From 1969 to 1970, I served as head of Community Services to the District of Columbia Department of Corrections. My responsibilities then included the supervision of all correctional halfway houses and the city's large parole system. Earlier I had worked as a psychiatrist at the large District of Columbia prison at Lorton, Virginia, and at the Norfolk prison in Massachusetts. As a result of these experiences, I have maintained an active interest in the criminal justice system. It was while in this work that I became convinced that the most effective correctional programs are not inside the prisons, but on the *outside*—in communities.

There are more than 1,000,000 Americans on probation and parole today. Vast numbers of that million are in desperate need of specific and effective programs for the prevention and treatment of drug and alcohol dependence. The key to making these preventive and treatment measures work—indeed for making any correctional program work (and, I concede, they often do not work well)—is the establishment of realistic, firm control over the behaviors of the convicted criminal law offender who, having been paroled and placed on probation, finds himself or herself in need of positive supervision and practical assistance in living crime-free.

Successful functioning in the community can be exceedingly difficult for the man or woman on parole and probation. The tendency to recidivism, to relapse into criminal behavior, is great. A leading cause of criminal recidivism in the United States today is drug and alcohol abuse. It follows, therefore, that a first priority of the parole and probation officers is to identify and, if possible, to prevent drug and alcohol problems from driving the parolee back into prison. This means close monitoring for drug use by frequent urine testing. It also means effectively educating both the correctional staff and the offenders. It means the development of comprehensive antidrug policies and programs. And, finally, it means imposing serious, strict, and clearly defined punishments for offenders who violate the rules against drug and alcohol use. If intelligently conceived and administered with the right balance of toughness and human concerns, a correctional program of this kind works.

At the same time, it must be noted, no matter how sound the basic correctional program may be, neither the staff nor the parolees can succeed in making it work "on their own." Almost always, they will need help. Fortunately, there are helpful resources which can be called upon; unfortunately, they are too often overlooked or ignored. The most incompletely used resources in helping these offenders achieve stable, crime-free lives in their communities are their families. Also too frequently underutilized are the unique services and guidance of such self-help groups as Alcoholics Anonymous and Narcotics Anonymous. To be effective, the parole or probation officer, like the effective sergeant in a military boot camp, must be a person who is both tough and fair and who bases both this toughness and fairness on shared goals and well-understood rules.

Combatting Drug Problems in Medical Practice

As a practicing physician, I strongly recommend that physicians and other health care professionals maintain a high level of suspicion as they encounter potential drug and alcohol problems among their patients, that they routinely conduct urine testing for illicit drugs—especially among adolescents—and that the results of positive test findings be reported both to the patient and to his or her family. Furthermore, I recommend that physicians assist families in monitoring the drug use of drug-dependent family members through the use of regular urine testing. This offers families an effective deterrent to drug dependence, and it offers drug-dependent patients on effective incentive to remain drug-free.

In addition, physicians and other health professionals can play a useful role by informing and educating the patient, the family, and the community about drug and alcohol problems and about the possible solutions to these problems. Traditionally, physicians have—for too long—considered drug-dependent people as hopeless and frustrating. Doctors should try to understand the phenomenon of drug and alcohol dependence. They should make full use of Family Action and the unique effectiveness of the Anonymous groups, as well as structured drug and alcohol treatment programs. If they do these things, physicians will find that the drug-dependent population actually constitute one of the most treatable of all patient groups.

Combatting Drug Problems with Religion

The role of religion in the prevention and treatment of drug dependence has been emphasized frequently in this book. Religious faith is a system of values which transcend the individual and his unique time on earth, to say nothing of the individual's momentary pleasure. Religious faith is a way of knowing who one is, where one came from, and where one is going, and what the purpose of life really is. In the context of drug abuse prevention, religion is a way to escape the limitations of the biologically based pleasure system for controlling behavior by seeing beyond the individualistic, present-tense pleasure to larger human values and purposes. As such, religion is, at the least, a helpful part of drug abuse prevention and, at most, an indispensable part of real recovery.

In this chapter on the community institutions dealing with drug problems, we consider not so much religious faith as the religious institutions in our society. Churches, synagogues, and temples are places of worship where one finds not only ideas but also people: a community of committed believers and, almost invariably, a staff of professional ministers. Worship is often a family activity. While churches in modern life have little of the harsh toughness of such institutions as the parole office (punishment, once a staple of religion, has gone out of style), they hold time-tested, postive values which are usually essential to solving drug problems.

My suggestions for churches are as simple as they are, by now, unsurprising. Involve the family and begin with a clear understanding of the nature and seriousness of the Drug Dependence Syndrome. It is no accident that Alcoholics Anonymous and churches go together: both are concerned with the process of turning problems over to God or, as it is called in AA, a Higher Power. Far more can be done by churches to involve families through education and support. The prevention and treatment of drug dependence should be integrated into the entire spiritual life of the church.

The church community can be a source of inspiration, education, and support for families struggling with drug and alcohol problems. All this, of course, is not easy for many modern American churches since it has become so difficult, if not impossible, to say no to individually chosen behaviors, however dangerous or "immoral" they may be. Just as the schools, the workplace, medical practice, and other modern institutions have to rethink their attitudes and their actions towards drug and alcohol problems, so do churches. When that is done, it is not necessary to return to the old fire-and-brimstone, judgmental zealotry of antialcohol values to be able to articulate and implement clear values promoting spiritual and physical health— values which reject drug dependence as one of the most common and debasing of human tragedies.

Religious institutions, which one might think are the most obvious places for drug abuse prevention to occur, are, in many ways, the last of our large social institutions to actively focus on the true nature of the drug problem and to employ the enormous potentials they have for positive solutions.

SUMMING UP

In this final chapter, we have dealt with the opportunities for community institutions to extend and reinforce the family-based drug dependence efforts that are the heart of this book. When it comes to the potential for community institutions to combat drug dependence, we developed four basic principles:

1. Drug and alcohol use is incompatible with successful functioning in communities. Therefore, a *Zero Tolerance* policy for intoxicating drugs is recommended for schools, the workplace, the criminal justice system, and on the highways.
2. The positive intervention of community institutions to prevent drug use is not a violation of individual rights. Such intervention is often essential for the full development of individual capacities—not only for achievement, but also for pleasure.
3. Community institutions need to team up with and to reinforce the primary site for all drug abuse prevention and treatment: the family.
4. When community institutions act to prevent drug dependence, their actions must be based on scientific facts, including a clear understanding of the Drug Dependence Syndrome and the specific effects of drugs (especially the GATEWAY DRUGS) on each particular institution. Furthermore, sustained and comprehensive actions, based on clearly articulated policies, need to be wisely disseminated and effectively enforced.

A Final Word

This book is a response to three questions:

- What Is the Drug Problem?
- What Are the GATEWAY DRUGS? and
- How Can Families Prevent and Treat Drug Problems?

The Drug Dependence Syndrome is a biologically based, understandable progression of drug experiences from experimentation to dependence, with predictable consequences at each stage for the drug user, his family, and his community. The most important fact to know about this syndrome is that initial drug use is mostly limited to the ages 12 to 20, with the peak incidence of first drug use occurring at about age 15. Experimentation with drugs is not only the first step in the Drug Dependence Syndrome; it is the principal focus of all drug abuse prevention, the goal of which is to help young people grow up through their teenage years *free of drug use*.

There has been an explosive increase in drug abuse in the United States during the last 20 years, with the primary victims being the Drug Epidemic Generation—Americans now aged 16 to 35. These are the children of the post–World War II Baby Boom.

There are three GATEWAY DRUGS in America today: alcohol, marijuana, and cocaine. They are the gateways, respectively, into all intoxicating drug use, into illegal drug use, and into intensified—often intravenous—drug use. Americans who do not use these drugs are virtually immune from the use of other mind-altering drugs. The GATEWAY DRUGS are uniquely dangerous and widely used precisely because their use is wrongly thought by users, and by many nonusers who relate to drug users, to be harmless and easily controlled. The GATEWAY DRUGS are, in reality, all dangerous and addicting.

321

Prevention and treatment of drug problems require the mobilization of the family and the community to promote drug-free lifestyles and to reject drug use. The most important goal is to help children grow up to be effective, contributing, self-supporting adults. The greatest threat to achieving this goal in modern America is also the greatest preventable cause of illness and death: drug dependence.

There are important drug abuse prevention roles for treatment programs and self-help groups, such as Alcoholics Anonymous, as well as in schools, in the workplace, and on the highways. There are positive roles for religion, the criminal justice system, and in medical practice.

Of all these, the most effective and most fundamental is the family. An educated and committed family is the nation's best defense against drug and alcohol problems.

This book has been written from my perspective as a practicing psychiatrist who sees drug-dependent people and their families in his office every day. I write out of my respect and concern for their pains, their hopes, and their needs.

I write also as a father of two teenage children, as my parents' son, as my wife's husband, as my relatives' relative, and as my neighbors' neighbor. As a person who feels deeply grateful for the successes I have had in my life (as well as my failures), a primary concern of mine is to return to others some of the blessings given to me by those who have loved me.

I have seen in my own family the tragedy of drug and alcohol dependence. I also know from my family the happiness that comes from preventing drug problems and from overcoming them.

It is my hope that this book can help families understand the drug problem and, working together, overcome it. Life is hard. For parents and for children. The joys of family life, however, fully justify the uncompromising effort required to prevent drug dependence. The pain of failure will not permit anything less than full commitment to that effort.

Additional Readings
and Resources

Readers interested in additional information about drug dependence, about the health effects of drugs of abuse including the GATEWAY DRUGS, and about strategies for successful prevention and treatment may find help by writing to the following:

The American Council For Drug Education (ACDE)
6193 Executive Boulevard
Rockville, Maryland 20852

The American Council is a national, nonprofit, private organization which is dedicated to informing the public about the negative health effects of a variety of drugs, particularly marijuana and cocaine. A wide variety of reliable and useful printed and film material is available.

Parent Resource Institute for Drug Education (PRIDE)
Georgia State University
University Plaza
Physical Education Building, Room 137
Atlanta, Georgia 30303
(800) 241-9746

PRIDE, founded by two of the leading parents in the Parents Movement, Dr. Thomas Gleaton and Dr. Keith Schuchard (who writes under the name Marsha Manatt, Ph.D.), provides support to families and communities in preventing drug abuse. PRIDE has an extensive range of printed and film materials and an apparently inexhaustible reservoir of well-informed, dedicated people ready to help.

323

The National Federation of Parents for Drug-Free Youth (NFP)
1820 Fanwall Avenue
Silver Spring, Maryland 20902

NFP is the national organization representing the many thousands of parent groups in the United States. They provide support and guidance to parent groups and do a first-rate job of reflecting parent and family views on drug-abuse prevention to the national Executive and Legislative bodies. NFP also distributes excellent publications and recommends speakers to help inform and mobilize families to combat drug dependence.

National Clearinghouse for Drug Abuse Information
The National Institute on Drug Abuse (NIDA)
Room 10A56, Parklawn Building
5600 Fishers Lane
Rockville, Maryland 20857

NIDA is the federal government's principal agency for drug abuse prevention, research, and policy development. They have a constantly expanding collection of scientifically accurate materials for the public and for professionals about drug abuse treatment and prevention.

PYRAMID PROJECT
Operated by the Pacific Institute for Research and Evaluation
Suite 612
7101 Wisconsin Avenue
Bethesda, Maryland 20814

PYRAMID PROJECT is the national technical assistance arm of NIDA. They have a substantial capacity to provide advice and support to organizations and programs in drug abuse prevention. They have, over the past decade, been the national leaders in technical assistance and support.

National Clearinghouse for Alcohol Information
National Institute on Alcohol Abuse and Alcoholism
1776 East Jefferson Street
Fourth Floor
Rockville, Maryland 20852

Like the information section of NIDA, this group has a wide range of free and low-cost publications regularly updated for the professional and for the public reader.

National Council on Alcoholism
733 Third Avenue
New York, New York 10017

The nation's leading private alcoholism educational agency has many useful publications.

Alcoholics Anonymous World Services, Inc.
Box 459
Grand Central Station
New York, New York 10163

AA has many useful publications available for the public.

Narcotics Anonymous World Services Office, Inc.
P.O. Box 622
Sun Valley, California 91352

Experts in the drug dependence process and the ways to recovery.

This listing of books for further reading must necessarily be brief and incomplete. Those seeking additional materials are referred to the organizations listed above and to their local public or university libraries. Several books, however, can be recommended, even on a short list. I believe the following books will prove interesting and useful to readers of this book:

Substance Abuse Disorders in Clinical Practice, by Edward C. Senay, M.D., is published by John Wright, PSG, Inc. of Boston. This is a book written for the practicing physician which has a wide usefulness in drug abuse treatment.

How to Talk to Kids About Drugs, by Suzanne Fornaciari, and *Strengthening the Family*, by H. Stephen Glenn, are both available from the Pacific Institute, which operates the PYRAMID PROJECT (address given above). They are concise and useful.

ToughLove, by Phyllis and David York and Ted Wachtel (New York, Bantam Books), is a useful handbook for parents and children who are facing drug and alcohol problems. It describes the formation of ToughLove groups based on the Ten Beliefs, such as "Parents are people too," "The essence of family life is cooperation, not together-ness," and "Blaming keeps people helpless."

Drugs, Drinking and Adolescents, by Donald Ian Macdonald, M.D., was published in 1984 by Year Book Medical Publishers of Chicago. Dr. Macdonald, one of the nation's most distinguished pediatricians, learned about drug abuse prevention as the result of his family's difficult but successful encounter with a drug problem. He has written a wise and useful book for families and professionals.

Love and Addiction, by Stanton Peele and Archie Brodsky, was pub-lished in 1975 by Taplinger Press in New York. Since then, it has also become available in paperback editions. These authors take an inter-esting approach to the problem of drug dependence.

Parents, Peers and Pot II: Parents in Action, by Marsha Manatt, Ph.D., is a sequel to the "bible" for parents seeking to overcome drug problems in their families and in their communities. It describes the personal tragedies of many leaders in the Parents Movement and how they overcame their problems and established a national counterattack on the drug epidemic. Their ultimate goal is a drug-free life for our children. The book is available in free single copies from the National Institute on Drug Abuse (address given above).

Two important books have been written by Richard Hawley, Ph.D. The first, *The Purposes of Pleasure: A Reflection on Youth and Drugs,* is published by The Independent School Press of Wellesley Hills, Massachusetts. The second book by Dr. Hawley, *A School Answers Back: Responding to Student Drug Use,* is published by ACDE (address given above). Both books are excellent.

ACDE, PRIDE, NFP, and NIDA all publish a wide range of continu-ously updated materials.

For those of you who are concerned about finding a good drug abuse treatment program, I recommend that you contact your local and/or state drug abuse agencies and your alcohol abuse prevention agencies for listings of local programs. Additional help can often be found from local or regional medical schools and from medical and psychiatric societies.

Index